CW01151

Palgrave Studies in Public Health Policy Research

Series Editors
Patrick Fafard
University of Ottawa
Ottawa, ON, Canada

Evelyne de Leeuw
University of New South Wales Australia
Liverpool, NSW, Australia

Public health has increasingly cast the net wider. The field has moved on from a hygiene perspective and infectious and occupational disease base (where it was born in the 19th century) to a concern for unhealthy lifestyles post-WWII, and more recently to the uneven distribution of health and its (re)sources. It is of course interesting that these 'paradigms' in many places around the world live right next to each other. Hygiene, lifestyles, and health equity form the complex (indeed, wicked) policy agendas for health and social/sustainable development. All of these, it is now recognized, are part of the 'social determinants of health'.

The broad new public health agenda, with its multitude of competing issues, professions, and perspectives requires a much more sophisticated understanding of government and the policy process. In effect, there is a growing recognition of the extent to which the public health community writ large needs to better understand government and move beyond what has traditionally been a certain naiveté about politics and the process of policy making. Public health scholars and practitioners have embraced this need to understand, and influence, how governments at all levels make policy choices and decisions. Political scientists and international relations scholars and practitioners are engaging in the growing public health agenda as it forms an interesting expanse of glocal policy development and implementation.

Broader, more detailed, and more profound scholarship is required at the interface between health and political science. This series will thus be a powerful tool to build bridges between political science, international relations and public health. It will showcase the potential of rigorous political and international relations science for better understanding public health issues. It will also support the public health professional with a new theoretical and methodological toolbox. The series will include monographs (both conventional and shorter Pivots) and collections that appeal to three audiences: scholars of public health, public health practitioners, and members of the political science community with an interest in public health policy and politics.

More information about this series at
http://www.palgrave.com/gp/series/15414

Marc C. Willemsen

Tobacco Control Policy in the Netherlands

Between Economy, Public Health, and Ideology

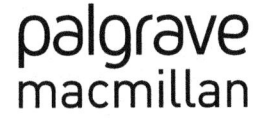

palgrave
macmillan

Marc C. Willemsen
Maastricht University
Maastricht, The Netherlands

Palgrave Studies in Public Health Policy Research
ISBN 978-3-319-72367-9   ISBN 978-3-319-72368-6   (eBook)
https://doi.org/10.1007/978-3-319-72368-6

Library of Congress Control Number: 2018937408

© The Editor(s) (if applicable) and The Author(s) 2018 This book is an open access publication
Open Access This book is licensed under the terms of the Creative Commons Attribution 4.0 International License (http://creativecommons.org/licenses/by/4.0/), which permits use, sharing, adaptation, distribution and reproduction in any medium or format, as long as you give appropriate credit to the original author(s) and the source, provide a link to the Creative Commons license and indicate if changes were made.
The images or other third party material in this book are included in the book's Creative Commons license, unless indicated otherwise in a credit line to the material. If material is not included in the book's Creative Commons license and your intended use is not permitted by statutory regulation or exceeds the permitted use, you will need to obtain permission directly from the copyright holder.
The use of general descriptive names, registered names, trademarks, service marks, etc. in this publication does not imply, even in the absence of a specific statement, that such names are exempt from the relevant protective laws and regulations and therefore free for general use.
The publisher, the authors and the editors are safe to assume that the advice and information in this book are believed to be true and accurate at the date of publication. Neither the publisher nor the authors or the editors give a warranty, express or implied, with respect to the material contained herein or for any errors or omissions that may have been made. The publisher remains neutral with regard to jurisdictional claims in published maps and institutional affiliations.

Cover illustration: Esben Klinker Hansen | Alamy Stock Photo

Printed on acid-free paper

This Palgrave Macmillan imprint is published by the registered company Springer International Publishing AG part of Springer Nature.
The registered company address is: Gewerbestrasse 11, 6330 Cham, Switzerland

For Jacqueline, Emma, and Julia

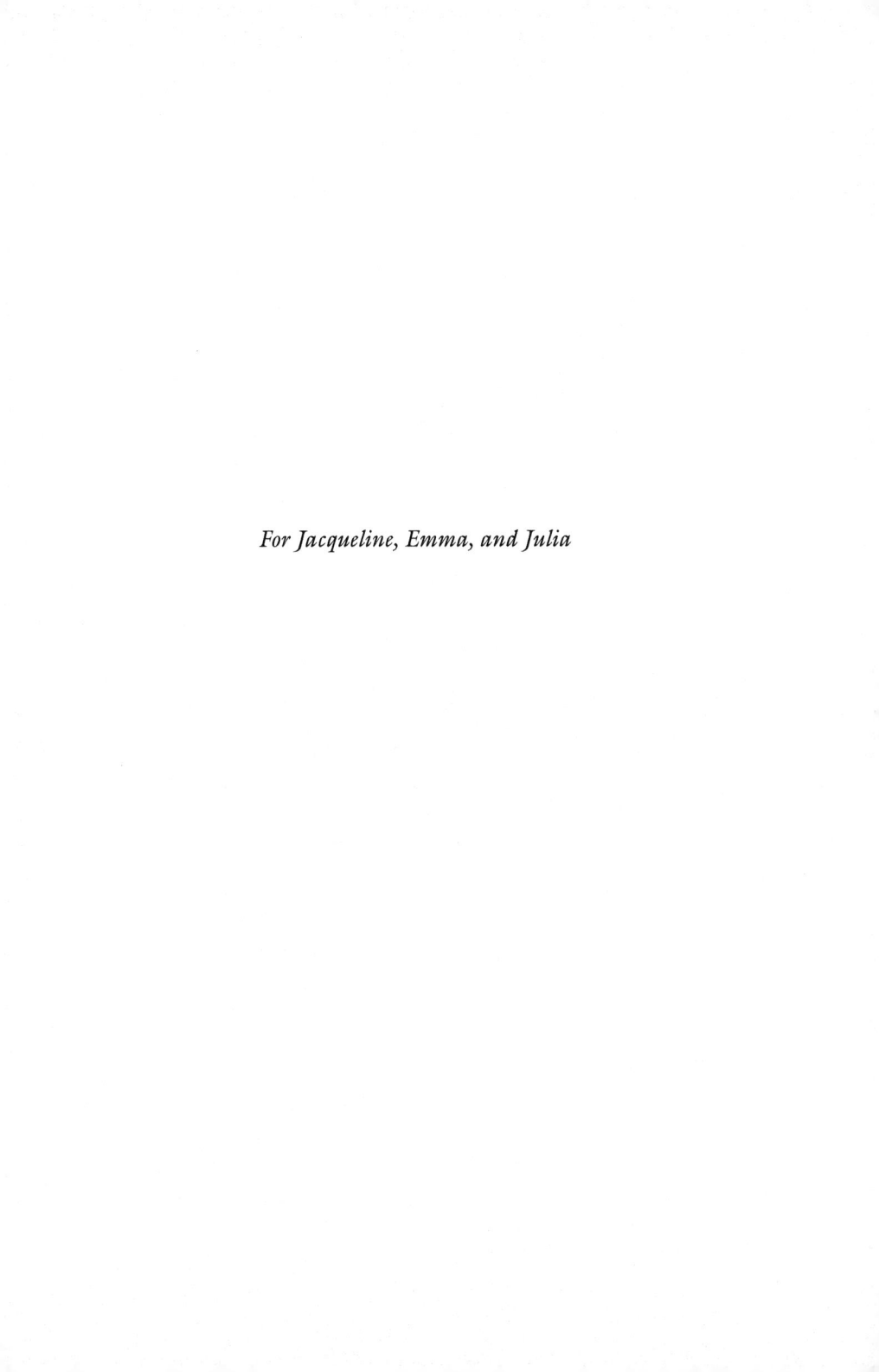

PREFACE

We doubt whether a man ever brings his faculties to bear with their whole force on a subject, until he writes upon it for the instruction or gratification of others.
—William Ellery Channing, 1890

If one is lucky, at some point in one's life, things fall into place. The process of writing this book and doing research for it was such an experience. For me, writing a book about Dutch tobacco control policy was the next logical step after more than a quarter of a century of research into tobacco control. I started my academic career developing and studying smoking cessation interventions. In the 1990s I became frustrated by the fact that regardless how much attention and counselling smokers who try to quit receive, the majority of quitters relapse within a year—most in the first month after treatment. Realising that even a combination of the best and most intensive treatment does not produce success rates much higher than 30%, I turned to more fundamental questions: what makes cigarettes so addictive, and what can be done to motivate whole populations to quit smoking? In 1998 I started to work for the *Stichting Volksgezondheid en Roken* (Dutch Smoking or Health Foundation) (STIVORO), the national expert centre on tobacco control. This gave me first-hand knowledge of tobacco control in practice, and I gradually learned about the political aspects of tobacco control. My appointment as Professor in Tobacco Control Research at the Department of Health Promotion at Maastricht University gave me the opportunity to cross the bridge from tobacco control research to tobacco policy research. I familiarised myself with the public policy literature, contacted political scientists, and attended the fifth Framework Convention on Tobacco Control Conference of the Parties (FCTC COP) in 2012 in Seoul to witness tobacco control politics and advocacy in action at the global level. I discovered that tobacco policy is an important topic for public policy scientists, but that insights from political science have not even begun to be absorbed by the tobacco control research community. I was thrilled when the opportunity arose for me to write a book about this. Most of the time the process of writing was a great pleasure, with many moments of excitement when I discovered new things and my understanding was deepened. The book has also turned into the first comprehensive historical account of tobacco control in the Netherlands, written for an international readership.

Inspiration for this work came from two sources. One was a book by Clavier and De Leeuw (2013) which drew attention to the fact that the health promotion field lacks a theoretical understanding of the adoption and implementation of health policies. The other was a book that presented an approach to the study of tobacco control policy that does justice to insights from public policy and political sciences while being accessible to those working outside the public policy field (Cairney, Studlar, & Mamudu, 2012). The first source made me realise that there is an under-recognised knowledge gap in the tobacco control field that needs to be filled, and the second presented me with a solution. There are so many public policy theories available that it can be quite overwhelming for a relative layperson, so I was pleased to stumble on to the general analytical framework provided by Cairney and his colleagues. It allowed me to focus on the basis elements of the policymaking process and to apply a logical structure to this book. I felt confident enough to borrow insights from two theories that I found particularly interesting, the Multiple Streams Approach (MSA) and the Advocacy Coalition Framework (ACF). However, I call on political scientists and public policy scholars to join me in studying the case of Dutch tobacco control. There is much more to learn from the enormous amount of information and data on Dutch tobacco control policy as I discovered, and it is available for further research.

I am most grateful for a grant from STIVORO, which made it possible to afford the necessary research and to dedicate working time to write this book. As part of STIVORO's science team, I had obtained first-hand knowledge of tobacco control and the workings of the broader tobacco control coalition in the Netherlands. In addition, from 2013 until 2017,

I worked for the Dutch Alliance for a smoke free society (ANR). These employments gave me relevant data and information—a clear advantage, given the complexity of the topic—but there was also the danger of bias. I distanced myself as much as possible from my own contribution to the processes I examined. I further reduced the risk of personal bias by having people critically comment on the work. I thank Paul Cairney, Pieter de Coninck, Sanne Heijndijk, Gera Nagelhout, Dewi Segaar, Fleur van Bladeren, Bas van den Putte, and Heide Weishaar for reading and giving feedback on draft versions of the book. Emma Willemsen was a great help with the coding and ordering of the large amount of text from the proceedings of parliament meetings and parliamentary papers. I am most grateful to each of the 22 people I interviewed for the book. The interviews were crucial for my understanding of Dutch tobacco control policy making and assured that I had identified the main events correctly. Regrettably, at the end, due to the need to be succinct and to stay within the word count, much of the interesting material from these, sometime lengthy, interviews did not make it to the book. My original plan was to write the book in Dutch, but Evelyne de Leeuw persuaded me to write it in English, offering to include it in the new series on public policy she was planning with Patrick Fafard. I am very grateful for her advice and for giving me the opportunity to publish my work as part of the new series. Book doctor Margaret Johnson did a truly wonderful job of proof reading and polishing the final manuscript. I thank Jacqueline and Julia for their patience and keeping things quiet around me during the many, many hours—much more than I had anticipated—that I needed to study and write.

This book was first and foremost written to find out what drives tobacco control policymaking and to understand its nuances and complexities from an academic vantage point—but if tobacco control advocates learn a thing or two from it, it will have served its purpose much better.

Maastricht, The Netherlands   Marc C. Willemsen

References

Clavier, C., & De Leeuw, E. (Eds.). (2013). *Framing public policy in health promotion: Ubiquitous, yet elusive*. London: Oxford University Press.

Cairney, P., Studlar, D. T., & Mamudu, H. M. (2012). *Global tobacco control: Power, policy, governance and transfer*. New York: Palgrave Macmillan.

Contents

1	Introduction	1
2	Dutch Tobacco Control Policy from the 1950s to the Present	19
3	The Tempo of Dutch Tobacco Control Policy	77
4	The Social and Cultural Environment	89
5	Making Tobacco Control Policy Work: Rules of the Game	113
6	The International Context: EU and WHO	145
7	Scientific Evidence and Policy Learning	165
8	Tobacco Industry Influence	183
9	The Tobacco Control Coalition	231

10 Problem Identification and Agenda Setting	271
11 Conclusions	305
References	319
Index	363

List of Abbreviations

This table gives English translations for Dutch abbreviations that appear multiple times in the text and provides explanations for the English abbreviations.

Abbreviation	Dutch	English
ACF	–	Advocacy Coalition Framework
ANR	Alliantie Nederland Rookvrij	Dutch Alliance for a smoke free society
ASH	–	ASH (Action on Smoking and Health)
BAT	–	British American Tobacco
BMA	–	British Medical Association
BVT	Bureau Voorlichting Tabak	Tobacco Education Bureau
CAN	Club for Active Non-smokers/Clean Air Nederland	Clean Air Netherlands
CDA	Christen-Democratisch Appèl	Christian Democratic Party
COP	–	Conference of the Parties
CU	Christen Unie	Christian Union (political party)
CVZ	College voor Zorgverzekeringen	Health Care Insurance Board
D66	Politieke Partij Democraten 66	Democrats 66 (political party)
ECTOH	–	European Conference on Tobacco or Health
FCA	–	Framework Convention Alliance
FCTC	–	Framework Convention on Tobacco Control
HORECA	Hotel, Restaurant, Café	The hospitality sector
ICBT	Interdepartementale Commissie Beperking Tabaksgebruik	Interdepartmental Committee for Reducing Tobacco Use
IGZ	Inspectie voor de Gezondheidszorg	Health Care Inspectorate

KHN	Koninklijke Horeca Nederland	Dutch trade association for the hotel and catering industry
KNMG	Koninklijke Nederlandsche Maatschappij tot bevordering der Geneeskunst	Royal Dutch Medical Association
LBT	Landelijke Belangenvereniging van Tabaksdistributeurs Nederland	National Association for Tobacco Distributors
LPF	Lijst Pim Fortuyn	Pim Fortuyn List (political party)
MSA	–	Multiple Streams Approach
NPT	Nationaal Programma Tabaksontmoediging	National Program Tobacco Control
NVWA	Nederlandse Voedsel en Waren Autoriteit	Netherlands Food and Consumer Product Safety Authority
PvdA	Partij van de Arbeid	Labour Party
PVV	Partij voor de Vrijheid	Freedom Party
RIVM	Rijksinstituut voor Volksgezondheid en Milieu	National Institute for Public Health and the Environment
RVZ	Raad voor de Volksgezondheid en Zorg	Council for Public Health and Health Care
SP	Socialistische Partij	Socialist Party
SRB	Stichting Rokers Belangen	Smokers' Right Group
SRC	Stichting Reclame Code	Advertising Code Foundation
SRJ	Stichting Rookpreventie Jeugd	Youth Smoking Prevention Foundation
SSI	Stichting Sigaretten Industrie	Dutch Cigarette Manufacturers Association
STAR	Stichting van de Arbeid	Labour Foundation
STIVORO	Stichting Volksgezondheid en Roken	Dutch Smoking or Health Foundation
TPD	–	Tobacco Product Directive
VNK	Vereniging Nederlandse Kerftabakindustrie	Dutch Fine Cut Tobacco Industry Association
VNO–NCW	Verbond van Nederlandse Ondernemingen en Nederlands Christelijke Werkgeversverbond	The Confederation of Netherlands Industry and Employers
VNS	Nederlandse Vereniging voor de Sigarenindustrie	Dutch Cigar Industry Association
VSK	Vereniging Nederlandse Sigaretten- en Kerftabakfabrikanten	Association for Dutch Cigarette and Fine Cut Tobacco Manufacturers
VTV	Volksgezondheid Toekomst Verkenning	Public Health Status and Foresight
VVD	Volkspartij voor Vrijheid en Democratie	People's Party for Freedom and Democracy

WARG	Wetenschappelijke Adviesraad Roken en Gezondheid	Scientific Advisory Council on Smoking and Health
WCPV	Wet Collectieve Preventie Volksgezondheid	Public Health Collective Prevention Act
WPG	Wet Publieke Gezondheidszorg	Public Health Act
WRR	Wetenschappelijke Raad voor het Regeerbeleid	Scientific Council for Government Policy

List of Figures

Fig. 1.1	Conceptual framework for understanding tobacco control making	10
Fig. 3.1	Tobacco Control Policy Index scores between 1969 and 2010 in 11 EU countries	84
Fig. 3.2	Dates of coming into force of key tobacco control policies in the Netherlands and in the United Kingdom	85
Fig. 4.1	The flywheel model of Tobacco Control (TC)	90
Fig. 4.2	Smoking prevalence in men and women since 1958	98
Fig. 4.3	Trends in adult smoking prevalence (men and women combined) in the Netherlands, the United Kingdom, and Canada	100
Fig. 4.4	Trends in youth smoking (10–19 year olds) between 1992 and 2013 in the Netherlands	101
Fig. 8.1	Number of workers employed in tobacco production in the Netherlands since 1939	204
Fig. 8.2	State revenues from tobacco taxation (excl. VAT) as a proportion of the total state income per year	205
Fig. 9.1	STIVORO's budget (× million Euro)	246
Fig. 10.1	Number of parliamentary questions since 1992 on tobacco policy, by year	297

List of Tables

Table 3.1	Tobacco control policy cycles	79
Table 3.2	Dates of coming into force of key tobacco control policies in the Netherlands and in the United Kingdom	81
Table 5.1	Members of cabinet who have held the tobacco policy portfolio	120
Table 8.1	Tobacco industry tolerance campaigns in the Netherlands	188
Table 10.1	Tobacco problem indicators in the Public Health Status Forecasts reports by the National Institute of Health and the Environment (RIVM)	274
Table 10.2	Quantitative goals for tobacco control in national prevention policy documents	277
Table 10.3	How smoking has been framed in the Netherlands by the tobacco control coalition, the government, and the tobacco industry	287

LIST OF BOXES

Box 2.1	Proposals in the 1975 Health Council report *Measures to reduce smoking*	25
Box 2.2	Major tobacco control policy events in the Netherlands	62
Box 5.1	Important pro- and anti-tobacco control parliamentary resolutions	127
Box 5.2	Dutch inspiration for a business-friendly policy agenda in Europe	132
Box 5.3	Municipalities and national tobacco control goals	136
Box 6.1	The Dutch blockade of the EU tobacco advertising ban	149
Box 7.1	Confrontational media campaigns to deter smoking	171
Box 8.1	Philip Morris' failed "cookies campaign"	189
Box 8.2	How the industry crushed the first Tobacco Act	197
Box 8.3	How the industry influenced the Dutch position on an EU Recommendation	201
Box 9.1	Robert Jasper Grootveld, "anti-smoke magician"	232
Box 9.2	STIVORO's great "smoke-outs"	244
Box 10.1	Smoking is an addiction	290

CHAPTER 1

Introduction

Twenty years ago I worked on an advisory report on the effectiveness of various tobacco control policy measures, commissioned by the Dutch Ministry of Health[1] as part of the process of presenting a revised Tobacco Act to the parliament (Willemsen, De Zwart, & Mooy, 1998). Soon after the report was finished I attended the World Conference on Tobacco or Health in Beijing, where I spoke with a civil servant from the Dutch Ministry of Health. I asked him what would happen with the report and was shocked when he told me that many of the conclusions were "not politically feasible" and could not be taken up.

This was the first time that I was confronted with the concept of "political feasibility." In hindsight this was rather naïve of me, but students and researchers who invest time and effort in understanding better ways of helping people to overcome tobacco addiction sooner or later come to realise that the tobacco problem has political roots. To do something about it on a societal level, one has to acknowledge what many people would describe as "nasty" politics. Many scientists shy away from this, just as I did then, because they believe that science is independent and politics-free or because they are intimidated by what they perceive as complexity, unpredictability, and irrationality in politics for which they are not prepared, being used to working from within an evidence-based science paradigm. A more effective strategy to address the tobacco problem on a

© The Author(s) 2018
M. C. Willemsen, *Tobacco Control Policy in the Netherlands*,
Palgrave Studies in Public Health Policy Research,
https://doi.org/10.1007/978-3-319-72368-6_1

societal level is to try to understand the policy process and why this process at times appears so irrational.

Since my professorship in tobacco control research, journalists, scientific colleagues from other countries, and students have asked me the same question: why is the Dutch government not doing more to control tobacco? This book is my attempt to formulate an answer. As an introductory text to the field, it seeks to provide an understanding of the full complexities of tobacco control policy. It further aims to offer a broad framework for thinking about tobacco control policymaking. Many of the understandings in the book can be applied to other public health areas, and lessons drawn from the analysis of the Dutch case may be of interest to other countries, particularly those with similar multi-party parliamentary democracies.

How does the trajectory of Dutch tobacco control compare with other developed countries? In the case of the Netherlands, there were nine years between the time that national data on the dangers of smoking were presented (1948) and the time that the government admitted there was a problem and the public should be informed (1957). It took another 25 years for the first regulative measure (health warnings on cigarette packs in 1982). Another six years passed before the Netherlands had a Tobacco Act (1988), and a further 14 years before effective measures such as an advertising ban and a workplace smoking ban were implemented (through a revision of the Tobacco Act in 2002).

This is an enormous period of time. Why was there such a delay between recognition of the tobacco problem and the policy response? Some might say this is a moralistic starting point for a book because it assumes that the government could have reacted sooner, faster, or more decisively. This is undoubtedly true—at least in theory, the government might just as well have reacted later, slower, and less decisively. In fact, the Netherlands has not done particularly badly in comparison with many other countries: the Netherlands is in some periods a laggard, and most of the time just struggles to keep up with the mainstream, but everywhere in the world there has been a wide gap between realising that there is a problem with tobacco and actually implementing effective solutions. Major tobacco control measures have had to be won in hard and long-running political battles, because tobacco control is a highly contested and politically sensitive topic. Even countries leading the way in tobacco control such as the United Kingdom, Australia, and Canada needed 20–30 years to come up with a comprehensive policy response (Cairney, Studlar, & Mamudu, 2012).

Idealists in the tobacco control field may expect that the presentation of scientific facts will automatically result in rational policy decisions, and when this does not happen a common explanation is that the tobacco industry has been successful in casting doubt on the evidence and in lobbying to delay regulation (Larsen, 2008). The industry is certainly well known for casting doubt on science, misleading politicians, and opposing or delaying tobacco control (Baba, Cook, McGarity, & Bero, 2005; Bornhauser, McCarthy, & Glantz, 2006; Costa, Gilmore, Peeters, McKee, & Stuckler, 2014; Lie, Willemsen, De Vries, & Fooks, 2016; Tobacco Free Initiative, 2008), but pointing to the tobacco industry as the sole reason for why governments do not take action is a gross simplification. Although efforts by the tobacco industry to prevent and delay tobacco policy making are important factors—and I will present many details on how this was done in the Netherlands—there are many other factors that one must take into consideration if one wants to understand the nuances and complexities of tobacco control policymaking.

With this book I move beyond the mainstream tobacco control literature which often assumes that knowledge on smoking risks leads, or should lead, to tobacco regulation. I want to explore what can be learned from insights from public policy research. I have already found a superficial glance at this rich literature rewarding, as it offers many insights that are immediately applicable to the tobacco control field. It can teach us, among other things, that public policymaking is not a rational, linear process starting with the identification of a problem, followed by selecting the best solution, finalised by adopting, implementing, and evaluating. Such models of knowledge transfer do not do justice to what happens in the real world. It is not so much that "knowledge plays no part in tobacco control, but that it is just one factor among many other policy determinants, and one that needs a political interpretation to have a policy effect" (Larsen, 2008, p. 764). Indeed, progress in tobacco control is a function of the internal dynamics of the policy process itself, and it has been argued that a more profound understanding of the political dimensions of health policy will help "to better anticipate opportunities and constraints on governmental action and design more effective policies and programs" (Oliver, 2006). Understanding these dimensions is crucial for those who want to contribute to more effective policies, including to so-called endgame strategies that may eventually eradicate the sale and consumption of tobacco products (Cairney & Mamudu, 2014; McDaniel, Smith, & Malone, 2016).

Understanding the Policy Process

A central tenet of public policy studies is that the relative influence of actors such as politicians, bureaucrats, and lobbyists on policy formation differs according to the policy sector (John, 2012, p. 5), so that a distinct sector such as tobacco control should be studied in its own right. However, to date there is not much understanding of politics in tobacco control. In 2014, I conducted a study where we searched scientific literature databases and counted the number of scientific publications in 31 European countries between 2000 and 2012 that had nicotine or tobacco as their main research topic (Willemsen & Nagelhout, 2016). Of the almost 15,000 papers identified, the proportion that had either "policy" or "politics" in their title was 0.9% and only half of these dealt with the determinants or impact of policies, leaving less than 0.5% of research that had the policy process as its main focus (unpublished data).

Despite some recent studies that have drawn on political sciences, most studies on tobacco control have paid little attention to policy processes. For example, one recent study tried to explain why smoking rates *increased* between 2005 and 2010 in France, which was "an unusual occurrence in countries in the 'mature stage' of the smoking epidemic" (McNeill, Guignard, Beck, Marteau, & Marteau, 2015). The research was a case study, comparing France with the United Kingdom, where smoking rates continued to decline in the same period. The main explanation was that in France there had been no tobacco price increases in that period, "stemming from the lack of a robust and coordinated tobacco control strategy." Furthermore, the French government had continued to financially compensate tobacconists (small tobacco shops) with more money than was spent on tobacco control, and was too permissive regarding tobacco control, resulting in violations of the French Tobacco Act. The researchers did not say *why* the French government, the first country in the European Union (EU) to ratify the World Health Organization's (WHO) Framework Convention on Tobacco Control (FCTC) in 2004, had no strong tobacco control strategy in the years 2005–2010, although they referred to a "lack of clear and consistent political will." When we look at the Netherlands, only one scientific publication has tried to explain Dutch tobacco control policy. It is a case study of the implementation of the smoking ban in the hospitality sector (Gonzalez & Glantz, 2013), but does not really answer the question of *why* a smoke-free policy failed in the Dutch context (De Leeuw, 2013).

The tobacco control field has come to realise that we need to know more about the policymaking process. In 2007 the US National Cancer Institute published the monograph "Greater than the sum: Systems thinking in tobacco control" (Best, Clark, Leichow, & Trochim, 2007) which concluded that slow progress in tobacco control "is likely due to many complex and overlapping factors that must be better understood if more effective action is to be taken." Fortunately, a small but growing body of literature emerging on the politics of tobacco control is slowly gaining attention (Cohen et al., 2000). In the past ten years or so, some useful attempts have been made to understand how and why specific tobacco policies have emerged in specific social, cultural, and political contexts (Albæk, Green-Pedersen, & Nielsen, 2007; Bryan-Jones & Chapman, 2008; Feldman & Bayer, 2004; Grüning, Strünk, & Gilmore, 2008; Kurzer & Cooper, 2016; Nathanson, 2005; Reid, 2005; Studlar, 2002, 2007a, 2007b; Young, Borland, & Coghill, 2010). To give one example, Nathanson (2005) examined differences in countries' political systems and cultures, and how these evolve over time. She explained the diversity in trajectories by pointing to differences in how policymaking is organised and structured (e.g., whether there is a federal or centralised government and how much executive power the government has), the resources and access to policymakers that anti- and pro-tobacco groups have, and the dominant ideologies regarding tobacco use and the role of the state versus individual responsibility.

The two theories that I find most useful in understanding tobacco control policy are the Advocacy Coalition Framework (ACF) (Sabatier, 1998, 2007; Sabatier & Weible, 2007) and the Multiple Streams Approach (MSA) (Kingdon, 2003; Zahariadis, 2007). ACF is the more ambitious of the two because it aims to describe the dynamics of the policy process within changing environments, using competition between two or more advocacy coalitions in a specific policy subsystem (in our case the subsystem of all people and organisations involved in tobacco control) as a starting point. External events, such as a new government, may shock the subsystem, and such shocks result in policy change when one of the coalitions is better at exploiting the opportunity to reinforce its position—usually by demonstrating that its belief system can solve the policy problem better than opposing coalitions can (Cairney, 2013). Whether this is successful depends on the coalition's resources and how good it is in framing its preferred solution, in exploiting public opinion, and in generating societal and political support.

What are "coalitions" in ACF theory? A network can be called an advocacy coalition when it is composed of people who share beliefs about the causes and solutions of a policy problem and have common core values. They must also engage in a "nontrivial degree of coordination" (Weible, Sabatier, & McQueen, 2009) and the stronger the coordination, the more efficient and successful their lobbying power can be. People in a pro- or anti tobacco coalition may have a variety of positions and may include interest group leaders, politicians, government officials, experts, researchers, and journalists. Shared beliefs act as the glue that binds them. The motivation to align with others in the same coalition is strengthened by what is called in ACF theory the "devil shift" (Sabatier & Weible, 2007): the tendency to perceive actors in opposing coalitions as more threatening and more powerful than they usually are. Some scholars make a distinction between purposive coalitions and material coalitions to acknowledge the fact that coalitions such as the tobacco industry coalition mainly exists because its members share material (economic) interests (Sabatier & Weible, 2007, p. 197). ACF theory assumes that, in most policy domains, two or more coalitions of policy actors can be identified (Sabatier & Weible, 2007). Often there is a dominant coalition of people who share a particular belief system, challenged by one or more competing coalitions.

Participants in a pro- or anti tobacco coalition share what ACF calls "policy core beliefs" about solutions to the problem. Such deeply ingrained beliefs remain stable within coalitions for long periods of time, explaining the resistance to change. Once a conservative coalition dominates the policy subsystem, policy change is unlikely. When one coalition's ideas about and framing of an issue resonate better with policymakers than with a competing coalition, there is a shift in the balance of power in relation to the new "core ideas." Subsystems contain "policy brokers," persons such as civil servants who communicate and deal with both sides. The ACF has been used to analyse the process of tobacco control policymaking at the national level: for example, in Japan (Sato, 1999) and Canada (Breton, Richard, Gagnon, Jacques, & Bergeron, 2008); in the EU (Smith, Fooks, Gilmore, Collin, & Weishaar, 2015); and at the global level (Farquharson, 2003).

The MSA is useful in identifying the defining moment when policy solutions have become accepted by policymakers as the answer to a policy problem. While the ACF can tell us what drives change and helps us understand how actors produce policy change over longer periods of time, the MSA tells us when change is most likely to happen. It distinguishes three policy domains, each having its own dynamics and actors (Kingdon, 2003; Zahariadis, 2007):

the domain of problems (is tobacco seen as a problem that needs a governmental response?), the domain of policy (which solutions are available for the problem?), and the domain of politics (is the government willing and able to act?). Substantial policy change is more likely to occur when problem appreciation, policy solution, and political opportunity align. Kingdon (2003) assigns a central role to "policy entrepreneurs" (lobbyists, activists, politicians, civil servants), who develop policy alternatives and couple these with problems at the right time (when ideological and political opportunities are favourable). In the political stream, a major electoral change may present an opportunity to advance or roll back government regulation. Changes in the perception of problems can also open up a window of opportunity: this might happen when activists point out that other countries have more advanced tobacco control policies and are more effective in tackling the smoking problem. It may then become clear to policymakers that there still exists a problem that can and should be tackled. Important changes in the policy stream can also open windows of opportunity. This may happen when new information is revealed about the feasibility and effectiveness of existing and novel policy options.

Kingdon (2003) developed his ideas after interviews with people involved with policymaking in the context of US health-care reform, regulation of transportation in the United States, and US tax changes, but not in tobacco control. The theory is nevertheless applicable and relevant, and is becoming more popular as a simple theoretical framework to understand tobacco policy (Asbridge, 2004; Barnsley, Walters, & Wood-Baker, 2015; Blackman, 2005; Bosdriesz, Willemsen, Stronks, & Kunst, 2014; Cairney, 2009; Mamudu et al., 2014; Schwartz & Johnson, 2010).

Almost ten years ago, Larsen (2008) noted that there was remarkably little interaction between mainstream tobacco control literature and public policy literature. This is slowly changing. For example, in a recent special issue of the scientific journal *Tobacco Control*, out of 20 contributions on the topic of "the tobacco endgame,"[2] most were from experts from the medical, public health or behavioural sciences, or from tobacco control advocates, but two were from public policy scholars. One discussed the political feasibility of various tobacco elimination endgame scenarios (Rabe, 2013), the other provided advice on how endgame solutions could be implemented and organised (Isett, 2013). Such interaction between political sciences and public health in tobacco control is welcome, but still rare. With this book I hope to contribute to this emerging literature, using the Netherlands as a case study.

A Multi-Lens Approach

Advanced tobacco control policies thrive within "policy environments" that are favourable to the implementation of tobacco control measures. Theories can inform the characteristics of such environments (Cairney & Mamudu, 2014), but a general problem in public policy is that there are almost as many models and approaches to the complex reality of policy formation as there are scholars. Each scholar takes a specific perspective, such as emphasising the context, or focusing on institutional factors, or emphasising the role of lobbyists as in the MSA, or starting with changes in policy core beliefs such as in the ACF. Discussions of the various approaches and accompanying theories can be found in textbooks on public policy (Birkland, 2011; Buse, Mays, & Walt, 2012; Cairney, 2012; John, 2012; Sabatier, 2007). Each theory offers a valuable but incomplete account of the policy process.

A complementary approach, using insights from multiple theoretical approaches, has the most chance to explain the complexity of policymaking. According to John (2012), "the approaches are not rivals; they can complement each other and be part of the explanation" (p. 14). Instead of selecting the most suitable theory for each policy problem or using multiple theories and determining which describes the data and the observations best, my book follows an approach advocated by Donley Studlar and Paul Cairney (Cairney, 2007; Cairney et al., 2012; Studlar, 2007b, 2015), who identified the core constructs from diverse theories that complement each other. They assumed that much might be gained from looking at the same policy case several times, each time from a different perspective and applying a different analytical lens.

Cairney et al. (2012) differentiated five fundamental ways of approaching tobacco control policy change, roughly coinciding with the major strands of thought within public policy science: looking at the context, at institutions, at the diffusion of ideas, at networks, and at agenda setting. John (2012) distinguished the same five elements and explained that policy change emerges from their interaction. These five ways of approaching the problem can be conceptualised as lenses through which the policy process can be analysed, and I will use these lenses in different chapters of this book. I interpret the five analytical lenses to mean the following:

1. *Context* refers to the social, cultural, and economic environment in which tobacco policymaking occurs. The social environment consists of factors such as public knowledge and concern about smok-

ing, and public support for policy measures. Cultural values lie at the core of ideological preferences and societal rejection of tobacco control measures. The economic aspect has to do with the economic importance of tobacco for the national economy, which relates to the tobacco industry's leverage to influence policy making.
2. *Institutions* refers to how policy is shaped by a country's specific policymaking system. What is the dominant policy system and what are its formal and informal rules? What is the role of bureaucracy and parliament, and what are the opportunities for and constraints on lobbying? Which part of government is responsible for tobacco policy? Which level of governance is responsible for tobacco: the sub-national, national, or supranational, or some combination of these?
3. *Diffusion of ideas* refers to the role of medical and scientific knowledge. To what extent is policymaking influenced by the transfer of information, knowledge, and ideas from within and from abroad? What is the level of knowledge that has accumulated within the political system, and how is this important when making decisions on tobacco?
4. *Networks* refers to the balance of power between policy "entrepreneurs" who are typically organised in policy coalitions. Networks become coalitions when network members share a common set of core beliefs and when there is a certain level of coordination. What changes can we see over time in how the tobacco control and the tobacco industry coalitions are organised, and how effective has their lobbying been? Has there been a shift in the balance of power?
5. *Agenda setting* refers to the process by which tobacco policy appears higher on the political agenda. This involves identifying at some point that there is a problem and that the government needs to do something about it. Ideological factors have to be taken into account: is it a responsibility for the government, or should the government leave it to citizens or to the free market to tackle the problem and find solutions? Problem and solutions need to be "sold" to politicians and policymakers.

To understand how the five elements fit together conceptually, and how they may either inhibit or promote tobacco control policy, I developed a conceptual framework (Fig. 1.1) that depicts the relationships between the five elements. They are congruent with the findings from the

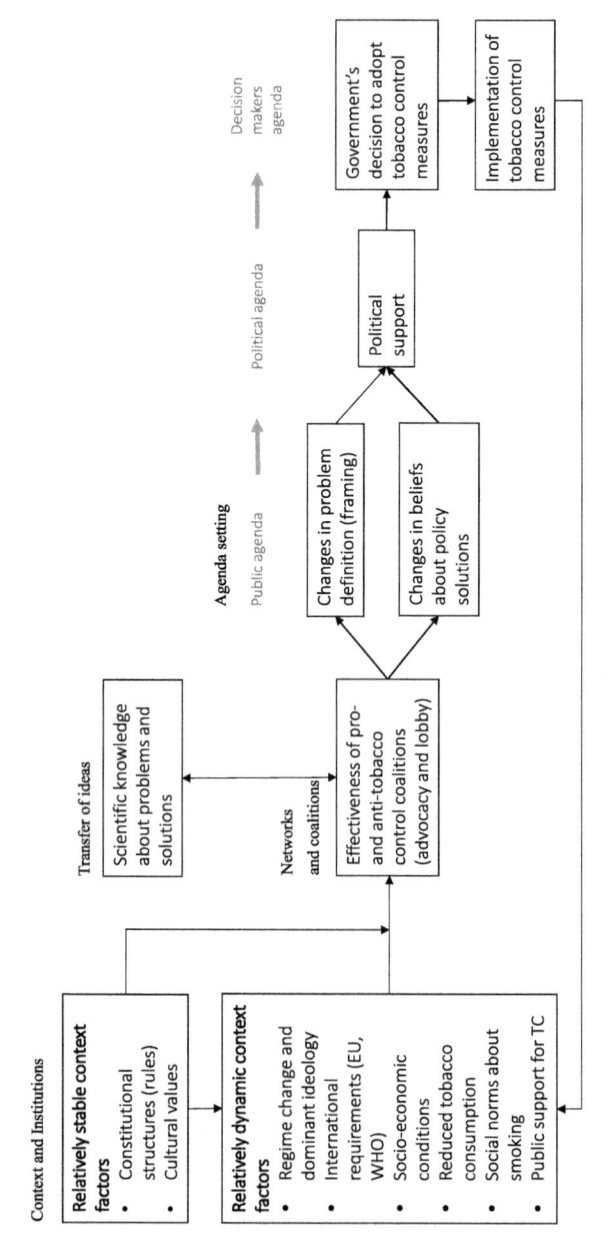

Fig. 1.1 Conceptual framework for understanding tobacco control making

research for this book, and are consistent with theoretical conceptualisations of the policy process. The distinction between relatively stable and relatively dynamic contextual factors is borrowed from the ACF (Sabatier & Weible, 2007; Weible et al., 2009) and, like the ACF, I award a central place in the framework to the competition between pro- and anti-tobacco coalitions and how effective they are at building supportive networks and setting up an effective lobbying apparatus. The model further reflects the basic idea from the MSA (Kingdon, 2003) that policy change is more likely to happen when advocates from coalitions succeed in bringing their conceptualisations of the problem and their preferred policy solution to the attention of politicians and policymakers. A topic's position on the policy agenda will be higher when both problem and policy solutions align with political opportunities. Opportunities result from changes in the policy environment, such as increased social support for tobacco control, new demands from the EU or the WHO, or a change of government with another dominant ideology. Ideology is particularly important in understanding tobacco policy (Cohen et al., 2000; K. Smith, 2013; Tesh, 1988). According to political scientist Silvia Tesh, "More powerful than vested interests, more subtle than science, political ideology has, in the end, the greatest influence on disease prevention policy" (Tesh, 1988, p. 155).

At the heart of the struggle for tobacco control is the almost universal fight between the economy, public health, and ideology. The model illustrates how new scientific information from domestic or international sources, about both problem and solutions, may feed into a coalition's repertoire, strengthening or broadening its lobbying capabilities. However, since statistical facts rarely speak for themselves and the making of facts may be commissioned by advocacy coalitions, the arrow between ideas and networks points in both directions. To have an effect, research findings need to be translated and "sold" to decision makers (Warner, 2005). The framework assumes that (at least in parliamentary democracies such as the Netherlands) a government's decision to adopt tobacco control measures depends on the presence of sufficient political support (majority positions in the parliament and cabinet), which is subject to the lobbying activities of the pro- and anti-tobacco control advocacy groups. In the background are the more stable and enduring contextual factors (notably cultural values), and institutional policymaking structures which directly or indirectly reinforce or inhibit the extent to which opposing coalitions can take advantage of new opportunities. Coalitions that are the best at taking advantage of opportunities arising from changes in the policy environment will be the most successful.

The framework provides for one large feedback loop. Tobacco control measures that are implemented by the government contribute to reductions in tobacco consumption at the population level. When there are fewer smokers and smoking is less visible, smoking becomes less popular and public opinion changes (smoking de-normalises), leading to more public support for further tobacco control measures and eventually contributing to new opportunities for the tobacco control coalition to advance its agenda. The empirical evidence for this loop is discussed in more detail in Chap. 4.

Outline

The next chapter is a detailed narrative of the events that shaped Dutch tobacco control policy: from when the government began to take the problem of smoking seriously in the 1960s until around 2014, when an era ended with the closure of the *Stichting Volksgezondheid en Roken* (Dutch Smoking or Health Foundation) (STIVORO), the national expert centre on tobacco control. Particular attention is given to the interaction between decision makers (ministers and state secretaries) and politicians in the parliament, to reveal what was done by governments in those years to tackle the smoking problem, and the struggles and politics involved. Chapter 2 structures the steps taken by the Dutch government to control tobacco, applying the idea of policy cycles, before comparing the pace of tobacco control policymaking in the Netherlands with other European countries. It will show that the Netherlands started relatively late, but caught up with mainstream Europe at the beginning of this century. Chapter 3 is the first chapter to apply one of the various analytical lenses, positioned so that we first look at policymaking from afar and gradually approach until we examine the internal dynamics of policymaking. The explanatory factors that are most distant from the actual policymaking process are external and relatively stable parameters, and serve as contextual structures that set the boundaries within which policymaking occurs. Chapter 4 first looks at the social and cultural environment. The government's willingness to consider tobacco control measures is influenced by social norms and societal support, and by the balance between the numbers of smokers and non-smokers. There is also a feedback loop, since these factors are also affected by the adoption of a new tobacco control policy. The way these factors influence each other over long periods of time at the population level is captured in the "flywheel model" of tobacco control. Chapter 5 examines the institutional structures and the "rules of the game" that make policymaking possible but also constrain it. Chapter 6 looks at how national tobacco control policy is increasingly determined by international institutions, particularly the EU and WHO. Chapter 7 examines the role of science and the diffusion of new ideas and knowledge about what works best in tobacco control at the national level. Chapters 8 and 9 respectively discuss pro- and anti-tobacco coalitions within the broader context of the tobacco control policy arena, and describe the failures and successes of advocacy efforts. The diminishing importance of the tobacco production and trade sector to the Dutch economy is also discussed in Chap. 8. Chapter 10 takes us to the core of public policymaking, which is problem definition and agenda setting by advocacy groups. The final chapter attempts to come to a synthesis of the main findings, answering the question of how tobacco control policy comes about in the Dutch context.

Research

As part of the research for this book, I examined several data sources. In addition to the scientific literature, I made extensive use of the database of parliamentary documents and proceedings of public debates on tobacco policy in both chambers of the Dutch Parliament, using NVivo software to facilitate the process of data ordering. This was a tedious task, given the large number of documents (more than 400), many of which were minutes of lengthy debates, but the documents proved most useful in presenting a detailed historical account of the policy process given in Chap. 3. The book further benefitted from interviews with key stakeholders and informants. I conducted 22 in-depth interviews with informants from the government, health organisations, and tobacco industry, focused on the five elements of public policymaking (context, institutions, agenda setting, ideas, and networks). Finally I examined documents made public through two freedom of information requests by investigative journalist Joop Bouma (Bouma, 2001). My research team added the Bouma documents to the Truth Tobacco Industry Documents database with help of the Maastricht University Library and the Dutch Cancer Society, so that the documents are now accessible for research.[3] They were most relevant in describing the lobbying practices of the Dutch tobacco industry network (Chap. 8). For the chapter on the tobacco control network (Chap. 9), I accessed documents from the archive of STIVORO to supplement what was learned in the interviews.

Notes

1. For the sake of simplicity I refer to the "Ministry of Health" and "Health Minister" throughout the book. However, this ministry had several names in the past. The Ministry was created in 1951 as the Ministry of Social Affairs and Public Health. It was the Ministry of Public Health and Environment (VoMil) between 1971 and 1982, when it was renamed into Ministry of Welfare, Public Health and Culture (WVC). Since 1994 its name is "Ministry of Public Health, Welfare, and Sport" (VWS).
2. See: "The end of tobacco? The tobacco endgame." Special issue. Tobacco Control, May 2013, vol. 22, Suppl. 1.
3. Accessible through https://industrydocuments.library.ucsf.edu/tobacco/collections/dutch-tobacco-industry/

References

Albæk, E., Green-Pedersen, C., & Nielsen, L. B. (2007). Making tobacco consumption a political issue in the United States and Denmark: The dynamics of issue expansion in comparative perspective. *Journal of Comparative Policy Analysis: Research and Practice, 9*, 1–20.

Asbridge, M. (2004). Public place restrictions on smoking in Canada: Assessing the role of the state, media, science and public health advocacy. *Social Science & Medicine, 58*, 13–24. https://doi.org/10.1016/S0277-9536(03)00154-0

Baba, A., Cook, D. M., McGarity, T. O., & Bero, L. A. (2005). Legislating "Sound Science": The role of the tobacco industry. *American Journal of Public Health, 95*, S20–S27. https://doi.org/10.2105/AJPH.2004.050963

Barnsley, K., Walters, H., & Wood-Baker, R. (2015). Bureaucratic barriers to evidence-based tobacco control policy: A Tasmanian case study. *Universal Journal of Public Health, 3*, 6–15.

Best, A., Clark, P., Leichow, S. J., & Trochim, W. M. K. (2007). *Greater than the sum: Systems thinking in tobacco control.* Tobacco control monograph. Bethesda, MD: U.S. Department of Health and Human Services, National Institutes of Health, National Cancer Institute.

Birkland, T. (2011). *An introduction to the policy process: Theories, concepts, and models of public policy making* (3rd ed.). Armonk, NY: M.E. Sharpe.

Blackman, V. S. (2005). Putting policy theory to work: Tobacco control in California. *Policy, Politics, & Nursing Practice, 6*, 148–155. https://doi.org/10.1177/1527154405276289

Bornhauser, A., McCarthy, J., & Glantz, S. A. (2006). German tobacco industry's successful efforts to maintain scientific and political respectability to prevent regulation of secondhand smoke. *Tobacco Control, 15*, e1. https://doi.org/10.1136/tc.2005.012336

Bosdriesz, J. R., Willemsen, M. C., Stronks, K., & Kunst, A. E. (2014). Tobacco control policy development in the European Union—Do political factors matter? *European Journal of Public Health*, 25(2), 190–194. https://doi.org/10.1093/eurpub/cku197

Bouma, J. (2001). *Het rookgordijn: De macht van de Nederlandse tabaksindustrie*. Amsterdam: Veen.

Breton, E., Richard, L., Gagnon, F., Jacques, M., & Bergeron, P. (2008). Health promotion research and practice require sound policy analysis models: The case of Quebec's tobacco act. *Social Sciences & Medicine*, 67(11), 1679–1689. https://doi.org/10.1016/j.socscimed.2008.07.028

Bryan-Jones, K., & Chapman, S. (2008). Political dynamics promoting the incremental regulation of secondhand smoke: A case study of New South Wales, Australia. *BMC Public Health*, 6, 192.

Buse, K., Mays, N., & Walt, G. (2012). *Making health policy* (2nd ed.). Berkshire: Open University Press.

Cairney, P. (2007). A 'Multiple Lenses' approach to policy change: The case of tobacco policy in the UK. *British Politics*, 2(2), 295–295.

Cairney, P. (2009). The role of ideas in policy transfer: The case of UK smoking bans since devolution. *Journal of European Public Policy*, 16(3), 471–488. https://doi.org/10.1080/13501760802684718

Cairney, P. (2012). *Understanding public policy: Theories and issues*. Basingstoke: Palgrave Macmillan.

Cairney, P. (2013). Policy concepts in 1000 words: The Advocacy Coalition Framework. Retrieved 20 July, 2017, from https://paulcairney.wordpress.com/2013/10/30/policy-concepts-in-1000-words-the-advocacy-coalition-framework/

Cairney, P., & Mamudu, H. (2014). The global tobacco control 'endgame': Change the policy environment to implement the FCTC. *Journal of Public Health Policy*, 35, 506–517. https://doi.org/10.1057/jphp.2014.18

Cairney, P., Studlar, D. T., & Mamudu, H. M. (2012). *Global tobacco control: Power, policy, governance and transfer*. New York: Palgrave Macmillan.

Cohen, J. E., Milio, N., Rozier, R. G., Ferrence, R., Ashley, M. J., & Goldstein, A. O. (2000). Political ideology and tobacco control. *Tobacco Control*, 9(3), 263–267. https://doi.org/10.1136/tc.9.3.263

Costa, H., Gilmore, A. B., Peeters, S., McKee, M., & Stuckler, D. (2014). Quantifying the influence of the tobacco industry on EU governance: Automated content analysis of the EU Tobacco Products Directive. *Tobacco Control*, 23(6), 473–478. https://doi.org/10.1136/tobaccocontrol-2014-051822

De Leeuw, E. (2013). Gezondheidsbeleidswetenschap: Tijd voor theorie. *Tijdschrift voor Gezondheidswetenschappen*, 91, 241–242.

Farquharson, K. (2003). Influencing policy transnationally: Pro-and anti-tobacco global advocacy networks. *Australian Journal of Public Administration, 62*, 80–92. https://doi.org/10.1111/j..2003.00351.x

Feldman, E., & Bayer, R. (2004). *Unfiltered: Conflicts over tobacco policy and public health.* Cambridge, MA: Harvard University Press.

Gonzalez, M., & Glantz, S. A. (2013). Failure of policy regarding smoke-free bars in the Netherlands. *European Journal of Public Health, 23*(1), 139–145. https://doi.org/10.1093/eurpub/ckr173

Grüning, T., Strünk, C., & Gilmore, A. B. (2008). Puffing away? Explaining the politics of tobacco control in Germany. *German Politics, 17*, 140–164.

Isett, K. (2013). In and across bureaucracy: Structural and administrative issues for the tobacco endgame. *Tobacco Control, 22*, i58–i60. https://doi.org/10.1136/tobaccocontrol-2012-050828

John, P. (2012). *Analyzing public policy* (2nd ed.). London: Routledge.

Kingdon, J. W. (2003). *Agendas, alternatives and public policies* (2nd ed.). New York: Addison-Wesley.

Kurzer, P., & Cooper, A. (2016). The dog that didn't bark: Explaining change in Germany's tobacco control policy at home and in the EU. *German Politics, 25*(4), 541–560. https://doi.org/10.1080/09644008.2016.1196664

Larsen, L. T. (2008). The political impact of science: Is tobacco control science- or policy-driven? *Science and Public Policy, 35*(10), 757–769. https://doi.org/10.3152/030234208x394697

Lie, J., Willemsen, M. C., De Vries, N. K., & Fooks, G. (2016). The devil is in the detail: Tobacco industry political influence in the Dutch implementation of the 2001 EU Tobacco Products Directive. *Tobacco Control, 25*, 545–550. https://doi.org/10.1136/tobaccocontrol-2015-052302

Mamudu, H., Dadkar, S., Veeranki, S. P., He, Y., Barnes, R., & Glantz, S. A. (2014). Multiple streams approach to tobacco control policymaking in a tobacco-growing state. *Journal of Community Health, 39*(4), 633–645. https://doi.org/10.1007/s10900-013-9814-6

McDaniel, P. A., Smith, E. A., & Malone, R. E. (2016). The tobacco endgame: A qualitative review and synthesis. *Tobacco Control, 25*(5), 594–604. https://doi.org/10.1136/tobaccocontrol-2015-052356

McNeill, A., Guignard, R., Beck, F., Marteau, R., & Marteau, T. M. (2015). Understanding increases in smoking prevalence: Case study from France in comparison with England 2000–10. *Addiction, 110*(3), 392–400. https://doi.org/10.1111/add.12789

Nathanson, C. A. (2005). Collective actors and corporate targets in tobacco control: A cross-national comparison. *Health Education & Behavior, 32*(3), 337–354. https://doi.org/10.1177/1090198105275047

Oliver, T. R. (2006). The politics of public health policy. *Annual Review of Public Health, 27*(1), 195–233. https://doi.org/10.1146/annurev.publhealth.25.101802.123126

Rabe, B. (2013). Political impediments to a tobacco endgame. *Tobacco Control*, 22, i52–i54. https://doi.org/10.1136/tobaccocontrl-2012-050799

Reid, R. (2005). *Globalizing tobacco control: Anti-smoking campaigns in California, France, and Japan.* Bloomington, IN: Indiana University Press.

Sabatier, P. A. (1998). The advocacy coalition framework: Revisions and relevance for Europe. *Journal of European Public Policy*, 5(1), 98–130. https://doi.org/10.1080/13501768880000051

Sabatier, P. A. (2007). *Theories of the policy process* (2nd ed.). Cambridge, MA: Westview Press.

Sabatier, P. A., & Weible, C. M. (2007). The advocacy coalition framework: Innovations and clarifications. In P. A. Sabatier (Ed.), *Theories of the policy process* (2nd ed.). Cambridge, MA: Westview Press.

Sato, H. (1999). The advocacy coalition framework and the policy process analysis: The case of smoking control in Japan. *Policy Studies Journal*, 27(1), 28–44. https://doi.org/10.1111/j.1541-0072.1999.tb01951.x

Schwartz, R., & Johnson, T. (2010). Problems, policies and politics: A comparative case study of contraband tobacco from the 1990s to the present in the Canadian context. *Journal of Public Health Policy*, 31(3), 342–354.

Smith, K. (2013). *Beyond evidence-based policy in public health: The interplay of ideas.* London: Palgrave Macmillan.

Smith, K. E., Fooks, G., Gilmore, A. B., Collin, J., & Weishaar, H. (2015). Corporate coalitions and policy making in the European Union: How and why British American Tobacco promoted "Better Regulation". *Journal of Health Politics, Policy and Law*, 40(2), 325–372. https://doi.org/10.1215/03616878-2882231

Studlar, D. T. (2002). *Tobacco control: Comparative politics in the United States and Canada.* Peterborough, ON, Canada: Broadview Press.

Studlar, D. T. (2007a). Ideas, institutions and diffusion: What explains tobacco control policy in Australia, Canada and New Zealand? *Commonwealth & Comparative Politics*, 45(2), 164–184. https://doi.org/10.1080/14662040701317493

Studlar, D. T. (2007b). *What explains policy change in tobacco control policy in advanced industrial democracies?* Paper presented at the European Consortium of Political Research, Helsinki.

Studlar, D. T. (2015). Punching above their weight through policy learning: Tobacco control policies in Ireland. *Irish Political Studies*, 30, 41–78.

Tesh, S. N. (1988). *Hidden arguments: Political ideology and disease prevention policy.* New Brunswick, NJ: Rutgers University Press.

Tobacco Free Initiative. (2008). *Tobacco industry interference with tobacco control.* Geneva: WHO.

Warner, K. E. (2005). The role of research in international tobacco control. *American Journal of Public Health*, 95(6), 976–984. https://doi.org/10.2105/AJPH.2004.046904

Weible, C. M., Sabatier, P. A., & McQueen, K. (2009). Themes and variations: Taking stock of the advocacy coalition framework. *Policy Studies Journal, 37*(1), 121–140. https://doi.org/10.1111/j.1541-0072.2008.00299.x

Willemsen, M. C., De Zwart, W. M., & Mooy, J. M. (1998). Effectiviteit van overheidsmaatregelen om het tabaksgebruik terug te dringen. In E. Roscam Abbing (Ed.), *Tabaksontmoedigingsbeleid: Gezondheidseffectrapportage*. Utrecht: Netherlands School of Public Health.

Willemsen, M. C., & Nagelhout, G. E. (2016). Country differences and changes in focus of scientific tobacco control publications between 2000 and 2012 in Europe. *European Addiction Research, 22*, 52–58.

Young, D., Borland, R., & Coghill, K. (2010). An actor-network theory analysis of policy innovation for smoke-free places: Understanding change in complex systems. *American Journal of Public Health, 100*(7), 1208–1217. https://doi.org/10.2105/AJPH.2009.184705

Zahariadis, N. (2007). The multiple streams framework: Structure, limitations, prospects. In P. Sabatier (Ed.), *Theories of the policy process* (2nd ed.). Boulder, CO: Westview Press.

Open Access This chapter is licensed under the terms of the Creative Commons Attribution 4.0 International License (http://creativecommons.org/licenses/by/4.0/), which permits use, sharing, adaptation, distribution and reproduction in any medium or format, as long as you give appropriate credit to the original author(s) and the source, provide a link to the Creative Commons license and indicate if changes were made.

The images or other third party material in this chapter are included in the chapter's Creative Commons license, unless indicated otherwise in a credit line to the material. If material is not included in the chapter's Creative Commons license and your intended use is not permitted by statutory regulation or exceeds the permitted use, you will need to obtain permission directly from the copyright holder.

CHAPTER 2

Dutch Tobacco Control Policy from the 1950s to the Present

Tobacco control policy is a long step from the neat theoretical path of identifying a problem, selecting the most effective strategy to tackle it, and then just implementing it. This chapter describes the many steps that were taken by the Dutch government to shape tobacco control policy. The description covers more than half a century and stays close to the timeline of events. The reader will learn how the government chose to combat smoking from the early years when it first became clear that smoking is not an innocent pleasure. At first the government was hesitant to react, but in the 1970s it became more active, culminating in a *Tobacco Memorandum* with far-reaching policy proposals, many of which were killed or toned down over subsequent years. The fight over tobacco policy then concentrated on two major national pieces of legislation: the 1988 Tobacco Act and its 2002 revision. These were not definitive laws but "framework" laws—meaning that they offered the basis for more specific decisions to be taken by the Council of Ministers (so-called orders-in-council) or by a minister (Ministerial Regulations) at a later stage. This opened up long periods of bargaining between interest groups, politicians, and the government about interpretations during the implementation phase.

Emerging Health Concerns (1950–1970)

Shortly after the Second World War, W.F. Wassink, a physician at the Antoni van Leeuwenhoek hospital in Amsterdam, published the results of a case-control study comparing the smoking habits of 137 male lung cancer patients with a control group of 100 "normal" men. He concluded that tobacco had to be the cause of the disease (Wassink, 1948). Two years later, a landmark study was published by British epidemiologists Richard Doll and Austin Bradford Hill (Doll & Hill, 1950). In the same year, a group of American epidemiologists concluded that the main cause of the rise in lung cancer death was smoking (Wynder & Graham, 1950). The international media quickly picked up the story. In 1952 the popular US-based *Reader's Digest* published an article entitled "Cancer by the Carton." This was the first mainstream publication that bluntly stated that smoking causes cancer, and blamed the high cancer rates on the tobacco industry's relentless promotion of tobacco. The effect was tremendous. Cigarette sales declined for the first time in over two decades in the United States.

In these years, the Netherlands was still a smokers' society, and in 1958 90% of men and 38% of women smoked (Gadourek, 1963, p. 66). Although *Readers Digest* was not distributed in the Netherlands at the time, the concern about smoking was felt. Alarming messages from the international studies that smoking can cause lung disease were summarised in a report from the Dutch Health Council (Wester, 1957) and attracted some attention in the Netherlands.

In March 1962 the British Royal College of Physicians of London published a landmark report that summarised the medical evidence and urged the UK government to take action (Royal College of Physicians, 1962a). It appeared in the same year in a Dutch translation (Royal College of Physicians, 1962b), and this attracted abundant media attention. From that moment, smokers' health was part of general public attention and tobacco use lost much of its innocence. In the summer of 1963, reports from the Dutch Central Bureau of Statistics about an alarming increase in lung cancer deaths among Dutch men were discussed extensively by the media and on national television, and this was a good reason for Senator Kranenburg (Christian Historical Union [CHU], a small protestant party) to ask the government whether it accepted that smoking causes lung cancer.[1] He also wanted to know what the government was going to do about it. Although the state secretary for health acknowledged that smoking was the leading cause of lung cancer, the government's response was restricted to education in schools, although it took the imposition of measures to reduce smoking under consideration. The Dutch Cancer Society received subsidies from the government in the order of a few hundred thousand guilders per year to execute these education campaigns. The Dutch government's minimal response was similar to the hesitant response of the UK government at the time (Berridge & Loughlin, 2005).

The next year, a report from the US Department of Health, Education, and Welfare (1964) (*Smoking and Health*), based on a review of over 7000 scientific articles, concluded unequivocally that there was a causative link between smoking and a 10- to 20-fold increase in the occurrence of lung cancer. This report had a lasting worldwide effect on how smoking was perceived. The year 1964 can be regarded as the year when serious concerns about smoking stirred the Dutch nation and health organisations like the Dutch Cancer Society got actively involved with tobacco control.

In 1965 tobacco manufacturers united in an effort to prevent government regulation of advertising, and reached a "gentlemen's agreement" in which they promised to stop marketing that suggested some brands were "better for health" than others (Tobacco Manufacturers' Association, 1971). They also promised to abstain from television commercials. Since tobacco commercials were not broadcast on Dutch television, this offer was not particularly impressive. Similar codes of conduct surfaced in Germany, Belgium, and Luxembourg (Pauw, 1971).[2] The UK-based manufacturers had agreed in 1962 to implement a code of advertising practice that would detract some of the glamour from cigarette advertisements (ASH, 2013). This strategy of self-regulation was successful in preventing governmental regulation of tobacco advertising for many years. The self-imposed restrictions in the Netherlands had no formal or legislative status, but were subject to scrutiny by the *Stichting Reclame Code* (Advertising Code Foundation) (SRC), an organisation founded in 1963 by the advertising sector to handle citizens' complaints about advertisements.[3]

In 1968 the US Department of State inquired through its embassies about tobacco control activities in 22 countries (National Clearinghouse for Smoking and Health, 1969; US Public Health Service, 1970). Few countries had taken action. Twelve had not started even rudimentary education in schools, and many were waiting for advice from their national health councils. However, some were already taking the first regulatory steps. Some had banned advertising on television (Italy,

Norway, Sweden), some had banned the sale of tobacco to minors (Austria, Norway), and some had initiated communication campaigns that went beyond youth education (Canada, the United Kingdom, Italy). Dutch tobacco control policy was restricted to providing subsidies for youth education, while the industry exhibited self-restraint regarding tobacco advertisements. In sum, at the end of the 1960s the Netherlands had no tobacco control legislation despite growing health concerns. The only action taken by the government was to provide a small yearly subsidy to the Cancer Society's youth education school programmes.

Ambitious Policy Intentions (1970–1977)

In 1970 Hans van den Doel, a Labour Party member of the lower house of the Dutch Parliament, asked whether the government was aware that US President Nixon had signed an intention to ban tobacco advertisement on radio and television and to put health warnings on cigarette packs.[4] Van den Doel wanted to know if the Dutch government intended to follow the American example. The government responded by setting up a working group with representatives from five governmental departments (the Ministries of Health, Social Work, Justice, Economic Affairs, and Finance), commissioned to examine the possibility of restricting tobacco advertisements.[5] This working group was called the Meulblok Committee after its Chairman J. Meulblok, head of the Public Health Department of the Ministry of Health.

Between 1971 and 1972 Dutch tobacco manufacturing organisations had several meetings with the Meulblok Committee about tobacco advertising. Meulblok actively sought input from the industry and felt that it was important that the committee and the industry were on the same wavelength (Interdepartementale Commissie Tabaksreclame, 1972a). The Committee's starting point was that it wanted "if possible, to prevent the necessity of interventions by the government" (Interdepartementale Commissie Tabaksreclame, 1972b). It struggled especially with the legal aspects of a ban on tobacco advertising, being under constant pressure from the tobacco industry to refrain from advising about advertising regulation. Meulblok thus wanted to first explore the option of self-regulation, because the committee expected that an advertising ban would be difficult to reconcile with constitutional rights of freedom of press and freedom of speech (Interdepartementale Commissie Tabaksreclame, 1972a). Meulblok wondered if this might show "where a small country such as the Netherlands can be great and be an example to other countries."

It was not only the lower house of the Dutch Parliament that was concerned about the smoking issue. In 1971 Upper House Senator Sidney Van den Bergh of the *Volkspartij voor Vrijheid en Democratie* (People's Party for Freedom and Democracy) (VVD), the conservative-liberal political party, read the second report from the UK Royal College of Physicians, "*Smoking and Health: Now*," which concluded that smokers were twice as likely to die by middle age than non-smokers and recommended health warnings on cigarette packs, advertising restrictions, and tax increases (Royal College of Physicians, 1971). When Van den Bergh asked the Dutch state secretary for health whether he was considering similar steps.[6] The state secretary responded by asking the Health Council for advice on how the government should inform the public about the risks of smoking. It is interesting to compare this reserved Dutch response to what was happening at the time in the United Kingdom. The English Health Education Council initiated a series of hard-hitting awareness campaigns in the beginning of the 1970s that shook up the public. Advertisements had texts such as, "The tar and discharge that collect in the lungs of the average smoker," "You can't scrub your lungs clean," and "Why learn the truth about lung cancer the hard way?" (Berridge & Loughlin, 2005). One advertisement showed smokers crossing London's Waterloo Bridge interspersed with images of lemmings throwing themselves off a cliff. A 1973–1974 campaign showed a naked pregnant smoking woman featuring the text, "Is it fair to force your baby to smoke cigarettes?" In 1978 the English Health Education Council attacked the industry's claim that safer cigarettes would be the solution, through an advertisement that had the line, "Switching to a substitute cigarette is like jumping from the 36th rather than the 39th floor of a building" (Berridge & Loughlin, 2005). Such campaigns paved the way for a more assertive and proactive governmental response to the smoking problem in the United Kingdom. The Dutch government did not take similar actions.

In 1975 the Health Council's report *Measures to reduce smoking* was published. A commission of 12 experts had worked on it for almost two and a half years, convening 16 times. Surprisingly, their conclusions were quite revolutionary at the time, and threatening to those with a vested interest in the tobacco sector. It stated as a starting point that "public health interests must prevail above economic interests" (Beernink & Plokker, 1975, p. 7). The report contained a comprehensive and integrated set of policy proposals.

The report concluded that "considering the large influence of smoking on the people's health, it is unjust and impossible for the government to look the other way much longer" (Beernink & Plokker, 1975). Interestingly, the report noted that full freedom of choice did not exist with respect to smoking because smokers had become pharmacologically and psychologically dependent on tobacco use after exposure to so much tobacco advertising. Tobacco control had to be "aimed primarily at the creation of a psycho-social climate in which smoking is negatively influenced and at stimulating a new attitude regarding smoking." The government was advised to communicate unequivocally to the public that smoking poses a serious danger to the health of smokers and non-smokers.

Measures to reduce smoking proposed a comprehensive programme of educational and regulative measures—and a 15-year action plan to tackle the smoking epidemic. The government was advised to consider a full tobacco advertising ban, restrictions on the availability of tobacco, removal of tobacco vending machines, increases in tobacco taxes to fund anti-tobacco advertising campaigns, and the banning of smoking in public places (see Box 2.1 for a more complete account of the commission's recommendations). Tobacco control policy was to be supported by financial means that were in fair proportion to the advertising budgets that tobacco companies had at their disposal and to the revenues that the government received from tobacco taxes.

Measures to reduce smoking could have been the starting point for the development of a comprehensive national tobacco control strategy or plan, but it did not translate into policy. Looking back at the report through modern eyes, it had all the necessary ingredients to propel the Dutch to leadership in the field. However, hardly any of the ideas was taken up. Some of the measures took many decades to materialise, others, such as a ban on vending machines and earmarked tobacco tax revenues, are still not realised. The progressive cabinet of the time (led by Labour Party leader Joop den Uyl) was not followed by a cabinet that put the policy intentions into action.

Box 2.1 Proposals in the 1975 Health Council report *Measures to reduce smoking*
- A ban on tobacco advertising
- Health warnings on cigarette packs
- Restrictions on smoking in public places, in combination with an educational campaign to explain the measure
- Smoking restrictions for specific occupations, such as doctors and teachers
- A smoking ban on public transport
- Restrictions on smoking in television shows and other programmes
- Restrictions on the number of points of sale of tobacco
- Removal of tobacco vending machines
- A ban on the sale of tobacco to minors (under 16 years of age). This measure was to be considered if the removal of vending machines was not effective enough
- Increasing tobacco taxes in tandem with neighbouring countries, the extra revenue to be allocated to anti-tobacco campaigns
- Consideration of a ban on the duty-free sale of tobacco products
- Mass media campaigns to stimulate interpersonal communication about the dangers of smoking, and to encourage the formation of group norms incompatible with smoking
- Health education programmes in schools, worksites and civil society organisations
- Motivation and training of health educators, doctors, and teachers to enable them to motivate and support patients, clients, and pupils not to smoke
- Developing effective behavioural counselling for smokers who wish to quit
- Foundation of a National Institute for the Reduction of Smoking, responsible for providing general information to the public, and for the coordination of education, campaigns, smoking cessation support, and research
- Development of a long-term scientific research program to include systematic monitoring of the smoking habits of the population and evaluation of the effectiveness of all current and future tobacco control measures, plus research into the psychological and sociological determinants of smoking, the best ways of supporting smokers to quit smoking, and the impact of smoking on health

One recommendation from the Health Council's report was taken up, though. This was the creation of a national institute for tobacco control, leading to the foundation of *Stichting Volksgezondheid en Roken* (Dutch Smoking or Health Foundation) (STIVORO). Since the core of the government's approach to tackling the smoking problem was health education, the new institute's tasks were to educate the public about smoking and to monitor national smoking habits through yearly surveys (see Chap. 9 for an account of STIVORO's role in tobacco control).

Soon after the publication of the Health Council's report, the Meulblok Committee presented its report to the cabinet, which sent it to the parliament in 1976. The Meulblok Committee stayed close to the Health Council's recommendations (Meulblok, 1975). It adopted the council's starting point: that the interests of public health must prevail above other interests. Meulblok pointed out that any negative impact on employment or tax revenues could not outweigh the necessity of protecting the public's health. Another starting point was that priority must be given to the protection of youth, and that this must not be restricted to education.

For the government, the Meulblok report was the starting point of a long process that eventually resulted in a "Tobacco Act." A particularly important recommendation from Meulblok was to start drafting a law to ban tobacco advertising. The committee's argument was that "advertising constantly confirms and reinforces the usual [positive] attitude in our society regarding smoking" (p. 28). The committee left open the possibility of a gradual approach, involving a series of restrictions, in the case that a full advertising ban was politically undesirable or unfeasible, but dismissed the idea of self-regulation by the industry. Frequent consultations with industry representatives had not convinced the committee to refrain from legislation. The industrial lobby had broken ranks and could not offer an acceptable, mutually agreed-upon alternative. Niemeyer, a local producer of cigarettes, no longer respected the gentlemen's agreement between manufacturers, part of which was that advertisements must not give the impression that one type or brand of tobacco was less harmful than others. Niemeyer, a market leader in brands of cigarettes with distinct harm reduction appeal, wanted to promote its brands Roxy Dual and Kelly Halvaret as low in nicotine and tar and relatively safe for consumers, and concluded that this was more profitable for them than adhering to the industry's mutual but non-binding caveats.

Since the industry was not able to present a convincing alternative, the Meulblok Committee advised the cabinet to start the process of drafting a

Tobacco Act that included advertising restrictions (Meulblok, 1975). The recommendations were threatening to the tobacco industry—which spent no less than 35 million guilders (about €40 million in current money) on tobacco advertising in 1977 (Algemene Rekenkamer, 1982).

The Meulblok Report was produced during the Den Uyl cabinet (1973-1977), the most progressive cabinet that the Netherlands has ever had. It comprised Christian Democrats and parties left of the political centre. Prime Minister Den Uyl (Labour Party) was credited for trying to free politics from corporatism. This was an era when the ideal of a better world dominated the political discourse, and many believed in the idea of a just and modifiable society (*maakbare samenleving*). In January 1977, just two months before Den Uyl's cabinet resigned, State Secretary for Health Jo Hendriks sent a letter to the parliament outlining the cabinet's strategy to combat smoking.[7] This *Tobacco Memorandum* (*Rookmemorandum*) put forth the recommendations from the *Measures to reduce smoking* report from the Health Council and ideas from the Meulblok Report that were felt would be the most feasible to implement.[8] Hendriks decided upon a "not too hasty approach" by not implementing all of the measures proposed by the Health Council at once, but by opting to do it gradually.[9] Health educational efforts had to be intensified, and accompanied by the three measures that the government felt it could implement on relatively short notice: bans on smoking in public venues, governmental buildings, and areas such as waiting rooms; labelling tobacco products (with health warnings and tar and nicotine yields); and a ban on tobacco advertising. Other measures were considered for the longer term.[10] The cabinet noted that smoking restrictions would help build a social climate in which non-smoking was the norm and that it might be a good idea, for each subsequent long-term measure, to estimate the extent to which the measure restricted the freedom of the individual. It was decided that a further analysis of the proposals was needed, including legal and political feasibility. A new committee was set up in July 1977 to do this. This *Interdepartementale Commissie Beperking Tabaksgebruik* (Interdepartmental Committee for Reducing Tobacco Use) (ICBT) consisted of delegates from six state departments, but mostly from the health and trade ministries (both had four seats at the table, but the Ministry of Health delivered the chair, vice-chair, and secretary). The committee's task was to formulate concrete proposals for regulative measures—other than education—to reduce tobacco use.[11]

Partly due to a change of government, it was almost two years (March 1979) before the committee was officially installed and started work. In the meantime, advice from the Meulblok Committee to introduce health warnings was followed through in a proposal for a law that was attached to the Food and Product Safety Act in 1981, ordering that from January 1982 onwards tobacco products had to carry the health warning, "Smoking threatens health. The Minister of Public Health and the Environment." Mandatory information about tar and nicotine content was also included. This was less confronting than the advice from Meulblok to use the text "Smoking damages yourself and others."

The Ministry of Economic Affairs Steps on the Brake (1977–1991)

In December 1977, the first cabinet under Christian Democratic leader Dries Van Agt came to power and changed the political landscape profoundly. This centre-right government was "fairly tolerant towards smoking," according to an internal industry memo (Colby, 1979). Philip Morris' analysis was that "the new government is favouring industry more than its predecessor. However, more legislation will probably be enacted, but in such a way as not to interfere with the economic situation; the Ministry of Finance and Economic Affairs carries considerable weight in Holland" (Unknown (Philip Morris), 1979). The government's position on tobacco from the first Van Agt cabinet until the third Lubbers cabinet (mid-1990s) can be characterised by the mantra "tobacco is an individual's own responsibility." Governments in these years were not happy with the Meulblok and Health Council reports and effectively bogged their recommendations in bureaucratic procedures.

One of the first things the new cabinet did was to tone down the ambitious tobacco control policy intentions of the previous cabinet. In a letter to Parliament, the new state secretary for economic affairs wrote that, "given the interests of businesses that are at stake here, I will make sure that tobacco control policy with respect to the supply side will be developed in a careful, gradual manner, in connection with the policy with respect to the demand-side."[12] Everything having to do with legally binding restrictions, including tobacco advertising and regulation of the sale of tobacco, was handled by the Ministry of Economic Affairs. The Ministry of Health controlled the demand-side. This division of tasks ensured that effective tobacco policy measures could not be made without the consent of the powerful Minister of Economic Affairs, who could step on the brake whenever the Ministry of Health moved too fast.

In March 1979, the ICBT committee began to work on its policy proposal report. The cabinet did not put much pressure on the commission, which was allowed to take its time. The new State Secretary for Health, Els Veder-Smit of the conservative–liberal VVD, regarded self-regulation by the industry as the best alternative to an advertising ban.[13] She believed that personal freedom and the responsibility of individuals for their own health were important aspects for the ICBT to keep in mind when considering appropriate measures. While the ICBT was working on its report, the tobacco industry presented a list of self-imposed advertising restrictions. This included old promises such as refraining from advertisements directed at youth and from making health claims, and ending the promotion of tobacco products through television and radio.[14] In 1979 the state secretary explained that "from our contacts with the tobacco manufacturing industry it is clear to us that they are prepared to ban health appeals from their advertising messages."[15] She trusted self-restraint by the industry, as long as this was supported by all manufacturers and backed by sanctions. The ICBT was requested to take the industry's proposals into account.

Parliament was more critical of the industry's self-regulative proposals. The *Christen-Democratisch Appèl* (Christian Democratic Party) (CDA) claimed that the industry had failed, and tabled a motion to urge the government to regulate tobacco advertising.[16] This resulted in a ban on advertising on radio and television in 1980 through the Media Act. Parliamentarians also became impatient with respect to smoking bans. Again the CDA tried to speed up the process[17] by tabling a motion to ban smoking in public places.[18] A year later this was followed by another motion from the CDA requesting the same, referring to the fact that France had implemented a ban on smoking in public places since July.[19] These motions were the start of an almost decade-long process leading to a public smoking ban, the main element of the Tobacco Act of 1988.

The ICBT reported to the state secretary for health in January 1981 (ICBT, 1981). The recommendations were more industry-friendly this time around than the previous reports; compromise was sought between health and economics. The committee identified four principles as starting points for tobacco control policy in declining order of significance: tobacco use is harmful for health; youth need to be protected; the right of physical integrity in non-smokers has to be balanced against the right of personal freedom of smokers; and undesirable societal and economic consequences must be taken into account. The committee underscored this last principle by writing that it was aware that the tobacco sector contributes significantly to the national economy. The idea of a tobacco advertising ban was postponed indefinitely because the commission felt that the industry must be allowed to use advertising as a means of "communicating" with their consumers about new products. The committee did criticise the existing self-regulation (the *Reclame Code*) for lack of sanctions and recommended that misleading advertisements should be sobered down, for example, through restrictions on the use of colours. The idea of deterring smoking through higher cigarette taxes (either by increasing general taxation levels or by linking the tax level to the level of harmful substances so that more harmful products would be taxed higher) was considered, but no concrete proposals were made. The most far-reaching recommendation was to restrict the number of tobacco selling points to specialty shops, but since this could have substantial consequences for the tobacco sector it was not to be done hastily, according to the committee. Other proposals were to ban tobacco vending machines and to ban smoking in public places and in government buildings. The ICBT report remarked that in a future Tobacco Act, regulation might be included to limit the quantity of substances that were harmful to health in tobacco products. In April 1981 the ICBT was asked by the state secretary for health to work out the details of a Tobacco Act, while parliament was disappointed that five years after the Meulblok Committee, nothing had been accomplished except further pointless deliberations and slow-down tactics by the industry.[20]

Piet van Zeil, the state secretary for economic affairs in the first Lubbers cabinet (1982–1986), discussed the idea of restricting the sale of tobacco products to specialty shops in parliament in August 1982. Van Zeil promised he would have another round of talks with the business community to hear their side of the argument.[21] He felt that for each measure (a ban on vending machines and restricting points of sale), costs and benefits needed to be balanced, and indications that measures could pose a burden on businesses had to be taken seriously. He pointed out that this cabinet was not likely to opt for a broad reduction of the number of sales outlets, nor even for a ban on vending machines. The Lubbers cabinet's motto was "more market, less government."

In July 1983 the cabinet gave the green light to the idea of promulgating a Tobacco Act. At the end of 1984, State Secretary for Health Joop van der Reijden and State Secretary for Economic Affairs Piet van Zeil sent a proposal to parliament for consideration.[22] In the introductory remarks of their clarification document, the two underlined the importance of economic considerations[23]:

> Against the interests of public health, that have to do with the reduction of smoking and the protection of non-smokers, are economic and fiscal interests that have to be taken into consideration as well. Thousands of citizens earn their daily bread, or at least part of it, from the production and distribution of tobacco products. Smoking is a deeply ingrained and socially accepted habit, although there are clear signs that this acceptance is diminishing. The state enjoys considerable revenues from tobacco taxes, which are used to finance many useful and necessary things.

The government gave the industry the benefit of the doubt by continuing the policy of self-imposed restrictions on tobacco advertisements. Only if this did not have the expected effect on youth smoking would the government consider imposing a ban by decree—but it did not specify how they would evaluate the effectiveness of self regulation.

The ICBT's proposal to reduce the number of tobacco selling points was not part of the proposal for the Tobacco Act, "because the harmful effects on the business community, especially middle and small businesses, cannot be sufficiently compensated."[24] Only the sale of tobacco in healthcare institutions and educational facilities was to be restricted. The proposal to ban the sale of tobacco to minors and to ban vending machines was also abandoned, because the government wished to follow the advice of a "deregulation" committee (see also Chap. 5 on the importance of deregulation committees), which made the point that such a ban would be difficult to uphold and easy for minors to circumvent. With respect to a smoking ban in public places, the government did not want a general ban, but instead left it to local administrators to decide on the best way to protect non-smokers from second-hand smoke and how to decide which local areas should be subject to smoking restrictions. The ban was restricted to government-owned buildings and buildings of organisations that worked for the government, such as hospitals, schools, and social welfare organisations. The government wanted to leave open the possibility of restricting smoking instead of banning it completely, for example, by tolerating smoking in designated sections or during designated hours. What was to be the centrepiece of the Tobacco Act became a disputable and vague instruction to the managers of public buildings, with no sanctions provided for violations. Borgman, the CDA parliamentarian behind the motion from 1980, summarised the general feeling of disappointment among parliamentarians: "the submitted Tobacco Act has, after going through the bureaucratic wheels of interdepartmental consultation, deregulation and so forth, more the appearance of a leaflet with suggestions and prescriptions than the ground-breaking law that the parliament has been asking for since 1977."[25] Parliamentarian Erwin Nypels (Democrats 66) proposed an amendment to include private workplaces in the smoking ban.[26]

In July 1986, when the second Lubbers cabinet (1986–1989) came to office, the new State Secretary for Health Dick Dees (VVD) at first was open to the amendment, but after some pressure from the employer organisation *Verbond van Nederlandse Ondernemingen en Nederlands Christelijk Werkgeversverbond* (Confederation of Netherlands Industry and Employers) (VNO–NCW),[27] advised against it.[28] In his national policy document on prevention of heart disease, State Secretary Dees did not announce further tobacco control measures.[29] The cabinet did not want to include smoking restrictions for private workplaces in the new act, and opted for the path of continued self-regulation instead. This meant reaching agreements with the business community through talks and negotiations with the "social partners" (the employee and employer organisations).

During the final debate in the senate, State Secretary for Health Dick Dees (VVD) admitted that he was still negotiating with the industry about a satisfactory code of conduct for tobacco advertising.[30] The industry accepted the conditions for self-regulation just before the Tobacco Act was published in the *Bulletin of Acts*. A new advertising code of conduct was decided upon and entered into force on 1 January 1989. It was agreed that this would last for another five years. Although the Tobacco Act included the threat of prohibiting advertising through an Order of Council, it did not come to this. Occasionally, the industry made small adaptations to the advertising code to accommodate calls for tighter restrictions by parliament and health organisations. This situation would continue for another decade. Protected by their code, tobacco industry spending on advertising increased from 21 million guilders in 1974 (Beernink & Plokker, 1975) to 35 million in 1977 (Algemene Rekenkamer, 1982) and to more than 200 million in 1996.[31] The Tobacco Act included a ban on tobacco advertising on radio and television, to comply with European Union (EU) regulations (Directive 89/552/EEC). This was no improvement, since advertising on TV and radio had already been banned since 1980.[32]

The final verdict of the senate in March 1988 was that the piece of legislation was too little, too late, and could not be expected to affect smoking rates. The senate supported it nevertheless, for lack of something better.[33] The Tobacco Act was approved on 10 March 1988 and went into effect on 1 January 1990, after four years of deliberations, debates, and amendments. It is a framework legislation, where specific details may be decided on at a later stage through ministerial decisions and governmental decrees. What was accomplished was that smoking was more or less banned (leaving open the possibility of smoking sections and smoking during designated times) in about 50,000 indoor venues in government-owned buildings and properties open to the general public.

In response to the general disappointment and discontent with the weak act, the government decided to intensify education, campaigns, and palliative measures to appease the health lobby for a while. A working group was installed to develop a multiple-year educational programme. The government's subsidy to STIVORO for campaigns increased somewhat from 1989 onwards, and STIVORO was commissioned to start a mass media campaign to motivate private companies to implement smoking policies on a voluntary basis.

During this time, the government asked the Health Council to reassess the harm from passive smoking in light of new evidence from abroad. The report was presented in 1990 but lacked firm conclusions about causal associations between prolonged exposure to passive smoking and the risk of lung cancer (Gezondheidsraad, 1990), which did not help put proposals for further restrictions on smoking on the political agenda (see Chap. 9 for a further discussion of this report and the relatively late official recognition that passive smoking is a public health problem in the Netherlands).

POLICY STAGNATION (1991–1994)

For some time the 1988 Tobacco Act remained the final governmental response to the tobacco problem. The third Lubbers cabinet (1989–1994) had a new state secretary responsible for tobacco control: Hans Simons (Labour Party). Simons commissioned Research For Policy, a commercial research firm, to evaluate the effectiveness of the Tobacco Act. He wanted to know whether the self-regulation of tobacco advertising and promotion by the industry was effective, and whether the new measures in the act were sufficient to protect youth and non-smokers. The conclusions of the report, published in September 1991, were that the code of conduct and the new Tobacco Act had had no detectable effect on the smoking habits of the Dutch (Dresscher, Elzinga, & Koldenhof, 1991). The researchers identified weak spots in the policy and considered it "ambivalent" because of the government's wish to accommodate the irreconcilable interests of health and economy. This resulted in advertising restrictions that were not comprehensive, smoking bans that offered little protection to non-smokers, and rules and regulations that were rarely adhered to. The industry spent more money on tobacco advertising than ever before and managed to sell more cigarettes per smoker, so that "the result is a policy that is neither fish nor fowl, its effectiveness largely depending on public norms" (Dresscher et al., 1991, p. 76). Despite these harsh comments, Research for Policy did not recommend a full advertising ban, anticipating attempts by the industry to circumvent any such ban. Instead they advised a middle way: extending the existing set of self-imposed measures and investing more in enforcement.

In a letter to parliament, State Secretary Simons, inspired by the report, was critical of the national tobacco policy of previous cabinets.[34] He noted that the Netherlands lagged behind other European countries and criticised the tobacco industry's attempts to circumvent their own advertising restrictions, saying that he wanted to intensify national tobacco control policy. He noted that the self-regulative measures of the tobacco industry in the United Kingdom and Denmark were stricter than in the Netherlands. For example, in the United Kingdom, the industry refrained from positive images in advertisements, such as Marlboro's tough cowboys. He proposed a substantial tightening of the advertising code of conduct, including more restrictions on advertisements and a ban on indirect advertising in radio and television programmes, and he wanted to examine the option of restricting smoking in private workplaces through legislative measures, as three quarters of private workplaces had no relevant smoking policy. These proposals were accompanied by two press releases. One carried the title "Self-regulation tobacco advertising insufficient" (VWS, 1991), the other "Tighter approach to tobacco policy" (WVC, 1991).

The tobacco industry was furious, and quickly commissioned a competing research firm to produce a detailed critique of Research For Policy's report, refuting the minister's accusations that the industry was not abiding with the code of conduct (Nederlands Economisch Instituut, 1991). The position of the Ministry of Economic Affairs was that Simons had to give the industry's advertising code the benefit of the doubt, and civil servants from that ministry suggested that if no agreement with their bureaucratic counterparts at the Ministry of Health was possible, Economic Affair's Minister Koos Andriessen would have to talk sense to Simons (Ministerie van Economische Zaken, 1991). Although Simons stated that tobacco control was a "very high policy priority,"[35] he gave in to the pressure and failed to make any advance in tobacco control policy.

The Dutch cabinet reconfirmed its preference for self-regulation over a legislative approach.[36] A compromise was reached between Hans Simons and the Minister of Economic Affairs that the government would not start the process of drafting a ban but would instead continue to work with the industry to increase their self-regulating efforts.[37] The initiative to protect non-smoking employees at the workplace was left to *Stichting van de Arbeid* (the Labour Foundation) (STAR), which decided not to consider a ban but to allow labour representatives and management of individual businesses to reach mutually satisfactory policies (Stichting van de Arbeid, 1992).[38] In practice this meant that if individual non-smoking employees had an issue with smoking at their workplace, and were unable to find a satisfactory solution with their colleagues and their employer, their only option was to take their employer to court. They would have to point to relevant passages in national occupational health and safety legislation—an almost impossible task for the average worker.

Heated fights and debates over the voluntary advertising agreements characterised the first part of the 1990s. While the ministries negotiated regularly with the industry about the advertising code of conduct, health organisations publicly declared its failure. Pressure on the government increased when the parliament tabled a motion for an advertising ban.[39] Simons started the process of drafting an amendment to the Tobacco Act that would open the door to an advertising ban, in case the industry's self-imposed restrictions were not satisfactory. The code of conduct was regarded as "the last chance that the cabinet offers to the industry in the way of self-regulation."[40] A new code went into effect on April 1994 and resulted in minor improvements, such as advertisements no longer depicting persons looking younger than 30, and no tobacco ads run in cinemas before 6PM. In addition, the industry agreed that it would not increase its total spending on tobacco advertisements above the level reached in 1990. It was agreed that the new code would be in place for another five years and would be evaluated every six months, not only for industrial compliance, but also for whether the industry was adhering to the spirit of the code, which was to keep all promotion of tobacco products away from children.

Protesters against the advertising code of conduct had support from the European (EC), which had proposed an EU-wide advertising ban in 1991. However, this had been successfully opposed by a group of member states, including the Netherlands, which raised legal objections and argued that EU legislation was not acceptable if an issue could be better addressed at the national level (the so-called subsidiarity principle; see Chap. 5). In 1994 the health warnings were improved slightly with "Smoking seriously harms health" replacing "Smoking threatens health."

Tobacco Control Proposals by Minister Borst (1994–1997)

In August 1994 the so-called Purple Cabinet came to power. This was a coalition between two liberal parties (VVD and Democraten 66 (D66), both "blue") and the "red" *Partij van de Arbeid* (Labour Party) (PvdA), hence the name "purple." It was relatively progressive, with only five VVD ministers against a prime minister from the Labour party, four additional Labour ministers and four D66 ministers. Els Borst (D66) was the first minister of health in Dutch history. Before her, state secretaries were responsible for public health. She had personal motives to fight smoking: she was the sister-in-law to a leading Dutch cancer specialist, and on entering office was already over 60 with a long career as a practising physician and director of an academic hospital. She had also been vice president of the Health Council. Borst had a strong position in the cabinet and a good working relationship with both the Prime Minister Wim Kok and with Hans Wijers, the Minister of Economic Affairs, who was from the same liberal-democratic party as she.[41] D66 had written in its election programme that the Netherlands was a European backbencher regarding restrictions on tobacco advertising, and that it should catch up as soon as possible.

Borst highlighted the urgency of tackling smoking in her disease prevention policy document, *Gezond en Wel*, launched in March 1995.[42] She characterised the Dutch tobacco policy as "mild" and made the point that anti-tobacco regulation had fallen behind other countries in Europe. She identified tobacco control as a priority for the government and announced her intention to "intensify" it. In a letter to parliament she explained that the "proven effectiveness" of a policy was an important criterion when choosing the right measures to tackle tobacco.[43] She wanted to limit the availability of tobacco products to minors, sharpen the smoking ban in public places by installing sanctions, intensify anti-tobacco youth education and smoking cessation efforts, and evaluate the current tobacco taxation level in light of European minimum standards. These proposals were not particularly ground breaking nor were they threatening to the industry—in her first years in office, Borst, a liberal politician and part of a coalition with the liberal–conservative VVD, was searching for measures that would have political support from liberals. Most parties in parliament, except VVD and CDA, rejected the weak proposals. Instead, they wanted the government to make the decision to ban advertising sooner and endorsed the need for the government to support stricter advertising regulation by the EU.[44]

Regarding advertising restrictions, Minister Borst was confronted with a major obstacle. The government had recently renewed its agreement with the industry for a new five-year period of self-regulation, promising that there would be no regulation as long as the industry adhered to the code of conduct. Borst ordered the state attorney to examine whether the government could unilaterally withdraw from these agreements with the industry, so that the route to an advertising ban would be open. This turned out to be very difficult, since the agreement had legal power and could only be overturned if the advertising code was not adhered to "in letter and in spirit" (De Landsadvocaat, 1995). Borst proposed a limited list of acceptable types of advertising, instead of working from the current extensive set of restrictions. This was because poorly formulated restrictions were relatively easy for the industry to circumvent, evidenced by a plethora of incidents in which the industry continued to promote its products to young people.

In January 1995, the industry refrained from advertising on billboards in the direct vicinity of hospitals and schools, and the fine for violating the code of conduct was increased from 50,000 to 100,000 guilders.[45] In 1996 the industry ended tobacco commercials on cinema screens. Despite these small improvements, tobacco advertising was still omnipresent—in magazines, on billboards, and through brand stretching and the promotion of brand logos at music festivals. The industry continued to broadcast commercials in cinemas for Mascotte cigarette-rolling paper and the Camel Trophy challenge. Tobacco promotion at the international Formula 1 Grand Prix racing in Zandvoort and the TT motor racing in Assen continued as well. During this period smoking rates went up, with a dramatic increase from 36% (1989) to 39% (1996) in the male population and from 29% to 32% in women (STIVORO, 1999).

In the autumn of 1995, Borst visited the Department of Health of the United States and was impressed by American tobacco control policy. Strengthened by the visit, she ordered her civil servants to write a comprehensive tobacco control policy. On 28 May 1996, she sent a letter to the parliament detailing her tobacco policy intentions (*nota Tabaksontmoedigingsbeleid*): "in light of the grave consequences of tobacco use, tobacco policy needs to be strengthened."[46] The document contained five major policy intentions. The first was to allocate more money to STIVORO's youth education activities, particularly to STIVORO's campaign "Smoking, a deadly sin,"[47] which confronted youth with the short- and long-term health consequences of smoking. A second intention was to tighten the existing tobacco promotion restrictions. The document contained a new set of detailed self-restrictions that had been agreed upon by cabinet and industry after extensive negotiations over half a year. They were intended to keep tobacco advertisements further away from children, including no advertisements in cinemas and in the vicinity of schools, nor in magazines read by children. A third policy intention was to extend the public smoking ban to institutions in the culture and art sector, and to private companies with a public function, such as public transport and post offices. This would bring Dutch regulation in line with EU Resolution 89/C189/01 that invited member states to implement smoking bans in public places, including public transport. In addition, the supervision of the smoking ban in public places, which was not well complied with, was to be tightened. The problem with the smoking ban was that the supervisory authority could impose neither sanctions nor fines for non-compliance (Verdonk-Kleinjan, 2014, p. 17). A further problem was that since the Tobacco Act had come into force, organisations were allowed to permit smoking in one-third of their space or one-third of the time. The fourth policy intention was to ban tobacco sales to youth under 18. The fifth was to use tobacco excise duties as a means to reach tobacco control goals. This was an important step: until then, levying tobacco excise duties had been regarded by the government solely as a means to generate revenue, but from 1996 it came to be considered a valid "secondary effect" of tobacco taxes (Visser, 2008, p. 157).

A working group with experts from the ministries of health, trade, and finance was commissioned to make a proposal for price increases. Three months after her *nota Tabaksontmoedigingsbeleid*, Borst announced in a letter to parliament that tobacco tax would be raised in such a way that the new price of a pack of cigarettes (25 sticks) and a pack of roll-your-own tobacco would be 50 cents higher,[48] and that "with this measure a comprehensive package of policy measures to discourage tobacco will be accomplished."

In 1997 Borst changed her position on tobacco advertising.[49] She no longer wanted to prolong the gentlemen's agreement between government and industry and announced a ban on all tobacco promotion, declaring that the Netherlands would no longer block the EU's advertising directive. The new Labour Government in the United Kingdom had stopped resisting the EU's advertising ban, and the Dutch government was able to follow the English example (see Box 6.1 in Chap. 6).

In the meantime, on 29 October 1996 the parliament adopted two resolutions.[50] One was proposed by parliamentarian Rob Oudkerk (Labour Party), requiring the government to make preparations for a ban on outdoor advertising; the other was by Jan Marijnissen (Socialist Party), requesting that the government restrict the sale of tobacco to specialty shops. Other motions were tabled in the same meeting: vending machines had just been banned in the United States, and Dutch parliamentarians mentioned this as an example for the Netherlands to follow. This resulted in a held motion (by Oudkerk and others) to ban vending machines in bars and cafés frequented by young people.[51] During the same plenary session, parliament also adopted a motion from the liberal–conservatives (VVD) to renounce tax increases.[52]

Drafting a New Tobacco Act (1998–2002)

In August 1998 the second Purple Cabinet was installed, with Els Borst again as Minister of Health. The coalition agreement contained an explicit goal to implement the European tobacco directive when the current code of practice ended in May 1999. Borst commissioned the Netherlands School of Public Health (NSPH) to examine the effectiveness of various policy options. Borst asked the NSPH to assess the full range of policy options, including education, sale restrictions, advertising restrictions, tobacco taxation, smoking bans and product regulation. She also wanted to know what the impact of tobacco policy would be on both public health and the economy. The report supported a comprehensive policy approach to tobacco control (Roscam Abbing, 1998). It made clear that isolated measures had little effect, and needed to be part of a comprehensive strategy so they could reinforce each other. An important conclusion was that "a specific combination of measures [would] give the government the ability to have the greatest impact." The NSPH report became an important building block for the new Tobacco Act. Borst's proposal for a revision of the Act was sent for first consideration to parliament in April 1999.[53] The main conclusion from the NSPH report, that a comprehensive approach was needed and that leaving out specific measures would weaken the policy, was repeated in the explanatory memorandum to the bill.[54] Borst remarked that considering that smoking trends were not going down, the WHO target of 20% smoking in 2000 was not feasible, "and because the situation in the Netherland does not compare favourably with our European partners, the researchers stress that a more intensive deployment of policy measures is required."

The NSPH report included a study on the societal costs and benefits of comprehensive tobacco policy (Van Leeuwen & Sleur, 1998). Borst learned from this that any negative economic effects on tobacco-production related sectors would be compensated by increased productivity in other sectors of the economy, and that the resulting macro-economic effect could even be positive. This conclusion was in line with the landmark *Curbing the Epidemic* report, published a month later by the World Bank, that concluded that tobacco control achieves unprecedented health benefits without harming national economies (World Bank, 1999). In a meeting with the minister of Finance, Borst used both reports to convince him that a tobacco tax increase in 2001 was a necessary part of the tobacco control policy package (Kalis, 2000). When comparing this 1998 explanatory memorandum to the 1984 one (which accompanied the proposal to the first Tobacco Act),[55] what stands out is the emphasis on public health and a lesser preoccupation with economic objections. Negative effects on the commercial activities of the tobacco industry were accepted as inevitable. Borst made this point clear again in 2000, in a reply to questions by the VVD about the economic effects of her tobacco control proposals.[56] She argued that tobacco control gradually leads to less consumption of tobacco products and more spending on other goods, resulting in a displacement of the production pattern in the economy in such a way that there would be a new equilibrium—much the same as the old situation in macro-economic terms—but far better for health: "less smoking is good for public health and certainly not bad for the economy: we will all gain."

In May 2000, Borst attended the annual meeting of the World Health Organisation (WHO) in Geneva and spoke at length with Gro Harlem Brundtland, its director. In an interview with a reporter of the Dutch morning newspaper *De Telegraaf*, Borst announced rigorous measures against tobacco (De Jong, 2000). Now that there had been a court decision in the Nooijen case, where an employee had successfully litigated for a smoke-free workplace (see Chap. 9), she felt that it was time for a legal prohibition on smoking in the workplace so that non-smoking employees no longer had to take their employers to court. She also wanted the sale of cigarettes restricted to specialty shops. In the interview she hinted at a complete end to tobacco, and threatened to ban tobacco production from Dutch soil: "This means that there will no longer be any future for Philip Morris in the Netherlands. If you don't want future generations to smoke, we shouldn't be producing cigarettes in this country." This declaration of war against the tobacco industry became headline news.

On 30 May 2000 Borst sent her proposal for a revision of the Tobacco Act for approval to Parliament.[57] This was four years after she had presented her policy intentions and two and a half years after her bill was debated upon in Parliament. In reply to displeased parliamentarians about why it had taken so long, she answered that it was because of consultations with the industry and discussions within the cabinet.[58] The proposal was subject to lengthy debates in parliament for another two years, in which it was changed several times because of amendments (nine in total) and motions (seven in total) from both chambers of parliament.

The original proposition for a revised Tobacco Act contained a proposal for a workplace smoking ban, but this was removed after discussion in cabinet. Instead, the proposal sent to parliament for approval included a conditional ban on smoking in shared workplaces in the private sector, which would only come to life if the social partners (employers and employees) were unable to come up with improved self-regulation measures. The government proposed to settle this through an order-in-council that would give the social partners another year to prove they could protect employees from tobacco smoke without needing a ban. Until then controls on smoking in private workplaces had been left entirely to labour and employer representatives who negotiated in STAR. In 1997 the Ministry of Social Affairs evaluated whether this arrangement still worked, and concluded that it did not: at the end of that year only 28% of private companies had some sort of policy in place to protect employees (Spijkerman & van den Ameele, 2001).

Borst proposed changing the Tobacco Act in such a way that it would include a complete ban on tobacco advertisements and sponsorship, improvements to existing sale restrictions, an age limit for the sale of tobacco products (18 years), and administrative monetary penalties for infringements. Since her proposal did not have a plan to phase out tobacco selling points, as requested by Socialist Party MP Jan Marijnissen, Agnes Kant (Socialist Party) tabled a new amendment to restrict the sale of tobacco to specialty shops.[59] When a motion with majority support from parliament is not acted on by the government, the government needs to explain why, and be prepared to confront parliament on the issue. Although Borst clearly wanted to restrict tobacco sales to specialty shops and felt she was supported by the NSPH report, which made a strong case for restrictions on tobacco sale, the cabinet could not come to an agreement about how to respond to the motion.[60] Borst translated the cabinet's stance in a rather cryptic answer to the parliament: "the government has not decided that it will not carry out the motion by Marijnissen and therefore it has not made this explicitly known." Sometime later, the Green–Left party (MP Corrie Hermann) tried to introduce into the act a gradual restriction on tobacco sales to specialty shops, cafés, and bars, with an amendment that proposed to do this through an order-in-council.[61] Neither amendment made it into the final text of the Tobacco Act. The idea of sale restrictions was postponed for consideration as part of a new tobacco control policy proposal (*Tabaksnota II*), by the next government.

On 31 May 2001, appropriately World No Tobacco Day, the proposal for the amendments to the Tobacco Act was discussed in the second chamber of Parliament.[62] The debate lasted almost 12 hours. The parties on the right flank (CDA, VVD) argued against a smoking ban and an advertising ban. The CDA called the bill "too detailed and patronizing." Several amendments were proposed, and led to two major changes to the bill. The first was to set the age limit for buying tobacco from 18 to 16 years (amendment by the Green–Left party and D66).[63] This may be considered a success for the tobacco industry network, because of their 1998 preemptive initiative to voluntarily implement a restriction not to sell to youth under 16 (slogan: "There is no excuse. We only sell above 16 years of age"), and initiatives to restrict the access of minors to vending machines. Following anecdotal evidence that an 18-year age limit was difficult to enforce, parliamentarians believed that 16 would be more effective—and at that time, the sale of beer and wine was also set at 16 years. The second change was the more important one: a direct smoking ban in private workplaces instead of continued self-regulation. This was the result of an amendment proposed by Corrie Hermann of the Green–Left party,[64] who was stimulated to table the motion by a strong lobby from the health network led by STIVORO, supported by Clean Air Netherlands (CAN) and the Lung Foundation. Part of the lobby was in the form of media attention to two court cases in 2000, the first initiated by an employee of the Royal Post (Nanny Nooijen) who successfully litigated for a smoke-free workplace. The other was by the mother of Nienke Hora Adema, a mentally disabled young woman. She had successfully demanded smoke-free living quarters for her daughter in the epilepsy institution Cruquiushoeve. The majority of parliament agreed with Borst that it should not require a court case each time an employee had a problem with tobacco smoke in the workplace, and the problem could better be resolved with a law. The revised Tobacco Act signified a breach with the long-term status quo where smoking restrictions in private workplaces were left to the discretion of STAR.[65] However, it also included a clause that made it possible to exempt certain categories of employers. This was primarily included with a view to exempting the hospitality sector, but it was possible for other categories as well, and further left open the option to stretch the time of implementation to give society ample time to adapt to the new law.

The CDA tabled a motion to the effect that the government would allocate 30 million guilders for education campaigns: only under this condition was CDA prepared to support the Act. The motion was not adopted. The amendments to the Tobacco Act were adopted in the lower house of parliament on 6 June,[66] but with CDA and VVD voting against. The CDA felt the act was "too elaborate and too paternalistic" and would fail to change smoking behaviour as it did not include the necessary funds for prevention and education. The VVD argued that it could not support a bill which made the government responsible for protecting people from tobacco smoke instead of leaving it to employer and employee organisations.

On 16 April 2002, after a lengthy and difficult debate, a majority in the senate adopted the bill as well. This was not an easy win for the minister, since the CDA and VVD together held a majority position in the senate, and both parties had voted against the bill in the lower house. In the senate the CDA voted in favour, but only on the condition that €15 million would be made available for mass media campaigns and support for smokers who wanted to quit smoking once the ban came into force. Most parties seconded a motion by Christian Democrat Jos Werner to this effect.[67] Another condition was that the government would agree to discuss exceptions to the smoking ban and exact enforcement dates with affected societal organisations. This resulted in agreements with the national sports federation (NOC x NSF) and *Koninklijke Horeca Nederland* (trade organisation for the hotel and catering industry) (KHN) on trajectories of self-regulation. Details of the implementation of the smoking ban were discussed with STAR, leading to the decision to implement in 2004 instead of 2003.

On 18 April 2002 the revised Tobacco Act was published in the Bulletin of Acts. On 28 June 2002, Borst signed an order-in-council stipulating when the different articles of the revised act would enter into force. The advertising and promotion ban went into effect in November 2002, although newspapers and magazines were granted a stay until January 2003. The 16-years age-of-sale was in effect from January 2003 as well. The legal right to a smoke-free workplace and smoke-free public transport took effect on January 2004, while the government allowed nursing homes and homes for the elderly to implement the smoking ban in 2005. Three weeks before the cabinet resigned, Borst managed to implement an important element of the first EU Tobacco Products Directive (TPD-1): cigarette packs had to carry warnings that covered 30% of the front of the pack and 40% of the back, with rotating texts. This came into effect on the first of May 2002—remarkable, as this was four months before the date required by the European Commission (EC) and sooner than any other EU country. Other aspects of TPD-1 could not be transposed in Dutch law through an order-in-council, but required a revision of the Tobacco Act itself. This was left to the new cabinet.

An Ambitious New Tobacco Control Policy Document That Never Made It

In 2000 Minister Els Borst had prepared a second tobacco control policy paper with significant new policy steps.[68] Details followed a year later, during long debates in both chambers of Parliament.[69,70] The ambitious new tobacco policy document, entitled *Together towards a Smokefree Society* (VWS, 2001), contained proposals for considerable increases in tobacco taxation, anti-tobacco marketing campaigns targeted at youth that were budgeted at 30 million guilders per year,[71] and a clear policy intention to restrict the distribution of tobacco products in such a way that tobacco would eventually be sold in specialty shops only (in line with Marijnissen's motion and the amendments by Agnes Kant and Corrie Hermann). This was discussed with representatives of the tobacco industry sector and the health sector in a meeting in The Hague, but never made it into a formal proposal for a new law. Although parliamentarians challenged Borst about

Tabaksnota II, as it was called in parliamentary debates,[72] she was unable to secure the necessary budget. She hoped that the next government would take it up, but this never happened.

Transposition of the EU Tobacco Product Directive into the Tobacco Act (2002–2003)

In July 2002, the first Balkenende cabinet came to power. This was a cabinet consisting of the CDA, VVD, and a new populist right-wing party *Lijst Pim Fortuyn* (LPF). The LPF was built around the legacy of Pim Fortuyn, a charismatic populist politician who had been assassinated the year before. This cabinet lasted 86 days and collapsed after internal conflicts in the LPF. In this cabinet, economist and former Labour Party member Eduard Bomhoff was minister of health for the LPF. He was not a tobacco industry-friendly minister, and after being bombarded with letters and requests for meetings by the industry when he took office, he publicly distanced himself from tobacco lobbyists. Once during a debate on tobacco policy in parliament he spotted a tobacco industry lobbyist in the public gallery sitting right across from him, which he felt intimidating.[73] He raised his voice and said, "I see a lobbyist at a distance of 30 meters from where I stand, and that distance seems a very good one to keep!"[74] Bomhoff, at his very first cabinet meeting, managed to make the weekly cabinet meeting smoke-free. Smoking had been banned in meeting rooms since 1990, but in the most important meeting room in the country the smoking ban was not yet complied with. Several ministers were ardent smokers, including Minister of Finance Gerrit Zalm, and Minister of Internal Affairs Johan Remkes (both VVD).

Eduard Bomhoff inherited two important tasks: implementing the new Tobacco Act and transposing the remaining elements of the TPD-1 into national law. He was not able to make significant steps regarding the first task as the cabinet had already disbanded, but the transposition of the TPD-1 was more pressing and could not wait. The final date on which all components of the directive had to be transposed into national law had been set by the EC as 30 September 2002. There were several obstacles. One was an issue brought forward by the CDA and VVD: the protection of tobacco industry company secrets in light of TPD's requirement that tobacco producers submit and publish lists of the ingredients in their products. The government remained steadfast that it would implement the TPD-1 requirements, despite industry protests. It accepted the risk of being taken to court by the industry, which eventually happened. Partly because of a change of government, the interim cabinet was unable to achieve the EU deadline. An additional problem was that the interim government failed to secure the €15 million for tobacco prevention education in the ministry's budget, despite Werner's motion to this effect and promises made to the parliament. This meant that the senate was not prepared to approve the amendments to the Tobacco Act that were necessary to transpose the TPD-1.[75] Acting Health Minister Clémence Ross-van Dorp, who stood in for Bomhoff in the interim cabinet, succeeded in scraping together €10 million from the budget,[76] still an unprecedented amount of money for tobacco prevention in the Dutch context. This was enough to satisfy the senate. The decision to make this a structural, yearly tobacco education budget was left to the new cabinet (Balkenende II), where it stalled. The revision of the Tobacco Act to accommodate the TPD-1 requirements was approved by the senate on 28 January 2003.

Implementing the Tobacco Act (2003–2005)

At the end of May 2003, the Balkenende II cabinet replaced the failed first Balkenende cabinet. Former Minister of Finance Hans Hoogervorst (VVD) succeeded Bomhoff as the minister of Health. Balkenende cabinet II wanted to diminish the role of the central government further and decentralise prevention and cure. In June 2003, during a debate with the second chamber of parliament, Hoogervorst said that *Tabaksnota II* would be part of his disease prevention policy paper.[77] This was a nondescript prevention programme with a few tobacco control policy intentions. In this way, the ambitious *Tabaksnota II* was silently killed without protest from politicians or from civil society.

Hoogervorst's prevention programme had a quantitative target for tobacco control: 25% smokers in 2007; but it announced no new tobacco control measures, nor was extra money set aside for tobacco prevention (VWS, 2003). It was assumed that the target of 25% smokers in 2007 could be reached by implementing the existing measures (smoking ban in workplaces in January 2004, implementation of mass media campaigns financed through the "Werner money," and strict enforcement of the age limit for the sale of tobacco and of the advertising and sponsorship ban), supplemented with a mass media campaign targeted at youth. For 2004, €5 million extra were allocated for educational campaigns, in addition to the ten million already set aside by the Werner motion.

A later date of implementation of the smoking ban in the hospitality sector was negotiated with employer and employee representatives through STAR, and with organisations representing employers and employees in the hospitality sector. The food and drinks catering sector was granted a period of self-regulation to make bars and restaurants smoke-free before the end of 2008. If this covenant failed, a ban would be implemented in bars and restaurants. This was one year sooner than Tony Blair's UK government's timeline. The UK Department of Health published a white paper on public health in November 2004, stating the intention to make workplaces, including restaurants and pubs which prepared and served food, smoke-free, through a staged approach ending in late 2008 (Department of Health, 2004). At that time very few countries in Europe had smoking bans in bars, or even in restaurants. In 2004 Ireland became the first European country with a comprehensive smoking ban in the hospitality sector, soon followed by Malta, Italy, and Norway (WHO, 2006). Most countries still had voluntary agreements, or limited or no restrictions.

The commercial sports sector in the Netherlands wanted exceptions similar to the smoking ban in sports canteens negotiated between the government and the hospitality sector. Hoogervorst came to an agreement with sportsfederation NOC × NSF to commence a two-year trajectory of self-regulation (until 2006) so that commercially run sports canteens would gradually become smoke-free.[78]

In November 2003, parliament debated the implementation of the workplace smoking ban with Hoogervorst,[79] shortly after the Health Council had published a second report on the health risks of passive smoking (an update of the 1990 report). The new report estimated that 2000 smokers were killed each year by passive smoking (Gezondheidsraad, 2003). Instead of underscoring the need for strict regulation without exceptions, parliament was sceptical of the report's conclusions, spurred by an attack on the report by a libertarian journalist in newsmagazine *HP/De Tijd* and parliamentary questions from the Socialist Party.[80]

VVD Member of Parliament Edith Schippers tabled a number of motions, together with the Socialist Party and the LPF, to weaken the smoking ban.[81] Seven out of nine received majority support.[82] There was support (including from the Labour Party and the Green–Left party) for a motion to give institutions in the mental health sector and other sectors where people lived in private accommodations, such as homes for the elderly and nursing homes, the possibility of self-regulation instead of a ban. Other motions receiving majority support from VVD, LPF, CDA, D66, and SP, requesting that the government come up with proposals to explore the viability of ventilation techniques and smoking sections as alternatives to bans in the food and drink sector, to extend the self-regulation to commercially run bars and canteens in sporting facilities, to choose a broader definition of "hospitality sector" so that amusement arcades and cinemas would be included, and to wait until the end of the self-regulation period for the hospitality sector before deciding if and when its exception status would come to an end. The government was requested to determine the success of self-regulation based on a set of "reasonable norms" for air quality and criteria for exposure to second-hand smoke. A motion to consider allowing smoking in coffee shops was supported both by the left (SP, Labour Party) and liberal parties (D66, VVD, LPF). The minister, however, rejected the motion.[83] He argued that coffee shops were part of the hospitality sector and already enjoyed the same lenient self-regulation trajectory as bars and cafés.

The smoking ban for workplaces and public transport came into force on 1 January 2004. The list of exceptions—the outcome of negotiations with civil society and pressure from parliament—was long: the hospitality sector (including theatres and music venues), tobacco specialty shops, amusement arcades, international trains, dedicated smoking rooms, private rooms in nursing homes and homes for the elderly, and penitentiary facilities. Hotels could reserve some of their rooms for smokers. Mental health institutions, old people's homes and institutions for the disabled were granted leeway so that smoking could be permitted in parts of the communal rooms, canteens, and waiting rooms. Dutch Railroads created smoking sections on train platforms to accommodate smoking travellers.

The implementation of the smoking ban was accompanied by a tax increase on February 2004 of €0.55 (including value-added tax [VAT]) per pack of cigarettes, a 14% increase. The tobacco manufacturers took this opportunity to also increase the price by €0.25, so that smokers were confronted with an effective increase of about €0.80. This undoubtedly encouraged the large number of quitters seen in 2004.

The Ministry of Health worked closely with STIVORO to make the most out of the introduction of the ban. One of STIVORO's smoking cessation specialists was seconded to the ministry to strengthen the collaboration between the two organisations. There was a long period of preparation, during which employers and employees were kept informed: employers received practical advice (e.g., a "7-step implementation plan" was sent by STIVORO to all employers), a new website (*Smoking and the Law*) was developed to inform employees and employers about their new rights and obligations, employees were offered smoking cessation programmes, and media campaigns accompanied the ban. A large-scale campaign ("The Netherlands starts quitting") to support smokers who wanted to quit around 1 January 2004 was run by STIVORO when the smoking ban came into force.

The efforts paid off. When the Netherlands went "smoke-free" in 2004 and it was no longer legal to light up in public transport and workplaces, there was a broad feeling of relief. To the surprise of many, there were very few problems. The ending of smoking in trains went smoothly, without noticeable disturbances, and journalists described it as a quiet revolution (Huisman, 2005). After one year around 70% of companies had successfully implemented smoking restrictions (VWS, 2005) and 75% of employers thought that the smoking ban was "fair" (VWA, 2005). Support among smokers for the idea that workers must not be bothered by tobacco smoke increased over the span of a year, from 56% before the ban to 79% after (VWS, 2005). A national survey showed that smokers became more concerned about their smoking, and more aware that passive smoking could be harmful to others (Willemsen, 2006). The mass media campaigns that accompanied the ban contributed to smoking becoming less socially acceptable (Van den Putte, Yzer, Ten Berg, & Steeveld, 2005). In the following years acceptance of smoking at work, in restaurants or bars, and on terraces further decreased (Hummel, Willemsen, Monshouwer, De Vries, & Nagelhout, 2016).

Despite the highly successful implementation of the smoking ban, problems remained with implementing the worksite ban in some sectors of society. One of the issues was the problem of smoking in health-care facilities where people lived permanently, such as psychiatric wards and homes for the elderly. These institutions had had to comply since 1990 with the Tobacco Act, but the Act lacked financial sanctions. This changed with the new, amended Tobacco Act, which made these facilities liable for fines when employees continued to work in smoke-filled rooms. This led to much unrest and media attention. Adherence to smoking bans in these types of home had dramatically worsened since the beginning of 2004. At the start of 2005, parliament debated the issue with the minister, voicing concerns from the mental health sector and workers in homes for the elderly where lifelong smokers could no longer smoke in their private rooms, so that workers were subject to all kinds of practical problems involved in escorting patients to smoking rooms.[84] The debate resulted in majority support for motions to—once again—consider ventilation as an alternative, to force mental health institutes to come up with a roadmap similar to the one in the hospitality sector as an alternative to a ban, and to insist that the KHN removes the goal of reducing the number of vending machines from their roadmap.[85] This latter motion was the result of incessant lobbying by British American Tobacco (BAT). The government responded by granting a one-year extension during which institutions would not be fined.

Parliament had repeatedly asked for better support for smokers with quitting smoking, especially financial reimbursement for costly pharmacotherapy for smoking cessation. Despite positive advice from the College voor Zorgverzekeringen (Health Care Insurance Board) (CVZ) (Kroes & Lock, 2003) and positive results from a pilot study in the province of Friesland commissioned by the government, which had shown that smokers who were reimbursed made more attempts at quitting and were more successful (Kaper, Wagena, & Van Schaijck, 2003), Hoogervorst did not want to make effective smoking cessation support for smokers illegible for financial reimbursement through the national health insurance system.[86] This was partly because of budgetary considerations (it would cost €45 million per year), but mainly because he felt that smokers were themselves responsible for quitting, and did not need to be compensated since they saved money when they quit smoking.

THE NATIONAL PROGRAM OF TOBACCO CONTROL (NPT) (2005–2010)

Since the Netherlands had implemented a comprehensive Tobacco Act, an important political question became whether this is sufficient for the time being or is more needed? In December 2004 Health Minister Hoogervorst started a round of consultations.[87] A total of 47 organisations from the tobacco industry network and the health network received invitations to comment on the way the government had tackled the tobacco problem so far, and to give suggestions for future steps. On 17

June 2005, Hoogervorst sent an evaluation of the government's tobacco control policy to parliament.[88] It presented data showing that about 70% of businesses had implemented measures to protect workers from tobacco smoke, and that most employers were positive about the new law and had had little trouble implementing the new rules (VWA, 2005). The ministry concluded that the new regulations in the revised Tobacco Act, in combination with the price increase and intensive campaigns, had been successful, and that smoking rates were finally going down after a long period of stagnation.[89] However, various breaches of the advertising and promotion ban had occurred as the tobacco industry continued to find loopholes. The report ended with the remark that other countries had much lower smoking rates and such results should be attainable in the Netherlands as well. However, instead of presenting a new governmental tobacco policy agenda, Hoogervorst made new policy intentions contingent on the tobacco control efforts of civil society and in particular the efforts of the three charities: Cancer Society, Lung Foundation, and Heart Foundation.

On 15 June 2005, the directors of the three charities and Hoogervorst signed a statement that they would join forces to intensify tobacco control: the *Nationaal Programma Tabaksontmoediging* (National Program of Tobacco Control) (NPT) (VWS, 2006).[90] STIVORO was appointed as the central coordinating organisation, responsible for implementing the programme. The government and the charities committed to a policy goal of 20% smokers in the population by 2010, even more ambitious than the goal of 25% in 2007, formulated in Hoogervorst's prevention paper. The ambitious goal was taken over from the *Nationaal Programma Kankerbestrijding* (National Program to Combat Cancer) (NPK), a collaboration between the Ministry of Health and Dutch cancer control organisations that had also started in 2005 (Jongejan, Hummel, Roelants, Lugtenberg, & Hoekstra, 2003). With the NPK programme, the government answered to calls from WHO and the European parliament to establish a national "comprehensive cancer control programme" geared towards optimisation of cancer control in the Netherlands.

Hoogervorst's decision to share responsibility for national tobacco control with non-governmental organisations must be seen against the backdrop of the cabinet's desire to reduce the role of the state, in line with the Balkenende II cabinet's intent to reinforce personal responsibility and sovereignty in civil society. Hoogervorst formally justified this by referring to a section in the text of WHO's 2003 Framework Convention on Tobacco Control (FCTC), in which the role of civil society is mentioned briefly[91]:

> The special contribution of non-governmental organisations and other members of civil society ... to tobacco control efforts nationally and internationally and the vital importance of their participation in national and international tobacco control efforts. (WHO, 2003)

The Dutch government hoped that the cancer, lung, and heart charities would contribute financially to the NPT programme. A five-year plan was to be developed "that contained collective and reinforcing efforts that would optimise the current tobacco control policy." Its main focus was smoking cessation, through how-to-quit campaigns and support for smokers, including patients and smokers from low socioeconomic groups.[92] While the 20% goal was taken from the NPK programme, the list of concrete policy actions for the government was not.[93] Instead, a number of optional measures were listed that were "possible" or "conceivable," including increasing the price of tobacco, having pictorial health warnings on packs, developing mass media smoking cessation campaigns, increasing the age for tobacco sale to 18, enforcing smoking bans in the Horeca (the hotel, restaurant and café industry), and restricting tobacco sales to specialty shops (STIVORO, 2005).

In 2006, Hoogervorst announced an intention to put graphic health warnings on cigarette packs through an adaptation of the Tobacco Act.[94] In addition, the old idea to restrict the sale of tobacco to specialty shops (Socialist Party member Jan Marijnissen's motion from 1996) was raised again. As a first step, Hoogervorst announced an increase in the legal age at which tobacco might be sold, from 16 to 18, and the ending of mobile tobacco sales at festivals.[95] These were policy intentions that required parliamentary approval. Parliament was informed on 18 May 2006[96] and a first debate followed a few weeks later.[97] The political reality was clear: the proposals had no chance. VVD, CDA, and LPF had a majority of 80 seats in parliament and were against. In June 2006, VVD parliamentarian Edith Schippers and Christian Democrat Siem Buijs tabled a motion condemning the government's prevention policy.[98] In it they wrote that current disease prevention policy was mainly based on "more control and repression, such as bans, commandments, reduction of selling points, increases in taxation on specific drugs and other matters that threaten the health of the people in the eyes of the government." They demanded that the government base its policy on "positive proposals and less on repressive measures that increasingly affect people's private life." Their bill received support from a majority of the Parliament,[99] signalling that there was no political support for tougher tobacco control.

From that moment the NPT programme was doomed. It was clear that the government had no political support for new policy measures, while the programme lacked a clear strategic plan and offered no ideas about how the ambitions and strengths of the four partners could best be accommodated and combined. The grim prospect of failing ambitions was confirmed when experts from the *Rijksinstituut voor Volksgezondheid en Milieu* (National Institute for Public Health and the Environment) (RIVM) calculated the likely impact of the NPT measures and concluded that even with very optimistic estimates, the 20% target could not be reached without new policy measures (Vijgen et al., 2007). The target would only be obtainable when the government imposed yearly tobacco tax hikes (between 10% and 20%) and substantially increased the reach of efficacious smoking cessation support, and when both government and charities allocated substantial sums of money to mass media campaigns. It was clear that this would not happen. Around the same time, another report by the RIVM concluded that the Netherlands did not have a strict tobacco policy compared to other countries, and that smoking rates would not go down without further measures (Van der Wilk, Melse, Den Broeder, & Achterberg, 2007). Policy steps that had been successful in other countries were recommended, such as a smoking ban in the hospitality sector, higher tobacco taxes, and better availability of smoking cessation services.

Parallel Interests and the Fight Over Smoking in Bars

In 2007 the fourth and last Balkenende cabinet was installed. This was a coalition of Christian Democrats, the Labour Party and the small Christian Union Party. The Minister of Health was Ab Klink (CDA), a liberal Christian Democrat *pur sang* and an influential party ideologist, having worked for many years at the scientific bureau of the CDA (between 1984 and 1992 as scientific staff member and from 1999 to 2007 as director). He re-introduced the idea of parallel interests as the leading concept for a prevention policy (Klink, 2007; VWS, 2007). This meant that such a policy was to be developed in concordance with the interests of societal organisations, including businesses and manufacturers, seeing "health as a justified interest in close connection with other justified interests," including those that were economic and social (VWS, 2007). The downside of this principle was that Klink de facto opened the door for tobacco industry lobbyists—and was far more receptive to industry contacts than previous ministers (see Chap. 8 for a detailed account of industry influence).

In 2007, the Netherlands was falling more and more behind other countries in Europe, as far as a policy to restrict smoking in pubs and bars was concerned. Seventeen countries had some kind of ban installed, including Germany (three states) and Belgium (albeit restricted to bars that serve food).[100] In February 2007, at his first public appearance a few days before the first cabinet meeting, Minister Ab Klink (CDA) surprised everyone by proclaiming that the hospitality sector must become smoke free within a year. This was not in line with the coalition agreement, which had 2011 as the final date (the end of the cabinet period), while former Minister Hoogervorst had agreed with the sector that the period of self-regulation would last until 2009. Klink saw injustice in the fact that workers in this particular sector were not yet protected against tobacco smoke while workers in others sectors were. His proclamation was headline news, framed in newspapers as revealing his "true nature." Klink was depicted in the media as a patronising Christian moral crusader, an image he detested since he regarded himself as a dyed-in-the-wool liberal. He was also an occasional smoker of cigars himself. However, he kept his promise under pressure from a strong health lobby, and in June 2007 the cabinet announced that it wished to make the sector smoke-free within 12 months.[101] The sports canteens and coffee shops, which also were still self-regulated, would be covered by the ban.

In the following months Klink set out to get approval from parliament. Between March and July the ministry organised consultation talks with representatives from the tobacco industry network, the hospitality sector, employer and employee organisations, the sports sector, and health organisations.[102] Parliament further requested a written consultation round, which was organised in September. While the health organisations unanimously applauded the ban, the industry-related network of organisations raised concerns, most of which were rebutted by the ministry; however, some resulted in a weakening of the ban, such as a more lenient definition of a smoking section as a room "specifically" dedicated to smoking instead of "exclusively" dedicated to smoking. This opened the possibility of having attractive smoking sections in pubs, receiving the same services as non-smoking sections. The only difference was that personnel could not serve drinks and food at a table.[103]

Parliamentarians from different parties attempted to soften the ban. For example, VVD parliamentarian Edith Schippers tabled (unsuccessful) motions to allow bar owners to eliminate tobacco smoke through ventilation techniques, and to exempt small pubs and bars with no personnel.[104] D66 and the Green–Left party drafted unsuccessful motions to exempt coffee shops from the ban.[105] In July 2008, the smoking ban was implemented in the hospitality sector, accompanied by a tax increase of €0.29 per pack of cigarettes, which translated to a consumer price increase of €0.35 per pack (including a price increase by the industry).

The Dutch bar smoking ban was one of the friendliest for smokers in Europe. Smoking was still allowed in designated areas with closed doors where personnel did not serve, and on covered terraces as long as one side was open. Smokers were not fined for non-compliance, only the bar owner. The ban was accompanied by a government-run mass media campaign that failed to explain the rationale for the ban. The campaign merely reinforced the image of pitiful smokers who were no longer welcome in cafés, and fanned the flames of discontent among bar owners and smokers' right groups. When the campaign was evaluated, it turned out that the proportion of people who were positive about a smoking ban in bars and restaurants (only 51% of the public) had not increased.[106] Despite its inept implementation, compliance to the ban was high at first, despite the low level of fines: first a warning, then €300 for the first violation, which was doubled for each repeated offence up to €2400. In the first three months, the Netherlands Food and Consumer Product Safety Authority (NVWA) undertook 7264 inspections and found that 94% of the hospitality sector complied.[107] This proportion was lower in pubs and bars, but was still 74%, with 15% having a smoking section.

With support and legal advice from the tobacco industry, small pubs began to deliberately provoke the government by openly showing disobedience (Baltesen & Rosenberg, 2009; Gonzalez & Glantz, 2013). The NVWA started to impose fines from October 2008 onwards and the public prosecutor began criminal prosecution for obstinate offenders. In two months 821 fines were imposed.[108] Tougher inspections, often accompanied by police officers, resulted in emotional responses from the smoking clientele of a small number of pubs. Some collected money from regular consumers to help pay fines. Newspapers ran headlines such as "Klink declares war on smokers pubs." The hospitality industry was quick to generate reports suggesting that the smoking ban had damaged the food and drink sector, which, it claimed, had suffered serious revenue declines and bankruptcies, leading to a series of parliamentary questions.[109]

In response to the pressure, parliamentarians from all parties declared themselves willing to explore pragmatic solutions to accommodate pub owners' concerns. Fleur Agema from the populist *Partij voor de Vrijheid* (Freedom Party) (PVV), the daughter of pub owners, called for several urgent debates on the matter, in which she attacked Minister Klink vehemently, demanding an end to the smoking ban for small pubs. Klink gave in to a request from the CDA to explore the possibility of using innovative air systems (such as curtains of air that prevented tobacco smoke from drifting from a smoking section to a non-smoking section) in bars, as an alternative to a full smoking ban.[110] VVD and CDA, with support from most other parties, convinced Minister Klink to attempt to define exact norms for air quality in pubs that would be acceptable for public health.[111] Until that moment, the government's stance was that there is no safe limit for exposure to second-hand smoke, in line with recommendations from the WHO and the RIVM. Chapter 8 discusses the industrial lobby for ventilation as an alternative to a smoking ban in more detail.

In the spring of 2009, successful legal procedures against the state by two small cafés (Victoria in Breda and De Kachel in Groningen) led to legal vagueness and uncertainty about whether the ban applied to small bars without personnel. Dutch courts considered the law discriminatory towards small bars without personnel on the grounds that the legislation was intended to protect employees from passive smoking, not visitors. This led to a new storm of media attention on the issue, and an escalation of the problem. Many pub owners reacted by replacing ashtrays on tables. In July 2009 Minister Klink responded by promising to rephrase the text of the Tobacco Act so that both employers and visitors would be protected.[112] Pending these alterations, smoking in bars without personnel was condoned and no fines were imposed, and existing penalties were put on hold. In November 2009 the industry organised a public protest in The Hague to put more pressure on the government to withdraw the ban; VVD and PVV added fuel to the flames by calling for an urgency debate on the issue.[113]

In December 2009, Klink presented the results of an assessment of the remaining issues and problems with the smoking ban.[114] The conclusion was reassuring: the ban was not responsible for reduced revenue for pubs and bars or for bankruptcies, as such effects could be explained by the long-term downward trend caused by the 2007–2008 global financial crisis, and financial compensation was therefore out of the question. Other potential problems, such as that small bars faced more technical obstacles in constructing smoking sections than did larger bars, and street disturbances when smokers went outside, remained within reasonable boundaries. About one-third of pubs had some sort of smoking section.[115] In the same month, further results of studies commissioned by the Ministry of Health and sent to parliament[116] showed that the smoking ban in bars and restaurants had improved the air quality (the concentration of fine dust particles), reduced exposure to second-hand smoke, had a beneficial effect on smoking cessation, and did not lead to more smoking in private homes (Dekker, Soethout, & Tijsmans, 2009). The government appealed the court decision and in March 2010 the Dutch Supreme Court ruled that the legislation was not discriminatory and applied to all bars, including those without personnel. By that time, however, compliance had dropped to the point where a little over half of all bars and cafés had replaced their ashtrays (Intraval, 2010).

In line with his policy focus of approaching the tobacco problem in a positive manner, and his wish to not be accused of paternalism, Klink approved the introduction of financial reimbursement for smokers who need smoking cessation counselling.[117] This would become available to smokers through the mandatory health-care insurance in the beginning of the next year (2011). This was a positive outcome, after a period of no less than 10 years of political hassle and many studies and advisory reports on this issue. The process had started in May 2001 with a motion by Labour and Socialist Parties (Rob Oudkerk and Agnes Kant) which requested the government to provide smokers with cessation support free of charge.[118]

Failure of the NPT Programme

Minister of Health Ab Klink put most of the NPT policy intentions initiated by Hoogervorst on ice.[119] He ignored the directors of the three health charities, who asked him to consider necessary measures such as pictorial health warnings on cigarette packs, increasing the age of sale to 18 years, and reducing the number of selling points (Rutgers, Hanselaar, Stam, & Van Gennip, 2007). Klink formulated his tobacco control strategy in 2009 as follows: "if it comes to tobacco control, I want to focus mainly on positive incentives."[120] He distanced himself from the previous government's intent to implement graphic health warnings on cigarette packs (unattractive warnings were "bad taste"),[121] said he did not want further regulation of tobacco sale outlets such as reducing their numbers or banning mobile sales of tobacco, and did not wish to pursue national regulations banning tobacco additives that increased attractiveness or addictiveness.[122] There was hardly a protest from parliament, which was too preoccupied with the issue of smoking bans in small pubs.

In 2010, by the end of the five-year NPT period, smoking prevalence was still high (27%) and had hardly decreased from when the NPT programme had started (28% in 2006). Smoking among women had gone up, and youth smoking had not gone down. Despite clear messages from experts that the NPT goals were unrealistic without new tobacco control measures, the government under the leadership of Klink remained unwilling to take the necessary steps. The charities were disappointed and were, in turn, not prepared to contribute sufficient sums to campaigns, leading to a complete failure of the NPT programme and tremendous feelings of disappointment among the health organisations (Zeeman & De Beer, 2012). STIVORO, which was responsible for execution of the programme, was scapegoated, and the three charities started to withdraw their financial support (further discussed in Chap. 9). Meanwhile, there was brief discussion within the government bureaucracy about starting a new five-year NPT programme, from 2011 to 2015 (Ministerie van Economische Zaken, 2010), but this was abruptly discarded when the Rutte cabinet came to power.

Sudden Reversal of Tobacco Control Policy (2010–2012)

On 20 February 2010, the Balkenende IV cabinet fell, over a dispute between the Labour Party and the Christian Democrats about continuing a military mission in the Afghan province of Uruzgan. The issue of smoking in pubs was declared controversial by the parliament, which meant that the resigning minister had to leave it to his successor to handle. In October 2010, the first Rutte cabinet took office. This was a minority cabinet formed by the VVD and the CDA, and had been made viable by support from the populist-libertarian PVV, which had enjoyed a tremendous election victory (from 9 to 24 seats). Support from the PVV put the Populist Party in a strong position to influence the new government's policy decisions, both through the coalition agreement and through parliament. Rutte's coalition agreement with the motto "freedom and responsibility" included few words on tobacco policy, but these few had far-reaching consequences. The coalition agreement included a firm commitment to ease the smoking ban by exempting bars without employees from the obligation to implement smoking restrictions. The criterion for a small bar was that it had less than 70 square metres of surface, modelled after the German smoking ban.

The main challenge for the new government was to deal with the aftermath of the economic crisis through a huge project to reduce government spending. The coalition agreement included large cuts to the Ministry of Health, including a €50 million reduction of spending on health education (Nagelhout & Fong, 2011). The new minister of Health was Edith Schippers (VVD) who since 2003 had been responsible for health issues as a member of the VVD parliamentary faction. Tobacco control advocates had long regarded her as one of their toughest opponents: she was known as a fighter for free-market principles and a strong adversary of the "nanny state," had opposed virtually every proposal for governmental regulation in the field of tobacco, and had been successful in softening the impact of the Tobacco Act and in limiting smoking bans. Schippers now saw an opportunity to execute a conservative–liberal agenda and reduce the government's involvement with tobacco to a minimum. She knew she had full support from the PVV, whose leader Geert Wilders was a smoker himself and had been a defender of tobacco industry interests in the Balkenende I cabinet when he was still a member of the VVD. When Schippers was the VVD spokesperson on tobacco in the Balkenende II cabinet, Minister Hoogervorst (also VVD) had repeatedly debated with her over tobacco and lifestyle. At one point Schippers characterised Hoogervorst's policy as "lifestyle inquisition."[123] When Hoogervorst was no longer minister, he looked back and commented on Schippers: "Edith is against a nanny state, while I had come to the conclusion that strict measures had to be taken. That debate between the two of us was very harsh sometimes" (Niemantsverdriet, 2011).

Like Klink, Schippers politicised prevention policy by taking ideological values as a starting point. It did not come as a surprise that Schippers, in her maiden speech as minister in parliament on 28 October 2010, announced that there was going to be a radical change: "From my point of view, from my personal conviction, it is absolutely disastrous if the government forces people into a straitjacket by all sorts of regulations, do's and don'ts, restrictions, images with doom scenarios, patronising and pedantic messages."[124] Schippers formulated the new political stance towards prevention as follows: "I don't think the government is a happiness machine, nor is it a lifestyle master. It is very important for me to make a change of policy which does justice to the motto of this cabinet, which is freedom and responsibility."

During a debate in parliament the Socialist Party (SP) and Christian Union (CU) noted that the proportion of smokers had stagnated and the government's aim to reduce smoking to 20% in 2010 had not been met.[125] They tabled two motions: one demanding that the minister present an effective package of measures to combat smoking as part of her prevention policy document, which was due later that year, and one requesting that the government take tobacco prevention seriously and reduce the number of tobacco sale outlets. Schippers rejected both. A few weeks later she confirmed the government's intention to exempt small cafés from the smoking ban[126]; but enforcement was postponed immediately in anticipation of a revision of the applicable order-in-council. In July 2011 smoking was officially allowed in small bars. To support the new regulation, fines were doubled for those who did not comply with the law.

Soon after her appointment Schippers announced that she was going to cut subsidies to disease prevention institutes. In May 2011, Schippers' health *nota* was published (VWS, 2011). Tobacco control was no longer a priority. She announced a three-year phasing down of subsidies to STIVORO, while smoking prevention was to be handed over to the Trimbos Institute (the Netherlands Institute of Mental Health and Addiction). This echoed parliamentary questions raised by Schippers in 2004 criticising alleged wastage of subsidies by STIVORO,[127] and again from 2008 questioning the necessity of the subsidies that STIVORO received and whether the government was financing its own political opposition.[128] Reimbursement for smoking cessation support was to be discontinued in 2012. Mass media campaigns were described as paternalistic and completely discarded. These swift and dramatic shifts were an unprecedented reversal of tobacco control policy decisions, and met with indignation and astonishment both from Dutch health and medical advocacy groups (NKI-AVL, 2012) and from international tobacco control experts (Arnott et al., 2011). The Network for Accountability of Tobacco Transnationals nominated the Dutch government for a "Marlboro Man Award," a "less-than-prestigious price for a government that is furthering Big Tobacco's interests and putting profit over people."[129] Ex-minister Hoogervorst commented: "Reversal of the smoking ban is a rear-guard action. The whole world is making its tobacco policy tougher, while the Netherlands is making its policy more lenient. I am a bit embarrassed"

(Niemantsverdriet, 2011). Schippers' tough position led to a strong polarisation between the Ministry of Health and tobacco control groups, especially STIVORO. This was aggravated when public television broadcasted a documentary in October 2011 entitled "Minister of Tobacco," revealing contacts between the Dutch tobacco industry network and Schippers.[130]

NORMALISATION OF RELATIONSHIPS (2012–2017)

In November 2012 the tension between government and health organisations over tobacco lessened when tobacco control became the task of State Secretary Martin van Rijn (Labour party) in the new Rutte–Ascher cabinet (a coalition between VVD and Labour Party). The Populist PVV party was no longer needed to support the government, and with its retreat from power there was less support for an extremely restrained tobacco control policy. Van Rijn normalised relationships between the ministry and health organisations by promising to follow the path of reason and by examining what could be done to strengthen tobacco control. Van Rijn had struck a deal with VVD and Schippers, who was still health minister, that no new tobacco regulatory measures would be taken in the next four years. Van Rijn moved cautiously, evaluating the effectiveness of a new measure before taking additional steps. He managed to retain this strategy until the end of the cabinet, arguing in parliament that he wanted policy measures that were enforceable, effective, based on science, consistent, and attracting sufficient societal support "while we constantly search for new methods to eliminate smoking."[131] In July 2014, Van Rijn sent a number of reports to the parliament, which examined new policy options such as restricting the number of selling points and point-of-sale restrictions, and promised to present a plan at the end of the year (Van Rijn, 2014).

In December 2013, the European parliament reached an agreement with the EU Council of Ministers about a new Tobacco Product Directive (TPD-2), which included pictorial health warnings covering 65% of the front and the back of tobacco packs, restrictions on the use of flavourings and dangerous additives in tobacco, and a ban on slim cigarettes. The new directive came into force on May 2014, and most provisions were implemented in the Netherlands by May 2016. Another policy measure that Van Rijn took did not follow his own initiative as well, but was the result of outside pressure: it had been decided that the age limit for drinking alcoholic beverages would rise from 16 to 18, to come into effect on 2014, and the parliament wanted a similar regulation for tobacco. After a parliamentary vote in October 2013, the legal age limit for selling tobacco was raised from 16 to 18, and went into effect in January 2014. Van Rijn further amended the Tobacco Act, so that small cafés were included again in the general smoking ban. This followed a successful legal action by CAN against the state that obliged the government to reconsider the exemption, and a successful motion from the Christian Union (CU) party that received majority backing (77 votes) in parliament. The motion requested the government to bring small cafés back under the smoking ban.[132] This came into effect in October 2014. In early 2017, parliament adopted an amendment to the Tobacco Act that included a ban on the display of tobacco products at point of sale, as part of the ban on advertising.

Conclusions

The main events of the narrative of how government and parliament shaped Dutch tobacco control policy are summarised in Box 2.2. The ambitions of the 1970s came to a virtual standstill in the 1990s, stuck in the political quagmire of the Dutch "polder."[133] Subsequent governments were reluctant to take decisive steps, sensing that this would meet with resistance from the tobacco industry, the business community, and the parliament, and they adopted a long-term approach of small steps. Tobacco policy was strengthened several times, often after long periods of self-regulation by the industry that was preferred over legally binding measures.

Box 2.2 Major tobacco control policy events in the Netherlands

Year	Event
1957	– Dutch Health Council advisory report *Smoking and health* confirms association between smoking and lung cancer
1965	– Start of "gentlemen's agreement" among tobacco manufacturers
1974	– Decision to create a national coordinating organisation for tobacco control, resulting in the foundation of STIVORO
1975	– Dutch Health Council report *Measures to reduce smoking* proposes a comprehensive tobacco policy
1976	– Advisory report by Meulblok Committee on tobacco advertising

Year	Event
1977	– State Secretary Hendriks presents the *Tobacco Memorandum*
1981	– STIVORO starts educational campaigns
1980	– Ban on tobacco advertisements on radio and television
1981	– Law on health warnings adopted
	– Industry-friendly advisory report from the second interdepartmental committee (ICBT) presented
1982	– Health warnings on cigarette packs ("Smoking threatens health")
	– New advertising code of conduct initiated by industry
1984	– Draft Tobacco Act (smoking ban in public places) presented to parliament
1988	– New advertising code of conduct (*Reclame Code*)
	– Tobacco Act adopted (smoking banned in public places)
1990	– First Health Council report on passive smoking
	– Tobacco Act implemented
1995	– "Healthy and Well" policy document (Minister Borst)
	– Advertising ban for billboards (self-regulation)
1996	– Advertising ban in cinemas (self-regulation)
	– "*Nota Tabaksontmoedigingsbeleid*" (Minister Borst)
1997	– The Netherlands supports the EU advertising ban
1998	– NSPH report advised on comprehensive national tobacco policy
2002	– Amendment to Tobacco Act adopted: smoke-free workplaces (with exception for hospitality sector), advertising and promotion ban, age limit for sale of tobacco set at 16 years
	– Self-regulation for hospitality sector until 2009
	– Large EU text health warnings on cigarette packs (30% front, 40% back)
2003	– Second Health Council report on passive smoking
2004	– Smoking ban in workplaces implemented
2005	– Netherlands ratifies FCTC
2006	– Start of the National Program of Tobacco Control (NPT) 2006–2010
2007	– Mister Klink announces to make hospitality industry smoke-free
2008	– Smoking ban extended to hospitality sector
2009	– Temporary suspension of smoking ban in small bars without personnel
2010	– Suspension overruled by supreme court (smoking ban again in place), then suspended again
2011	– Smoking cessation treatment reimbursed
	– Smoking again allowed in small bars with no personnel
	– Minister Schippers stops subsidy to STIVORO while transferring tobacco education to the Trimbos Institute
2012	– Smoking cessation treatment no longer reimbursed

Year	Event
2014	– Ban on tobacco sale extended to all under 18 years – Smoking ban extended to all bars, including small bars with no personnel
2016	– EU Tobacco Product Directive II implemented: pictorial warnings on cigarette packs
2017	– Ban on the display of tobacco products at point of sale adopted by parliament

The 1988 Tobacco Act did not contain measures strong enough to affect smoking rates, and until the end of the 1990s health considerations were subordinate to economic interests. This changed when Health Minister Borst amended the Tobacco Act in 2002 and brought it up to international standards. None of Borst's successors has taken comprehensive tobacco control initiatives remotely similar to hers.

The Dutch governments' approach to tobacco control can be characterised as reactive and cautious, resulting in incremental change instead of radical steps. With the exception of Health Minister Borst (1994–2002), none of the state secretaries or health ministers who were responsible for tobacco control took much interest in the topic; none showed strong leadership. Official documents did not outline bold ambitions; nor did they testify to a vision of tobacco control that might inspire the nation. The bureaucracy seemed to react to incidents rather than initiate them, and to feel most comfortable with a technical, non-visionary approach. Even Minister Borst realised that she could not make great strides. During a debate in the senate in 2002, she lamented: "How does one handle things in such a way that individual freedom of adults is respected while at the same time trying to reduce the harm [of smoking]? It is a struggle. That is why we take it one step at a time and do not try to make some sort of enormous victory in one smash."[134]

One important observation is that Dutch politicians and government officials consistently tried the least controversial option first and gradually progressed to more stringent measures. Policies often metamorphose in such a way. According to John (2012, p. 20), policy change is often limited to "minor variations in a pattern of continuity." These have been called first, second, and third order policy changes (Hall, 1993). A first order change is when a policy remains the same but is adjusted to new circumstances and new experiences. In the case of the Netherlands, smoking bans were broadened from public places to workplaces and eventually to the hospitality sector. Another first order change concerned the age limit for the sale of tobacco, which increased from 16 to 18 years.

Second order change is when the instrument of policy is altered while the overall goals remain the same. The oldest example was the realisation that education alone would not solve the problem, and that regulation of the product and how it was sold and marketed were necessary as well. Another second order change occurred when self-imposed advertising restrictions were broadened several times and eventually replaced by an advertising and promotion ban.

A third order change is characterised by a more radical shift in the goal of the policy. This is more politically or ideologically inspired than based on the appearance of new facts about what works or experiences with failed policy. The change from regarding tobacco use as an economic benefit to seeing it as a public health threat can be regarded as a radical shift (Studlar & Cairney, 2014). In the Netherlands this process started in the 1960s with the growing recognition of the seriousness of the health problems of tobacco, and eventually evolved into the current dominant public health perspective. The key alteration of the status quo occurred between 2002 and 2004 when the Tobacco Act was amended and Minister Borst successfully took tobacco policy out of the sphere of influence of the trade ministry and under the control of the Ministry of Health, resulting in tobacco control measures that had a huge impact on society. However, this was not a guarantee of consistent strong tobacco control in subsequent years. Later health ministers assigned such low priority to tobacco control that it stagnated under Minister Klink (2007–2010) and even temporarily reversed under Minister Schippers (2010–2012).

In the next chapter, a comparison will be made between the trajectory of tobacco control in the Netherlands and those of other European countries. Subsequent chapters explore in more detail some of the explanatory factors that have already been briefly alluded to in the current chapter: changes in governance (decentralisation, power shift to Brussels), institutional changes (more control ceded to the Ministry of Health at the expense of the Ministry of Economic Affairs), the importance of the judiciary, the role of ideology (neo-liberalism and small government), rules of the game (*polderen*), and the influence of the anti- and pro-tobacco control lobbies.

Notes

1. Appendix Proceedings I, 1963–1964, nr. 14.
2. In 1971 this code of conduct was weakened by agreeing that "it is not against the rules if information is given in a positive way, either in word or illustration, about the way of smoking and how a maximum of smoking satisfaction can be derived" (Van Vliet, 1971).
3. Philip Morris drafted mission and action plans for the *Stichting Reclame Code* (Advertising Code Foundation) (SRC) so that it would have maximum additional value (Philip Morris, 1996).
4. Proceedings II, 1969–1970, Annex 1074.
5. Proceedings II, 1971–1972, Annex 707.
6. Proceedings I, 1970–1971, Annex 40.
7. Parliamentary Papers II, 1976–1977, 14,360, nr. 1.
8. It also referred to the WHO report *Smoking and Its Effects on Health* (WHO, 1975).
9. Parliamentary Papers II, 1976–1977, 14,360, nr. 2.
10. These were regulations to limit the sale of tobacco to specialty shops (including a ban on vending machines) and to use tobacco taxation as a means to improve health.
11. Parliamentary Papers II, 56ste meeting, 1 March 1979, p. 3781.
12. Parliamentary Papers II, 1982–1983, 17,600, nr. 36.
13. Parliamentary Papers II, 1977–1978, 14,800 XVII, nr. 34.
14. A ban on advertising through television and radio was effectuated in 1980 by an order-in-council to the existing Broadcasting Act (Ministry of Culture, Recreation and Welfare).
15. Parliamentary Papers II, 56ste meeting, 1 March 1979, p. 3780.
16. Parliamentary Papers II, 1978–1979, 15,426, nr. 12.
17. Proceedings II, 29 October 1980.
18. Parliamentary Papers II, 1979–1980, 15800 XVII, nr. 37.
19. Parliamentary Papers II, 1980–1981, 16400 XVII, nr. 32.
20. Proceedings II, 1980–1981, 15,426, nr. 24.
21. Parliamentary Papers II, 1981–1982, 17,100 Chapter XIII, nr. 149.
22. Parliamentary Papers II, 1984–1985, 18,749, nrs. 1–3.
23. Parliamentary Papers II, 1984–1985, 18,749, nr. 3.
24. Parliamentary Papers II, 1984–1985, 18,749, nr. 3.
25. Proceedings II, 48ᵉ meeting, 11 February 1985, pp. 48–46.
26. Parliamentary Papers II, 1986–1987, 18,749, nr. 14; Parliamentary Papers II, 1986–1987, 18,749, nr. 35.
27. Interview, on 24 August 2016.
28. Proceedings II, 1 July 1987, 94-4839.
29. Parliamentary Papers, 1987–1988, 20,259, nrs. 1–2.

30. Proceedings I, 17ᵉ meeting, 8 March 1988, pp. 17–562.
31. 200 million guilders in 1996 is comparable to €300 million (current value); Parliamentary Papers II, 1998–1999, 26472, nr. 3.
32. Promotion of tobacco products on TV and radio was banned on 22 February 1980, based on Article 50.2 of the Broadcasting Act (ICBT, 1981).
33. Proceedings I, 17ᵉ meeting, 8 March 1988.
34. Proceedings II, 1991–1992, 22,300 XVI, nr. 7.
35. Parliamentary Papers II, 1992–1993, 22,684, nr. 4. p. 34.
36. Parliamentary Papers II, 1991–1992, 22300 XVI, nr. 36, pp. 9–10.
37. Parliamentary Papers II, 1991–1992, 22300 XVI, 7, p. 13.
38. The STAR, founded in 1945, is where employers and employees negotiate social-economic topics such as wages, pensions, employability and workers safety. It comprises the main employer representatives organisations (such as VNO–NCW) and the main employee representatives organisations. It represents the cornerstone of Dutch "polderen."
39. Proceedings II, 22 December 1993, 41, 3246–3247.
40. Proceedings II, 1993–1994, 23400 XVI, 78, p. 5.
41. This changed in the second cabinet Kok, when Annemarie Jorritsma (VVD) became Minister of Economic Affairs.
42. Parliamentary Papers II, 1994–1995, 24,126, nr. 2.
43. Parliamentary Papers II, 1995–1996, 24,126, nr. 7, p. 5.
44. Proceedings II, 1995–1996, 24,126, nr. 10.
45. 100,000 guilders in 1995 is comparable to about €67,000 in 2017.
46. Parliamentary Papers II, 1995–1996, 24743, nr. 1.
47. In Dutch: "Roken, dood en doodzonde."
48. Parliamentary Papers II, 1996–1997, 24,743, nr. 2.
49. Proceedings II, 1997–1998, 21, 501–519, nr. 29.
50. Proceedings II, 1996–1997, 18, 1266–1268.
51. Parliamentary Papers II, 1996–1997, 24,743, nr. 19.
52. Proceedings II, 29 October 1996, 18–1266.
53. Proceedings II, 1998–1999, 26,472, nr. 3.
54. Proceedings II, 1998–1999, 26,472, nr. 3, pp. 12–13.
55. Parliamentary Papers II, 1984–1985, 19,749, nr. 3.
56. Parliamentary Papers II, 1999–2000, 26,472, nr. 6, p. 45.
57. Parliamentary Papers II, 1999–2000, 26,472, nr. 6.
58. Parliamentary Papers II, 1999–2000, 26,472, nr. 6, p. 6.
59. Parliamentary Papers II, 1998–1999, 26,472, nr. 4.
60. Parliamentary Papers II, 1999–2000, 26,472, nr. 6, p. 24.
61. Parliamentary Papers II, 2000–2001, 26,472, nr. 8.
62. Proceedings II, 31 May 2001, 82, 5175–5239.
63. Parliamentary Papers II, 2000–2001, 26,472, nr. 12.

64. Parliamentary Papers II, 2000–2001, 26,472, nr. 13.
65. http://www.trouw.nl/tr/nl/5009/Archief/article/detail/2496082/2001/03/29/Borst-wil-betere-positie-niet-roker.dhtml
66. Proceedings II, 6 June 2001, 83, 5258–5260.
67. Proceedings I, 2001–2002, 26,472, nr. 59^c.
68. Parliamentary Papers II, 1999–2000, 26,472, nr. 6.
69. Proceedings II, 31 May 2001, 82, 5175–5239.
70. Parliamentary Papers I, 2001–2002, 26,472, nr. 59a.
71. This is equivalent to €18 million in 2015.
72. Proceedings I, Tabakswet, 26 March 2002, 24–1236.
73. Interview, on 22 March 2016.
74. Proceedings II, 26 September 2002, 6, 343–356.
75. Proceedings I, 17 December 2002, 13, 406–417.
76. Parliamentary Papers I, 2002–2003, 28,401, nr. 60c.
77. Proceedings II, 2002–2003, 28,600 XVI, nr. 146.
78. Proceedings II, 2002–2003, 28,600 XVI, nr. 154.
79. Proceedings II, 2003–2004, 29,200 XVI, nr. 158.
80. Proceedings, 2003–2004, Annex 619.
81. Proceedings II, 25 November 2003, 28, 1963–1967.
82. Proceedings II, 2 December 2003, 31, 2176.
83. Ibid.
84. Proceedings II, 2004–2005, 29,800 XVI, nr. 98.
85. Proceedings II, 1 February 2005, 44–2845.
86. Proceedings II, 2004–2005, 29,800 XVI, nr. 136, p. 6.
87. Parliamentary Papers II, 2004–2005, 22,894 en 29,800 XVI, nr. 55.
88. Parliamentary Papers II, 2004–2005, 22,894, nr. 61.
89. Parliamentary Papers II, 2004–2005, 22,894, nr. 61.
90. Parliamentary Papers II, 2005–2006, 22,894, nr. 83.
91. Proceedings II, 2004–2005, 22,894, nr. 61.
92. Parliamentary Papers II, 2006–2007, 22,894, nr. 114.
93. The NPK programme listed a number of actions: to classify tobacco smoke as a carcinogenic substance, to recognise that smoking is an addictive disease, to provide financial reimbursement for smoking cessation support, to introduce a full smoking ban in hospitality establishments as soon as possible, and to increase tobacco tax levels by at least €50 cents above inflation every two years (Jongejan et al., 2003).
94. Parliamentary Papers II, 2005–2006, 22,894, nr. 78.
95. Parliamentary Papers II, 2005–2006, 22,894, nr. 83.
96. Parliamentary Papers II, 2005–2006, 22,894, nr. 86.
97. Parliamentary Papers II, 2005–2006, 22,894, nr. 104.
98. Proceedings II, 2005–2006, 22,894, nr. 94.

99. The bill was supported by D66, the *Groep Wilders*, de VVD, CDA, LPF en the *Groep Nawijn*; voting was on 27 June 2006.
100. Parliamentary Papers II, 2006–2007, 31, 200-XVI-7-b1.
101. Parliamentary Papers II, 2006–2007, 30,800 XVI, nr. 149.
102. Parliamentary Papers II, 2007–2008, 31,200 XVI, nr. 8.
103. Parliamentary Papers II, 2007–2008, 31,200 XVI, nr. 8.
104. Proceedings II, 5 July 2007, 90–5101.
105. Proceedings II, 18 October 2007, 15–1021.
106. Parliamentary Papers II, 2009–2010, 32011, nr. 5.
107. Parliamentary Papers II, 2008–2009, 22894, nr. 206.
108. Parliamentary Papers II, 2008–2009, 22,894, nr. 206.
109. Proceedings II, 2008–2009, Annexes 570, 1648, 1867, 2267, and 3169.
110. Proceedings II, 2008–2009, 22,894, nr. 216; Parliamentary Papers II, 2008–2009, 32,011, nr. 1.
111. Proceedings II, 2 April 2009, 72–5691.
112. Parliamentary Papers II, 2008–2009, 32,011, nr. 1.
113. Proceedings II, 2008–2009, 22,894, nr. 207.
114. Parliamentary Papers II, 2008–2009, 22,894, nr. 206.
115. Parliamentary Papers II, 2008–2009, 22,894, nr. 212.
116. Parliamentary Papers II, 2009–2010, 32,011, nr. 3.
117. Parliamentary Papers II, 2009–2010, 22,894, nr. 280.
118. Proceedings II, Tabakswet 31 mei 2001, TK 82-5220.
119. Parliamentary Papers II, 22894, nr. 154.
120. Parliamentary Papers II, 2008–2009, 22,894, nr. 226.
121. Parliamentary Papers II, 22,894, nr. 167.
122. Parliamentary Papers II, 2007–2008, 22,894, nr. 153.
123. Proceedings II, 2003–2004, 29,200 XVI, nr. 158.
124. Proceedings II, TK 15, 28 October 2010.
125. Proceedings II, TK 15, 28 October 2010.
126. Parliamentary Papers II, 2010–2011, 22,894, nr. 289.
127. Proceedings II, 2003–2004, Parliamentary Questions 2030408200.
128. Proceedings II, 2007–2008, 22,894, nr. 167.
129. https://www.stopcorporateabuse.org/press-release/netherlands-nominated-%E2%80%9Cmarlboro-man-award%E2%80%9D
130. In the investigative journalistic series "Zembla."
131. Proceedings II, 2 October 2013, TK 8, 8-6-1.
132. Parliamentary Papers II, 2012–2013, 33,400 XVI, nr. 78.
133. "Polder" refers to the Dutch version of consensus-based policymaking (see Chap. 5).
134. Proceedings I, 26 March 2002.

References

Algemene Rekenkamer. (1982). Verslag van een onderzoek naar de gesubsidieerde activiteiten verband houdend met het tegengaan van het roken en daarmee samenhangende aangelegenheden. *Truth Tobacco Industry Documents*, Bates No. JB2303. Retrieved from https://industrydocuments.library.ucsf.edu/tobacco/docs/#id=kpdp0219

Arnott, D., Berteletti, F., Britton, J., Cardone, A., Clancy, L., Craig, L., ... Willemsen, M. C. (2011). Can the Dutch Government really be abandoning smokers to their fate? *The Lancet, 379*, 121–122. https://doi.org/10.1016/S0140-6736(11)61855-2

ASH. (2013). Key dates in the history of anti-tobacco campaigning. Retrieved August 29, 2014, from http://www.ash.org.uk/files/documents/ASH_741.pdf

Baltesen, F., & Rosenberg, E. (2009, June 22). Big tobacco pays Dutch opposition to smoking ban. *NRC Handelsblad*. Retrieved from http://vorige.nrc.nl/international/article2278646.ece/Big_tobacco_pays_Dutch_opposition_to_smoking_ban

Beernink, J. F., & Plokker, J. H. (1975). Maatregelen tot beperking van het roken. Advies van de Gezondheidsraad. *Verslagen, Adviezen, Rapporten* (Vol. 23). Leidschendam: Ministerie van Volksgezondheid en Milieuhygiëne.

Berridge, V., & Loughlin, K. (2005). Smoking and the new health education in Britain 1950s–1970s. *American Journal of Public Health, 95*, 956–964. https://doi.org/10.2105/AJPH.2004.037887

Colby, F. G. (1979). Summary of the PR program of the Dutch Cigarette Manufactures Association. *RJ Reynolds Records Collection*, Bates No. 500877429–500877431. Retrieved from https://industrydocuments.library.ucsf.edu/tobacco/docs/#id=jrpj0096

De Jong, A. (2000). Complete prohibition on smoking in the workplace. *British American Tobacco Records*, Bates No. 322075711–322075712. Retrieved from http://legacy.library.ucsf.edu/tid/llp14a99

De Landsadvocaat. (1995). Verbod tabaksreclame. *Dutch Tobacco Industry Collection*, Bates No. JB1037. Retrieved from https://www.industrydocumentslibrary.ucsf.edu/tobacco/docs/gtcp0219

Dekker, H., Soethout, J., & Tijsmans, N. (2009). *Even uitblazen. Eén jaar rookvrije horeca*. Amsterdam: Regioplan Beleidsonderzoek.

Department of Health. (2004). *Choosing health: Making healthy choices easier*. London: UK Department of Health.

Doll, R., & Hill, A. B. (1950). Smoking and carcinoma of the lung: Preliminary report. *British Medical Journal, 2*, 739–748.

Dresscher, I., Elzinga, A., & Koldenhof, E. (1991). *Evaluatie tabakswet en zelfregulering tabaksreclame*. Zoetermeer: Research voor Beleid.

Gadourek, I. (1963). *Riskante gewoonten en zorg voor eigen welzijn*. Groningen: J.B. Wolters.
Gezondheidsraad. (1990). *Passief roken: Beoordeling van de schadelijkheid van omgevingstabaksrook voor de gezondheid*. Den Haag: Gezondheidsraad.
Gezondheidsraad. (2003). *Volksgezondheidsschade door passief roken*. Den Haag: Gezondheidsraad.
Gonzalez, M., & Glantz, S. A. (2013). Failure of policy regarding smoke-free bars in the Netherlands. *European Journal of Public Health, 23*(1), 139–145. https://doi.org/10.1093/eurpub/ckr173
Hall, P. (1993). Policy paradigms, social learning, and the state: The case of economic policymaking in Britain. *Comparative Politics, 25*, 257–296.
Huisman, C. (2005). Uit de walm. *Volkskrant*. Retrieved from http://www.volkskrant.nl/archief/uit-de-walm~a643849/
Hummel, K., Willemsen, M. C., Monshouwer, K., De Vries, H., & Nagelhout, G. E. (2016). Social acceptance of smoking restrictions during 10 years of policy implementation, reversal, and reenactment in the Netherlands: Findings from a national population survey. *Nicotine & Tobacco Research, 19*, 1–8. https://doi.org/10.1093/ntr/ntw169
ICBT. (1981). *Advies inzake maatregelen ter beperking van het tabaksgebruik*. Den Haag: Interdepartementale Commissie Beperking Tabaksgebruik (ICBT), Ministerie van Volksgezondheid en Milieu.
Interdepartementale Commissie Tabaksreclame. (1972a). Verslag van een Hearing op 24 januari 1972 over het onderwerp reklame voor tabaksprodukten, gehouden door de Interdepartamentale Commissie. *Dutch Tobacco Industry Collection*, Bates No. JB1936. Retrieved from https://industrydocuments.library.ucsf.edu/tobacco/docs/mhbp0219
Interdepartementale Commissie Tabaksreclame. (1972b). Verslag vergadering Interdepartementale Werkgroep Tabaksreclame 13 juli 1972. *Dutch Tobacco Industry Collection*, Bates No. JB1858. Retrieved from https://www.industrydocumentslibrary.ucsf.edu/tobacco/docs/hkgp0219
Intraval. (2010). *Inventarisatie naleefniveau rookvrije horeca najaar 2010*. Groningen: Intraval.
John, P. (2012). *Analyzing public policy* (2nd ed.). London: Routledge.
Jongejan, B. A. J., Hummel, H., Roelants, H. J., Lugtenberg, G., & Hoekstra, G. A. (2003). *National Cancer Control Programme. Part I—NPK vision and summary 2005–2010*. Den Haag: NPK Steering Group.
Kalis, A. W. (2000). Tabaksaccijns. *Dutch Tobacco Industry Collection*, Bates No. JB2028. Retrieved from https://www.industrydocumentslibrary.ucsf.edu/tobacco/docs/lpfp0219
Kaper, J., Wagena, E. J., & Van Schaijck, O. (2003). *Het effect van het vergoeden van ondersteuning voor stoppen met roken: Resultaten van een gerandomiseerd experiment*. Maastricht: Universiteit van Maastricht.

Klink, A. (2007). *Kaderbrief 2007–2011 visie op gezondheid en preventie*. Den Haag: Ministry of Health.
Kroes, M. E., & Lock, A. J. J. (2003). *Stoppen met roken ondersteuning: Zeker weten!* Diemen: College voor Zorgverzekeringen (CVZ).
Meulblok, J. (1975). Advies inzake maatregelen tot beperking van de reclame voor sigaretten en shag en tot het aanbrengen van aanduidingen op de verpakkingen van sigaretten en shag. *Dutch Tobacco Industry Collection*, Bates No. JB2105. Retrieved from https://www.industrydocumentslibrary.ucsf.edu/tobacco/docs/ztbp0219
Ministerie van Economische Zaken. (1991). Nota Mondeling Overleg 17 oktober 1991 met vaste Commissie voor de Volksgezondheid van de Tweede Kamer inzake tabaksontmoedigingsbeleid. *Dutch Tobacco Industry Collection*, Bates No. JB2777. Retrieved from https://industrydocuments.library.ucsf.edu/tobacco/docs/lxfp0219
Ministerie van Economische Zaken. (2010). Dossier voor kennismakingsgesprek met tabaksindustrie. *Dutch Tobacco Industry Collection, Ministerie van Economische Zaken*, Bates No. JB0533. Retrieved from https://industrydocuments.library.ucsf.edu/tobacco/docs/lxxb0191
Nagelhout, G. E., & Fong, G. T. (2011). Netherlands: Plan to cut all health education. *Tobacco Control, 20*(4), 253–254.
National Clearinghouse for Smoking and Health. (1969). Smoking and health programs in other countries. *Philip Morris Records*, Bates No. 2016003319–2016003331. Retrieved from http://legacy.library.ucsf.edu/tid/jdh68e00
Nederlands Economisch Instituut. (1991). *De evaluatie van het tabaksontmoedigingsbeleid nader beschouwd*. Rotterdam: NEI.
Niemantsverdriet, T. (2011, November 9). Minister Edith Schippers: De vrouw van 75 miljard. *Vrij Nederland*. Retrieved from http://www.vn.nl/Archief/Politiek/Artikel-Politiek/Minister-Edith-Schippers-De-vrouw-van-75-miljard.htm
NKI-AVL. (2012). *Artsen zeggen NEE tegen tabak: Wij vragen de politiek om een effectief tabaksontmoedigingsbeleid*. Amsterdam: NKI-AVL.
Pauw, P. M. (1971). Televisiereclame en anti-reclame. *Dutch Tobacco Industry Collection*, Bates No. 2501265710–2501265713. Retrieved from http://legacy.library.ucsf.edu/tid/pwr22e00
Philip Morris. (1996). Corporate Affairs 1996/1997 The Netherlands. *Philip Morris Records*, Bates No. 2501076006–2501076023. Retrieved from https://www.industrydocumentslibrary.ucsf.edu/tobacco/docs/nzjl0112
Roscam Abbing, E. W. (1998). *Tabaksontmoedigingsbeleid: Gezondheidseffectrapportage*. Utrecht: Netherlands School of Public Health (NSPH).
Royal College of Physicians. (1962a). *Smoking and health*. London: Royal College of Physicians of London.
Royal College of Physicians. (1962b). *Roken en gezondheid. Een rapport van de Koninklijk Genootschap van Londense artsen over roken in verband met longkanker en andere aandoeningen*. Amsterdam: Strengholt.

Royal College of Physicians. (1971). Smoking and health now. A new report and summary on smoking and its effects on health. *Annals of Internal Medicine, 75*(1), 147–148. https://doi.org/10.7326/0003-4819-75-1-147

Spijkerman, R., & van den Ameele, A. N. (2001). *Roken op het werk 2000 (een herhalingsonderzoek).* Den Haag: Arbeidsinspectie.

Stichting van de Arbeid. (1992). Aanbeveling over de bescherming van de niet-roker op het werk. *Dutch Tobacco Industry Collection*, Bates No. JB2035. Retrieved from https://www.industrydocumentslibrary.ucsf.edu/tobacco/docs/khdp0219

STIVORO. (1999). *25 jaar STIVORO: een goed begin [year report].* Den Haag: STIVORO.

STIVORO. (2005). *Nationaal Programma Tabaksontmoediging 2006–2010.* Den Haag: STIVORO.

Studlar, D. T., & Cairney, P. (2014). Conceptualizing punctuated and non-punctuated policy change: Tobacco control in comparative perspective. *International Review of Administrative Sciences, 80*(3), 513–531. https://doi.org/10.1177/0020852313517997

Tobacco Manufacturers' Assocation. (1971). Gentlemen's agreement. *Philip Morris Collection*, Bates No. 2501265714–2501265715. Retrieved from http://legacy.library.ucsf.edu/tid/qwr22e00

U.S. Department of Health, Education, and Welfare. (1964). *Smoking and health: Report of the Advisory Committee to the Surgeon General of the Public Health Service (Vol. DHEW publication no. (PHS) 64-1103).* Washington, DC: Public Health Service.

Unknown (Philip Morris). (1979). *Smoking & health—Five year plan*, Bates No 2501020542–2501020686. Truth Tobacco Industry Documents.

US Public Health Service. (1970). Smoking and health programs around the world. *American Tobacco Records*, Bates No. 968012023–968012038. Retrieved from http://legacy.library.ucsf.edu/tid/cob34f00

Van den Putte, S. J. H. M., Yzer, M. C., Ten Berg, B. M., & Steeveld, R. M. A. (2005). *Nederland start met stoppen/Nederland gaat door met stoppen. Evaluatie van de STIVORO campagnes rondom de jaarwisseling 2003–2004.* Amsterdam: Universiteit van Amsterdam, ASCOR.

Van Gennip, E. M. S. J. (2007). Brief STIVORO aan Ministerie van Algemene Zaken over beleidsvoornemen om de horeca-rookvrij te maken. *Dutch Tobacco Industry Collection*, Bates No. JB0344. Retrieved from https://www.industrydocumentslibrary.ucsf.edu/tobacco/docs/snhb0191

Van Leeuwen, M. J., & Sleur, D. G. (1998). De economische effecten van maatregelen ter bestrijding van het roken. In E. Roscam Abbing (Ed.), *Tabaksontmoedigingsbeleid: Gezondheidseffectrapportage.* Utrecht: Netherlands School of Public Health (NSPH).

Van Rijn, M. (2014). Onderzoeken naar effecten verkooppunten en leeftijdverificatiesystemen tabaksproducten. *Kamerbrief 626288-122861-VGP*.

Van Vliet, G. F. W. (1971). Gentlemen's agreement manufacturers on publicity vs. smoking and health. *Philip Morris Collection*, Bates No. 2501265716. Retrieved from http://legacy.library.ucsf.edu/tid/rwr22e00

Verdonk-Kleinjan, W. M. (2014). *Impact assessment of the tobacco legislation: Effects of the workplace smoking ban and the tobacco sales ba to minors*. PhD, Maastricht University, Maastricht.

Vijgen, S. M. C., Gelder, B. M. v., Baal, P. H. M. v., Zutphen, M. v., Hoogenveen, R. T., & Feenstra, T. L. (2007). *Kosten en effecten van tabaksontmoediging*. Bilthoven: RIVM.

Visser, W. M. G. (2008). *Accijnzen : Een onderzoek naar de rechtsgronden van de Nederlandse accijnzen aan de hand van 200 jaar parlementaire geschiedenis (1805–2007) en naar de werking van het Europese accijnsregime binnen de interne markt in het licht van deze rechtsgronden*. PhD, University of Amsterdam, Amsterdam. Retrieved from http://dare.uva.nl/document/98972

VWA. (2005). *Evaluatie van de handhavingervaring van de Tabakswet 2002–2004: Een kwantitatieve en kwalitatieve analyse*. Utrecht: NVWA.

VWS. (1991). Zelfregulering tabaksreclame voldoet niet. *Press release 15 Oktober 1991, no 68*.

VWS. (2001). Tabaksnota "Samen naar een rookvrije samenleving" *Truth Tobacco Industry Documents*, Bates No. JB2316. Retrieved from https://industrydocuments.library.ucsf.edu/tobacco/docs/rfgp0219

VWS. (2003). *Langer Gezond Leven: Ook een kwestie van gezond gedrag*. Den Haag: Ministerie van VWS.

VWS. (2005). *Evaluatie Tabaksontmoediging*. Den Haag: Ministerie van VWS.

VWS. (2006). *Nationaal Programma Tabaksontmoediging*. Den Haag: Ministerie van VWS.

VWS. (2007). *Gezond zijn, gezond blijven. Een visie op gezondheid en preventie*. Den Haag: Ministerie van VWS.

VWS. (2011). *Gezondheid dichtbij. Landelijke nota gezondheidsbeleid*. Den Haag: Ministerie van VWS.

Wassink, W. F. (1948). Ontstaansvoorwaarden voor longkanker. *Nederlands Tijdschrift voor Geneeskunde, 92*, 3732–3747.

Wester, J. (1957). Roken en gezondheid. Rapport van de Gezondheidsraad. *Nederlands Tijdschrift voor Geneeskunde, 107*, 459–464.

WHO. (1975). *Smoking and its effects on health*. Report of a WHO expert committee No. 568, Technical Report Series. Geneva: World Health Organization.

WHO. (2003). *WHO framework convention on tobacco control*. Geneva: World Health Organization.

WHO. (2006). *Legislating for smoke-free workplaces*. Copenhagen: WHO Regional Office for Europe.

Willemsen, M. C. (2006). *Rokers onder vuur? Invloed van de gewijzigde Tabakswet op rokers, met speciale aandacht voor verschillen tussen sociaal-economische klassen*. Den Haag: STIVORO.

World Bank. (1999). *Curbing the epidemic: Governments and the economics of tobacco control.* Washington: The World Bank.
WVC. (1991). Scherpere aanpak van tabaksontmoedigingsbeleid. *Press release 16 Oktober 1991, no 69.*
Wynder, W. L., & Graham, E. A. (1950). Tobacco smoking as a possible etiological factor in bronchiogenic carcinoma: A study of six hundred and eighty-four proved cases. *Journal of the American Medical Association, 143,* 329–336.
Zeeman, G., & De Beer, M. A. M. (2012). 50 jaar GVO en Gezondheidsbevordering: Geschiedenis van de tabaksontmoediging in Nederland; succesverhaal met een droevig einde. *Tijdschrift voor Gezondheidswetenschappen, 90,* 253–261.

Open Access   This chapter is licensed under the terms of the Creative Commons Attribution 4.0 International License (http://creativecommons.org/licenses/by/4.0/), which permits use, sharing, adaptation, distribution and reproduction in any medium or format, as long as you give appropriate credit to the original author(s) and the source, provide a link to the Creative Commons license and indicate if changes were made.

The images or other third party material in this chapter are included in the chapter's Creative Commons license, unless indicated otherwise in a credit line to the material. If material is not included in the chapter's Creative Commons license and your intended use is not permitted by statutory regulation or exceeds the permitted use, you will need to obtain permission directly from the copyright holder.

CHAPTER 3

The Tempo of Dutch Tobacco Control Policy

This chapter considers the tempo at which the Dutch government took steps to control smoking by comparing the moment of adoption of policy measures in the Netherlands with the United Kingdom and with the rest of Europe. Before we embark on comparisons, it will be useful to define what 'tobacco control policy' is. It is not straightforward, since it refers to various actions that governments may take. Scholars (e.g., Birkland, 2011) distinguish between "types" of policy: *laws, services, incentives* (spending, grants, reimbursement), *taxation*, and *persuasion* (education, campaigns). These differ in effectiveness, timelines (a quick or a slow effect), cost, efficiency, flexibility, visibility, accountability, and degree of citizen choice (Levine, Peters, & Thompson, 1990). Effective tobacco control is comprehensive in that it is a combination of many policy instruments. At its core are laws that restrict the availability of and exposure to tobacco products. Such regulations tend to become increasingly restrictive over time and are supported by various degrees of education, cessation support, incentives, and taxation.

Experts have identified elements of effective tobacco control policy by considering evidence from countries across the world (Warner & Tam, 2012). There is international consensus that the main building blocks of comprehensive tobacco control are:

1. Restrictions on the sale of tobacco to minors
2. Health warning labels and package descriptors

3. Ban on tobacco advertising and promotion
4. Smoke-free legislation
5. Educational programmes to raise awareness
6. Support for smoking cessation
7. Taxation of tobacco products (WHO, 2003, 2004)

Note that the first four are regulations involving lasting improvements in tobacco control, requiring a process of law making that involves formal parliamentary voting, while 5 and 6 are more dependent on the political will to set aside the needed budgets. Measures 5, 6, and 7 may be adjusted every year. The building blocks are sometimes simplified to five measures plus monitoring of tobacco use and prevention policies, and referred to as the MPOWER package (WHO, 2008).

Policy Cycles

In the previous chapter a detailed account was given of the stages that Dutch tobacco control policy has gone through. It is helpful to restructure the events according to the stages of the policy process. According to the "stages heuristics approach" (Moloughney, 2012; Sabatier, 2007), the following stages can be distinguished:

- Agenda setting (recognising a problem that requires government's attention)
- Policy formulation (considering various policy options)
- Policy adoption (making the decision)
- Policy implementation (assuring that the policy decision is carried out, and establishment of rules and procedures)
- Policy evaluation (assessing whether the policy achieved its objectives)

The stages form cycles. A policy cycle starts when the problem is put on the political agenda and ends when impact is evaluated (Moloughney, 2012). After evaluation, a new policy process starts, depending on the outcomes of the evaluation or the recognition of a new or continued problem on the agenda.

The stages heuristic approach has been criticised for its simplistic depiction of the policy process, which in reality rarely follows a linear course. A more realistic representation is that there is an ongoing process in which policymakers consider ideas, negotiate, try out, move away, and come back when new opportunities arise. John (2012, p. 20) noted that "There is no beginning and end to public policy; for the most part there is only the middle." Despite such critical comments I use the policy stages, because categorising the process into distinct stages is useful for descriptive purposes in this chapter (Moloughney, 2012).

Tobacco control policy does not change gradually or evenly, but there are periodic bursts of activity, with intermediate periods where little seems to happen. To date the Dutch government has gone through a full policy cycle four times (Table 3.1); the cycles have become shorter over time. The first one lasted for 23 years, the next two for 10 years; the latest was 7 years. There were interims of a few years when tobacco control was almost off the political agenda.

The first cycle began in 1954, when the government started to investigate the health concerns of smoking. The first choice of policy was education, and STIVORO was founded to coordinate and professionalise education. In the 1970s an ambitious policy agenda was brought to the attention of the government, but only one option, health warnings on tobacco products, was adopted and implemented, and when the right-wing Van Agt Cabinet came to power in 1977 tobacco control disappeared from the political agenda. The first policy cycle was terminated in 1977 before it could come to blossom.

Table 3.1 Tobacco control policy cycles

Period	Policy cycle	Accomplished policies, initiated by government or parliament
1954–1977	1. Education	• Educational programmes targeted at youth • Health warnings on cigarette packs
1978–1980	Interim period	
1981–1991	2. Self-regulation	• Tobacco Act: – Smoke-free public places
1992–1994	Interim period	

1995–2005	3. Regulation	• Revision of the Tobacco Act:
		  – Advertising and promotion ban
		  – Smoke-free workplaces
		  – Ban on tobacco sales to those under 16

2006–2007	Interim period	
2007–2014	4. Decentralisation and shared responsibility with civil society	• Smoking ban in pubs and restaurants • Reimbursement for smoking cessation • Ban on tobacco sale to those under 18
2014–present	Interim period	

From 1981 until 1991 a second policy cycle emerged from proposals set out in the *Interdepartementale Commissie Beperking Tabaksgebruik* (Interdepartmental Committee for Reducing Tobacco Use) (ICBT) report. This was a long period in which anti-tobacco policy was successfully kept off the political agenda by the tobacco industry network, which had a strong presence in and around government. The government chose to rely on self-regulation by the industry. In this period economic interests trumped health interests. The cycle resulted in the adoption of the Tobacco Act in 1990 with smoke-free public places and ended when it was evaluated in 1991.

The third policy cycle started in 1995, when the government realised that smoking rates were still high compared to other countries and were unlikely to go down without further measures. Minister Borst gave the reduction of tobacco-related harm high priority and accomplished an important institutional shift, giving the Ministry of Health a more central role in the policy process at the expense of the Ministry of Economic Affairs. The tobacco industry became foe instead of friend. Just before the end of her term in office, Borst succeeded in getting parliament to adopt a substantial amendment to the Tobacco Act, resulting in smoke-free workplaces, a full advertising and promotion ban, and a lower age limit for the sale of tobacco. This cycle ended in 2005 when Minister Hoogervorst evaluated the government's policy and concluded that the goal of 28% smokers had been reached.

In 2007 Hoogervorst started work on a new tobacco control policy plan based on consultation with health organisations and the industry. He assessed the political viability of new measures and concluded that there was insufficient political support to achieve any of these. The process was abruptly terminated and replaced by the *Nationaal Programma Tabaksontmoediging* (National Programme of Tobacco Control) (NPT). His successor, Ab Klink, was occupied with securing a smoking ban in the hospitality sector, a headache "dossier" that he had inherited from previous governments. Instead of further regulation, the government continued along the path of decentralisation and sharing responsibility with civil society. The policy cycle ended in 2014 when all involved concluded that the NPT had failed. The government decided against starting a second NPT. As it has not yet committed to a new tobacco control programme, the current period must be regarded as the interim.

Adoption of Tobacco Control Policy in the Netherlands Compared with the United Kingdom

The United Kingdom has not always been the leader in tobacco control. Scandinavian countries like Norway already had a Tobacco Act in 1975, requiring health warnings on tobacco packs and a ban on advertising of tobacco products, and banned smoking in workplaces in 1988. For many years the Netherlands and the United Kingdom roughly had the same timing for implementation of policies, as shown in Table 3.2, which compares the coming into force of key Tobacco Acts in both countries. For many decades the United Kingdom and the Netherlands relied on voluntary agreements with the industry instead of statutory measures. Both countries had a strong tobacco industry presence.

Table 3.2 Dates of coming into force of key tobacco control policies in the Netherlands and in the United Kingdom (**bold** indicates fastest date)

	Netherlands	UK
Ban on tobacco advertising on television	1980	**1965**
Ban on tobacco advertising on the radio	1980	**1978** (voluntary)
"Smoking damages health" warning on cigarette packs	1982 (voluntary)	**1971** (voluntary)
Smoking ban in public places	**1990**	1992 (voluntary)
Ban on tobacco advertising in cinemas	1996	**1986** (voluntary)
Removal of misleading descriptors such as "light" and "mild" from cigarette packs	**2002** (EU)	2003 (EU)
Large-text health warnings covering 30% of the front and 40% of the back of cigarette packs	**2002** (EU)	2003 (EU)
Ban on advertising and promotion (via billboards, direct mail, internet)	**2002** (EU)	2003 (EU)
Ban on sales to those under 16	2003	**1908, 1986**
Ban on advertising in print media	2003	2003
Smoking ban in private workplaces	**2004**	2007
Smoking ban in the hospitality sector	2008	**2007**
Smoking ban in small bars	2014	**2007**
Ban on sale to those under 18	2014	**2008**
Picture warnings on cigarettes packs	2016	**2008**
Ban on sales through vending machines	–	2011
Ban on tobacco displays in large stores	–	2012
Ban on smoking in cars in the presence of children	–	2015
Ban on tobacco display in small shops	–	2015

Source for United Kingdom: ASH (2013)

The Netherlands was slow in restricting sales to minors (2003), which the United Kingdom had implemented in 1908 and reconfirmed in the 1986 Protection of Children (Tobacco) Act. The United Kingdom introduced the first voluntary health warnings on cigarette packs in 1971, much sooner than the Netherlands, but the Dutch were faster to implement smoking bans in public places and private workplaces. When the Netherlands adopted its Tobacco Act in 1988, there did not yet exist an equivalent piece of legislation in the United Kingdom. From 1999 the United Kingdom made policy either for the kingdom as a whole (tobacco advertising) or separately for devolved governments (England, Wales, Scotland, Northern Ireland), as in the case of smoking bans. In 2005 the United Kingdom still had no ban on smoking in public places. The 2006 UK Health Act governed smoking in workplaces, but its workplace smoking ban, introduced in 2007, was comprehensive. The Netherlands retained an exemption for restaurants and bars until 2008, and for small bars until 2014, and still allows separate smoking sections.

Both countries have a long history of self-regulation by the industry of advertising restrictions, with England leading the way. In the United Kingdom, the industry banned advertising on radio already in 1978 and in cinemas in 1986. However, a comprehensive advertising and promotion ban was discussed in the same year (2001) in both parliaments. By then no fewer than seven other EU countries had already adopted this regulation and, outside the EU, so had Norway, Iceland, Poland, and Hungary.[1] The first European Advertising Directive stipulated that misleading descriptors such as "light" and "mild" must be removed from packages, and large health warnings became mandatory. The Netherlands was a year faster in transposing this EU directive into national law (2002) than the United Kingdom (2003).

Table 3.2 only compares the coming into force of regulative measures that involved lasting improvements in tobacco control and require a process of law making and formal voting in parliament, but not measures such as tax increases, campaigns, and smoking cessation support. In 2000, following the *Smoking Kills* white paper, the United Kingdom introduced smoking cessation services (Department of Health, 1998) and from that moment embarked on a different course than the Netherlands. A combination of high tobacco taxes (not included in Table 3.2), made reasonably enforceable by the United Kingdom's island status, substantial investment into smoking cessation services and awareness-raising mass media campaigns, and consistent commitment by the government to reduce tobacco's appeal to children through legislation, propelled the United Kingdom into the league of world leaders in tobacco control. In contrast, the allocated budget for tobacco control in the Netherlands was cut by the government, after a relatively high level of spending in the beginning of the 2000s. It went from €0.93 per capita in 2003 to €0.12 in 2012 (Heijndijk & Willemsen, 2015). The second UK white paper published in 2010 (Department of Health, 2010) was an extension of the comprehensive UK tobacco control strategy and resulted in several measures that have not yet been taken in the Netherlands.

The Netherlands Compared with Europe

Various attempts have been made to compare countries within Europe. Studlar and Cairney (2014) looked at the pace of tobacco policy adoption in 23 countries by identifying the average year by which 24 tobacco control instruments had been adopted. The Netherlands was relatively slow, with 1994 as the median year of adoption: 1986 was the median for the 23 countries. Another attempt to compare progress across Europe was made by a group of experts in 2003 (Thyrian & John, 2006) who drafted a 40-item questionnaire which covered a long list of tobacco control measures that the group identified as having the most influence on smoking. Data was gathered from 142 participants from 14 EU member states to the World Conference on Tobacco or Health in Helsinki, who were asked to assess the level of tobacco control in their own country. Fourteen Dutch delegates participated. The assessment came very soon after the implementation of the amended Dutch Tobacco Act, and this was reflected in the data: the Netherlands came out higher than average, ranking just below Finland, Sweden, Ireland, and the United Kingdom. According to the 14 Dutch respondents, the Netherlands was particularly good at providing smokers with effective smoking cessation treatment (highest rank, together with the United Kingdom).

The most widely cited effort to compare the strength of tobacco control between countries in Europe was undertaken by tobacco control experts Luk Joossens and Martin Raw in 2004 (Joossens & Raw, 2006). Their Tobacco Control Scale (TCS) is a composite scale with points allocated by a group of experts to the six tobacco policies considered most effective according to a report from the World Bank (World Bank, 2003): tobacco taxation level, smoke-free laws, public information campaigns, advertising bans, health warning labels, and cessation support (Joossens,

2004). The scoring reflected best practice at the time the scale was developed and did not capture early interventions considered ineffective, such as self-regulation by the industry and bans on tobacco sales to minors. Data have been published for six distinct years. The Netherlands ranked 7th (among 28 countries) in 2004, 10th (30 countries) in 2005, 14th (30 countries) in 2007, 13th (31 countries) in 2010, 13th (34 countries) in 2013, and 9th (35 countries) in 2016 (Joossens & Raw, 2017). Since 2006 the United Kingdom and Ireland have received the highest scores, mainly due to relatively high tobacco taxes and relative large budgets allocated to media campaigns and smoking cessation treatment.

Various research groups have used the TCS to study different aspects of tobacco control policy change. Nguyen, Rosenqvist, and Pekurinen (2012) created a Tobacco Control Policy Index (TCPI) based on four of the six policy components of the TCS: smoke-free laws, bans on tobacco advertising, health warnings on tobacco packaging, and smoking cessation treatment services. They recalculated the TCS scores into a composite score ranging from 0 to 100.[2] J.R. Bosdriesz, Willemsen, Stronks, and Kunst (2014) calculated TCPI scores for 11 European countries in each year from 1969 onwards. This showed that the cumulation of policy measures follows an approximate S-curve (Fig. 3.1). It also showed that the Dutch government managed to keep up with other countries in Europe, indicating that the Netherlands is neither a leader nor a laggard in tobacco

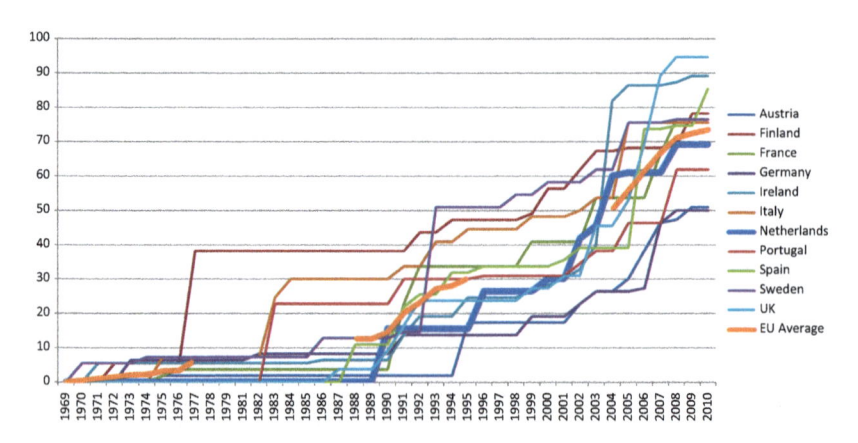

Fig. 3.1 Tobacco Control Policy Index scores between 1969 and 2010 in 11 EU countries

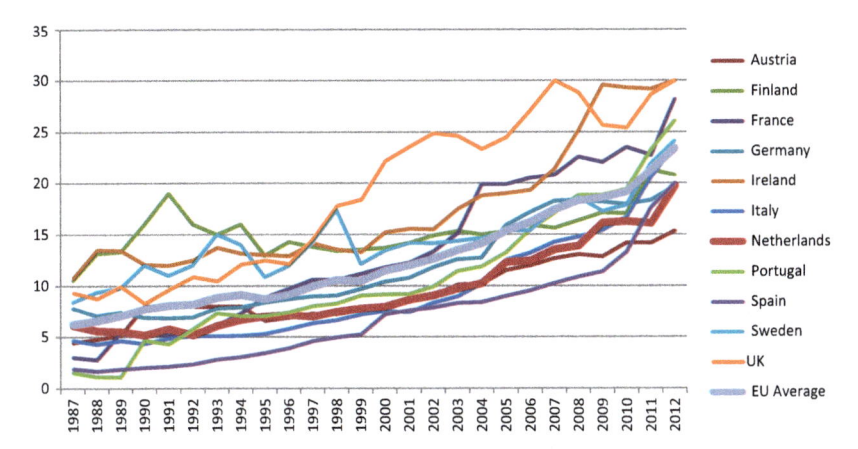

Fig. 3.2 Dates of coming into force of key tobacco control policies in the Netherlands and in the United Kingdom

control. However, it was a particularly slow starter. All countries had a zero score in 1969, but the Netherlands kept its zero the longest, after Austria. With the implementation of the Tobacco Act in 1990, the Netherlands caught up and received an average score. Between 1991 and 2002, the Netherlands again was below average, but caught up through improvements in smoking cessation treatment in the middle of the 1990s. With the adoption of the amendments to the Tobacco Act in 2002, Dutch tobacco control strength was again on a par with other countries.

With respect to tobacco taxation levels, the Netherlands can be characterised as a follower. Figure 3.2 shows TCPI scores for the level of tobacco taxation, indicated by the real price of cigarettes (Nguyen et al., 2012): this is the actual price corrected for purchasing power. Scores range from 0 to 30, with 15 points for the highest price for a pack of Marlboro Red and 15 points for the highest rank regarding the price of a pack of cigarettes in the most popular price category. Prices are relative to the highest score (30), which was allocated to the United Kingdom in 2007 (Joossens & Raw, 2011). The Netherlands consistently keeps its real price of cigarettes in tandem with the European average, with a price level somewhat lower than average, while the United Kingdom and Ireland have the most expensive cigarettes.

Although Dutch cigarette prices are among the highest in the EU (only France, Ireland, and the United Kingdom are higher) (Blecher, Ross, &

Leon, 2013), cigarettes in the Netherlands are more affordable to the average smoker than in most European countries (Blecher et al., 2013). While it took 28 minutes for the average Dutch smoker to work for one pack of cigarettes in 2010 (the same as in Germany and Belgium), it took 42 minutes in the United Kingdom and as much as 61 in Hungary (Bogdanovica, Murray, McNeill, & Britton, 2012). Indeed, Dutch smokers are less concerned about how much money they spent on cigarettes compared with smokers in other countries (23% compared with, e.g., 61% in France and 49% in the United Kingdom) (ITC Project, 2015).

Conclusion

Compared to most other high-income European countries, the Dutch government was relatively late in its move to regulate tobacco. It took until 2004 to catch up with the rest of Western Europe, and currently just manages to keep up with other EU countries, neither lagging nor trying to be a leader in the field. Tobacco taxation levels are kept in line with the EU average, with real price levels just below average.

Notes

1. Proceedings II, 31 May 2001, 82–5212.
2. Changes in tobacco taxes were presented separately. The other missing component of the TCS is spending on information campaigns. This was left out in the TCPI, because reliable information on spending was not available for each year for each country.

References

ASH. (2013). *Key dates in the history of anti-tobacco campaigning*. Retrieved August 29, 2014, from http://www.ash.org.uk/files/documents/ASH_741.pdf

Birkland, T. (2011). *An introduction to the policy process: Theories, concepts, and models of public policy making* (3rd ed.). Armonk, NY: M.E. Sharpe.

Blecher, E., Ross, H., & Leon, M. E. (2013). Cigarette affordability in Europe. *Tobacco Control, 22*, e6. https://doi.org/10.1136/tobaccocontrol-2012-050575

Bogdanovica, I., Murray, R., McNeill, A., & Britton, J. (2012). Cigarette price, affordability and smoking prevalence in the European Union. *Addiction, 107*, 188–196. https://doi.org/10.1111/j.1360-0443.2011.03588.x

Bosdriesz, J. R., Willemsen, M. C., Stronks, K., & Kunst, A. E. (2014). Tobacco control policy development in the European Union—Do political factors matter? *European Journal of Public Health, 25*(2), 190–194. https://doi.org/10.1093/eurpub/cku197
Department of Health. (1998). *Smoking kills. A white paper on tobacco.* London: Department of Health.
Department of Health. (2010). *A smokefree future: A comprehensive tobacco control strategy for England.* London: Department of Health.
Heijndijk, S. M., & Willemsen, M. C. (2015). *Dutch tobacco control: Moving towards the right track?* FCTC Shadow Report 2014. Den Haag: Alliantie Nederland Rookvrij.
ITC Project. (2015). ITC Netherlands National Report. Findings from the Wave 1 to 8 Surveys (2008–2014). Waterloo, ON, Canada: University of Waterloo.
John, P. (2012). *Analyzing public policy* (2nd ed.). London: Routledge.
Joossens, L. (2004). *Effective tobacco control policies in 28 European countries.* Brussels: ENSP.
Joossens, L., & Raw, M. (2006). The tobacco control scale: A new scale to measure country activity. *Tobacco Control, 15*(3), 247–253. https://doi.org/10.1136/tc.2005.015347
Joossens, L., & Raw, M. (2011). *The tobacco control scale 2010 in Europe.* Brussels: Association of European Cancer Leagues.
Joossens, L., & Raw, M. (2017). *The tobacco control scale 2016 in Europe.* Brussels: Association of European Cancer Leagues.
Levine, C. H., Peters, B. G., & Thompson, F. J. (1990). *Public administration: Challenges, choices, consequences.* Glenview, IL: Scott, Foresman/Little Brown.
Moloughney, B. (2012). The use of policy frameworks to understand public health-related processes: A literature review. Retrieved from https://www.peelregion.ca/health/library/pdf/Policy_Frameworks.PDF
Nguyen, L., Rosenqvist, G., & Pekurinen, M. (2012). *Demand for tobacco in Europe: An econometric analysis of 11 countries for the PPACTE project.* Tampere: National Institute for Health and Welfare.
Sabatier, P. A. (2007). *Theories of the policy process* (2nd ed.). Cambridge, MA: Westview Press.
Studlar, D. T., & Cairney, P. (2014). Conceptualizing punctuated and non-punctuated policy change: Tobacco control in comparative perspective. *International Review of Administrative Sciences, 80*(3), 513–531. https://doi.org/10.1177/0020852313517997
Thyrian, J. R., & John, U. (2006). Measuring activities in tobacco control across the EU. The MATOC. *Substance Abuse Treatment, Prevention, and Policy, 1,* 9. https://doi.org/10.1186/1747-597X-1-9
Warner, K. E., & Tam, J. (2012). The impact of tobacco control research and policy: 20 years of progress. *Tobacco Control, 21,* 103–109.

WHO. (2003). *WHO framework convention on tobacco control.* Geneva: World Health Organization.
WHO. (2004). *Building blocks for tobacco control: A handbook.* Geneva: World Health Organization.
WHO. (2008). *MPOWER.* Geneva: World Health Organisation.
World Bank. (2003). *Tobacco control at a glance.* Washington, DC: World Bank.

Open Access This chapter is licensed under the terms of the Creative Commons Attribution 4.0 International License (http://creativecommons.org/licenses/by/4.0/), which permits use, sharing, adaptation, distribution and reproduction in any medium or format, as long as you give appropriate credit to the original author(s) and the source, provide a link to the Creative Commons license and indicate if changes were made.

The images or other third party material in this chapter are included in the chapter's Creative Commons license, unless indicated otherwise in a credit line to the material. If material is not included in the chapter's Creative Commons license and your intended use is not permitted by statutory regulation or exceeds the permitted use, you will need to obtain permission directly from the copyright holder.

CHAPTER 4

The Social and Cultural Environment

Policy is not made in a vacuum. Disputes over tobacco control are fought within changing policy environments. This chapter explores key population-level factors that influence a national government's decision to adopt tobacco control policy measures. These factors include social norms about smoking, the proportion of smokers in the population, societal support for tobacco control, and cultural values. These factors are interrelated in a specific way and to understand this, we will take a short detour into what is sometimes called "system thinking in tobacco control." Ten years ago, the US National Cancer Institute (NCI) published a monograph on this topic (Best, Clark, Leichow, & Trochim, 2007), which acknowledged the complexity of tobacco control at the national level, involving as it does the interplay of factors over long periods of time, including feedback loops. According to experts from the NCI, a government's willingness to acknowledge and address the smoking problem follows from its level of awareness that tobacco is a problem, and from the balance of lobbying forces that propose or hold back policy solutions. A government's awareness of the problems associated with tobacco is further affected by specific population factors that are amenable to change. A country's smoking rate is one of these: as long as the proportion of smokers is high, the government is more likely to be aware that there is a public health risk that needs to be addressed. Changes in the number of smokers also affect public support for tobacco control, which increases when adult smoking rates go down—a process which was believed to be mediated by social norms. Reduced smoking (people quitting or fewer people starting) shifts the balance between smokers and non-smokers, increasing the level of anti-smoking norms and altering public opinion. There is also evidence for the reverse effect, in that people quit smoking when social norms become less accommodating. Together, these population factors determine the context within which national tobacco control policymaking takes place. I have put the main factors together in a simplistic model, which I have called the flywheel model of tobacco control (Willemsen, 2011).

The flywheel model (Fig. 4.1) assumes that population-level factors interact in a circular feedback manner over long periods. The term "flywheel" reflects the notion that the process that moves a population in the direction of a smoke-free society is difficult to set in motion but once begun continues for some time on its own until it loses speed and eventually comes to a stop in the absence of a new impetus (i.e., new tobacco control interventions). The model assumes that as long as the wheel keeps

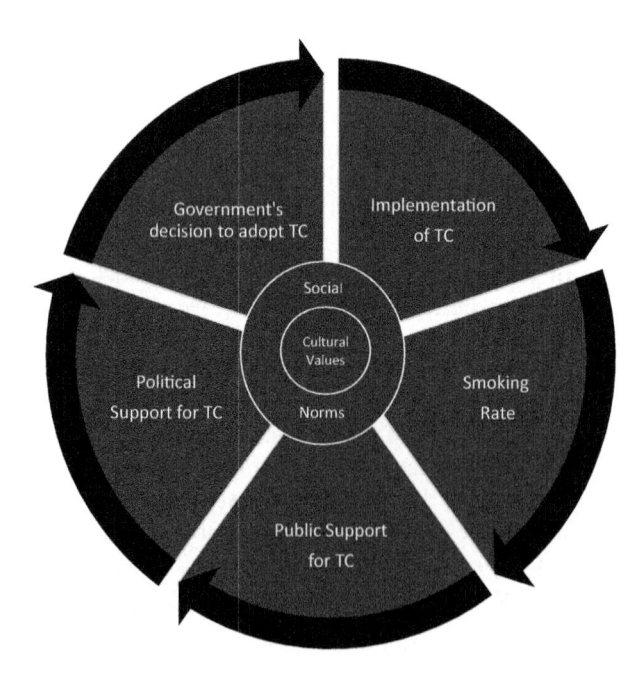

Fig. 4.1 The flywheel model of Tobacco Control (TC)

turning, either through new policy input or because the process of denormalisation of tobacco use in society continues, smoking rates will go down. It predicts that policymakers are more willing to introduce tobacco control measures when they are supported by politicians, when the general public and civil society are supportive, when the public thinks more negatively about smoking, and when the prevalence of smoking is low. It assumes a gradual reduction of the proportion of smokers in the population, but eventually will reach its "destination" when smoking rates are at a level that is acceptable to society and government.

Interest groups can influence each element of the flywheel model, with the exception of cultural values. Tobacco control proponents may give the wheel a spin by influencing any of its five sectors, while tobacco interest groups attempt to slow, stop, or reverse the wheel through the same access points. For example, the tobacco industry may develop campaigns to normalise smoking, apply strategies to lower the price of cigarettes in an attempt to offset the effect of tax increases, or present arguments that reduce political support for tobacco control.

The reader is invited to compare the flywheel model with the general conceptual framework in Chap. 1, which includes the same long-term feedback loop as the flywheel model. The flywheel is another way of conceptualising the dynamics of tobacco control, differing from the general conceptual framework in Fig. 1.1, in that it focuses on the population-level sociological factors that drive down smoking rates, resulting from the implementation of tobacco control measures, while ignoring the dynamics of the policymaking process itself.

The flywheel model starts with the implementation of tobacco control measures (TC). Depicted as one factor, in reality it consists of many possible policy solutions to the smoking problem. For example, tax increases make smoking less affordable, directly affecting tobacco consumption, while improvements in the smoking cessation infrastructure and smoking cessation campaigns build confidence in being able to quit and prompt smokers to quit. Tobacco control measures, when properly implemented, can have an impact on population smoking rates (Gravely et al., 2017; Ngo, Cheng, Chaloupka, & Shang, 2017). Some measures work indirectly through social norms (Rennen et al., 2014), particularly smoking bans (Betzner et al., 2012) and mass media campaigns that denormalise smoking (Durkin, Brennan, & Wakefield, 2012). A more detailed discussion of the effectiveness of different tobacco control measures appears in Chap. 7. In the current chapter I discuss the four factors of the flywheel that make up the sociological environment in which tobacco control policymaking takes place: cultural values, social norms, smoking rate, and public support for tobacco control.

Cultural Values

Some of the differences in acceptance and reaction to tobacco control between countries can be explained by cultural values (Hosking et al., 2009; Vogel, Kagan, & Kessler, 1993), which have been found to influence perceptions of tobacco products and smoking (Helweg-Larsen & Nielsen, 2009; Unger et al., 2003). Dominant cultural values and aspects of national culture are stable and relatively insensitive to outside influence, and are therefore located at the heart of the flywheel. Culture is revealed through a set of unique shared values and beliefs that exist for the majority of a population and distinguish it from other populations (Pasick, Onofrio, & Otero-Sabogal, 1996; Schwartz, 2006). According to S. Schwartz (2006), cultural values "shape and justify individual and group beliefs, actions, and goals. Institutional arrangements and policies, norms, and everyday practices express underlying cultural value emphases in societies." In our context, cultural values determine whether specific tobacco control policy initiatives may fall on fertile soil.

According to a landmark study by Geert Hofstede, who analysed cultural values in more than 50 countries (Hofstede, 1980), Dutch national culture can be characterised as extremely individualistic. People value their freedom to make personal decisions. They expect people to look after themselves and be independent. Personal choice is highly valued. Dutch culture is also a typical example of a "feminine" cooperative culture, according to Hofstede's research, meaning that negotiation and compromise are considered more appropriate than conflict. The combination of high individualism and high feminism has been proposed as an explanation for why the Dutch smoking ban in bars rested on the assumption that smoking customers would be cooperative, complying for the benefit of the employer who would be fined for non-compliance (feminine value orientation), while resistance to the ban reflected a high individualistic value orientation (Dechesne, Dignum, & Dignum, 2013).

Interestingly, the Dutch also score high on the dimension of indulgence, defined as "the extent to which people try to control their desires and impulses" (Hofstede Centre, 2015). A high score means that the Dutch recognise and respect other's desires to enjoy life and have fun, which may help explain the recurring wish from policymakers to be considerate to smokers. When Health Minister Ab Klink opened a British American Tobacco (BAT)-financed smoking area in the Dutch parliament building in September 2008, he announced, "this smoking area is a symbol for our two-pronged policy. On the one hand, protection; on the other hand, we don't want to go so far with regulating that we take away people's pleasures." The high score of the Dutch on individualism, femininity, and indulgence was confirmed by S. Schwartz (2006), who used similar orientations, albeit differently worded (respectively, intellectual autonomy, egalitarianism, and affective autonomy). The combination of these values is very alive today, illustrated by the still popular lines of the "alternative" national anthem *Fifteen million people*: "Fifteen million people/On that tiny strip of earth/You don't patronize them with laws/You take them for what they are."[1]

The Dutch version of smoking bans further typify the libertarian and individualistic approach to smoking and the egalitarian, "feminine" value orientation. The bans are more smoker-friendly than in other countries. Many exemptions were included in early formulations, such as providing smoking rooms to accommodate smokers and setting up transitional regimes for sectors where smoking was considered more difficult to enforce. Smokers who disobeyed were not prosecuted, but instead the owner or administrator of the venue or property where the violation took place risked a fine. In one study we compared smoking bans in bars in the Netherlands, Germany, France, and Ireland (Nagelhout et al., 2011). After the implementation of the ban, reports of smoking remained fairly common in the Netherlands and Germany, two countries with lenient policies. In contrast, in Ireland and France where comprehensive bans were introduced with no exceptions and where fines for smokers were in place, smoking was reduced to almost zero, making these policies national successes.

Social Norms

At the core of comprehensive approaches to tobacco control are attempts to "denormalise" smoking rather than merely "controlling" it. By positioning social norms between cultural values and the other factors in the flywheel model, I want to express that societal norms regarding smoking are central to tobacco control. They reflect the deeply held cultural values, and in turn determine the preferences of groups of people for types of policy (Dechesne, Dignum, & Tan, 2011). Tobacco control evolves around how smoking is perceived in society. Normative factors explain why populations differ in their susceptibility to change (Chaiton, Cohen, & Frank, 2003). The famous British social epidemiologist Geoffrey Rose (1992) said, "Social norms rigidly constrain how we live. (...) We may think that our personal life-style represents our own free choice, but that belief is often mistaken. It is hard to be a non-smoker in a smoking milieu, or vice versa." (p. 90) Smoking rates are indeed lower in constituencies that have an unfavourable "smoking climate" (Kim & Shanahan, 2003).

Changes in social norms have been found to be a driver of tobacco control (Hammond, Fong, Zanna, Thrasher, & Borland, 2006). Denormalisation of smoking reduces tobacco consumption (Alamar & Glantz, 2006; Baha & Le Faou, 2010; Biener, Hamilton, Siegel, & Sullivan, 2010; Hosking et al., 2009) and may result in more smokers quitting (Baha & Le Faou, 2010; Bosdriesz, Kunst, Muntaner, Willemsen, & O'Campo, 2017). Indeed, the second most frequently mentioned reason to quit smoking (after health concerns) is social concerns (McCaul et al., 2006). Best et al. (2007) proposed a feedback loop between social norms and smoking rates to acknowledge an independent process whereby when smoking becomes increasingly unpopular within the wider society, it leads to more people quitting and fewer young people starting, which make smoking even less popular.

The crucial role of social norms in tobacco control was already recognised in the 1970s. At the opening speech of the fourth World Conference on Smoking or Health in Stockholm in 1979, the director of WHO said that tobacco control advocates should try harder to reduce the social acceptance of smoking. Several tobacco industry representatives were present at the session. One of the industry observers wrote a memo, made public by the Norwegian Association on Smoking and Health, revealing that the centrality of social norms as mentioned by the WHO director was not new to the industry but was "just a confirmation of our own analysis that the social acceptability issue will be the central battleground on which our case in the long run will be lost or won" (Clairmonte, 1983, p. 85). More than a decade later, Philip Morris complained in an internal memo that smoking bans were not only hurting business, but that they had "a more important effect (...) on the social acceptability of smoking. Attempts to depict tobacco use as anti-social get a powerful boost when its use is banned in social settings. This impact on our business, whilst slower, is just as real" (Goldberg, 1999). Philip Morris' PR firm formulated this in 1990 as follows: "Social acceptability is ultimately the bedrock upon which the industry's long run survival depends" (Burson-Marstellar, 1990). Indeed, in the 1990s the tobacco industry fought relentlessly with governments over the right to smoke in public.

The centrality of social norms in tobacco control has long been known to Dutch policymakers as well. In 1975 the Dutch Health Council advised that "activities against smoking must primarily aim at the creation of a psycho-social climate in which smoking is perceived negatively and a new attitude towards smoking emerges" (Beernink & Plokker, 1975). In 2000, Health Minister Borst defined her approach to tobacco control in parliament as follows:

> At the core of the [tobacco control] policy is the objective that few young people start smoking and that smoking is increasingly seen as an abnormal behaviour. Tobacco needs "denormalisation" in our society. This and other measures must lead to a social climate where non-smoking is the social norm and not starting or quitting smoking is the result.[2]

It is one thing to recognise that social norms are important, but it is another thing to have good data on how a country's social norms compare with those of other countries. For decades the tobacco industry had an information advantage. The big tobacco multinationals were able to organise worldwide comparison studies, cleverly exploiting the fact that they were present in a large number of countries across the world. In 1979 researchers who worked for tobacco manufacturer Philip Morris International analysed the social and political environment of that business in 27 countries (Unknown (Philip Morris), 1979). They remarked of the Dutch, "As the personal freedom concept is widely accepted and supported in Holland, the anti-smoking cause is not exceptionally strong. ... Members of the medical profession and government appear to have highly individual opinions and the consensus is that smoking is a matter of personal choice." Twenty years later, Philip Morris' analysts remarked that "the Dutch resent government interference, [and] the public debate is more and more balanced," and they characterised opinion as tolerant towards smoking (Philip Morris, 1996). Population survey data collected for Philip Morris further showed that social acceptance of smoking in the Netherlands was still high in 1997 (GfK Great Britain, 1998). Only 19% of non-smokers believed there was any element of risk about being around smokers in bars or pubs, or of "living with a smoker" or "working with a smoker." This was one of the lowest results in Europe. The report also noted the low demand for government action against smoking among the Dutch.

It is only fairly recently that not only the tobacco industry but also the Dutch tobacco control community has come to realise that social norms regarding smoking are still more lenient than in other countries. Since 2008 the Netherlands participates in the International Tobacco Control (ITC) evaluation study. ITC data revealed that Dutch smokers were less often aware of societal disapproval of smoking than smokers in other high-income countries, at 63% compared to between 72% and 89% (ITC Project, 2015). Furthermore, only 22% of Dutch smokers often thought about the harm they did to themselves, while 33% of smokers in Germany, and between 43% and 56% in other high-income countries, did. The percentage of smokers who often thought about the harm they might inflict on others was extremely low in the Netherlands too (9%), and the Netherlands had the second-lowest percentage (21%) of smokers with a "negative" or "very negative" opinion of smoking, among the 13 ITC countries where this was measured (the German figure was 20%). All other countries scored between 45% and 62%.

How can the low concern among Dutch smokers and relatively tolerant norms towards smoking be explained? One explanation is the previously discussed "feminine" cooperative culture in the Netherlands that supports a tolerant approach towards smokers, which does not go well with confrontational media campaigns. For example, in the 1980s, the "Meinsma approach" (relentlessly hammering on health risks; more on Lenze Meinsma in Chap. 9) was replaced by a "more positive approach, where the advantages of non-smoking as part of an attractive lifestyle, are promoted" (WVC, 1984). In 1986, the government stated that awareness campaigns were important, but it wanted non-governmental organisations to run them, because the government said it was "handicapped," hinting to the societal and political sensitivity of paternalistic lifestyle campaigns (WVC, 1986, p. 174). Since the 1950s, when the serious health consequences of smoking became clear, only one health risk campaign has ever been run in the Netherlands. This was part of a EU-funded project that made it possible to adapt the Canadian campaign *Joanne* for use in Dutch cinemas, featuring a young girl looking in a mirror, watching in horror as her face wrinkles and turns grey because of lifelong smoking. This campaign made a tremendous impression on smokers, who still recalled the campaign, many years later, when asked to give examples of anti-smoking campaigns.

The lack of hard-hitting media campaigns to deter smoking is a remarkable aspect of Dutch tobacco control, since many countries run confrontational anti-smoking media campaigns. They are an integral part of national tobacco control strategies and not regarded as particularly problematic in other countries. There is abundant evidence that, at least in the field of tobacco control, campaigns that make an emotional appeal can be effective (Biener et al., 2006; Borland & Balmford, 2003; Durkin et al., 2012; National Cancer Institute, 2008; Timmers & Van der Wijst, 2007; Wakefield, Loken, & Hornik, 2010). The Australian "Every cigarette is doing you damage" campaign targeted at adult smokers to quit is notorious in this regard. Campaign exposure has been associated with increased negative thoughts about smoking (Borland & Balmford, 2003) and contributed to reductions in smoking prevalence in Australia (Wakefield et al., 2008). This campaign was adapted for use in other countries as well, for example, in 2003 in Norway. Box 7.1 (Chap. 7) discusses the Dutch government's reluctance to run such national media campaigns to deter smoking, which has to do with the belief that media campaigns offer expensive but ineffective ways to influence lifestyle.

Smoking Rates

When the ratio of smokers to non-smokers changes in favour of non-smokers, public support for policy restrictions increases. For example, when Health Minister Els Borst introduced her revision of the Tobacco Act in the parliament, she legitimised this by referring to the fact that already two-thirds of the adult population was non-smoking by then.[3] Countries with relatively few smokers, like Finland, the United Kingdom, and Australia, have the most comprehensive tobacco control policies. "Policy follows prevalence" said Kenneth Warner, an international tobacco control expert (quoted in D. J. Reid, Killoran, McNeill, and Chambers (1992)), and several ecological studies which used the country as a unit of analysis found that European countries with more stringent tobacco policies have fewer smokers—although the association is not very strong (Martinez-Sanchez et al., 2010; Willemsen, Kiselinova, Nagelhout, Joossens, & Knibbe, 2012). The direction of causality is not clear and obviously goes in two directions, as is captured in the flywheel model. In any case, within the problem stream of policymaking, data on the proportion of smokers among adults and adolescents constitute a crucial element in policymakers' appreciation of the tobacco problem (see Chap. 10 on problem identification).

From an epidemiological perspective, tobacco's worldwide spread is, as depicted by WHO, an epidemic (Roemer, 1982). The tobacco epidemic took many decades to unfold and will take even more time to resolve. Countries progress through the various stages of the epidemic in remarkably similar ways. A widely acclaimed model describes how the epidemic diffuses through populations (Lopez, Collishaw, & Piha, 1994; Thun, Peto, Boreham, & Lopez, 2012). In developed countries during the 1950s and 1960s, more than half of the population smoked, while in the higher strata of these societies almost all men smoked. High-income and male subpopulations were the first to become addicted to smoking, followed by lower income groups and females two decades later. After a period of gradual increase in smoking, prevalence reached a peak 40–50 years after onset, then slowly diminished. This pattern is clearly discernible in the Netherlands. In 1958 the cigarette epidemic had already reached its peak in the male population: 90% of men and 29% of women smoked. The proportion of male smokers in the Netherlands was exceptionally high: for example, in the United Kingdom 60% of the male population smoked in the 1950s and 1960s (Reid et al., 1992). Figure 4.2 shows how the proportion of smokers in the population has gone down since 1957.[4] The decline follows a similar pattern as in other developed countries, marked by a fast decline in the 1960s and 1970s and a slower

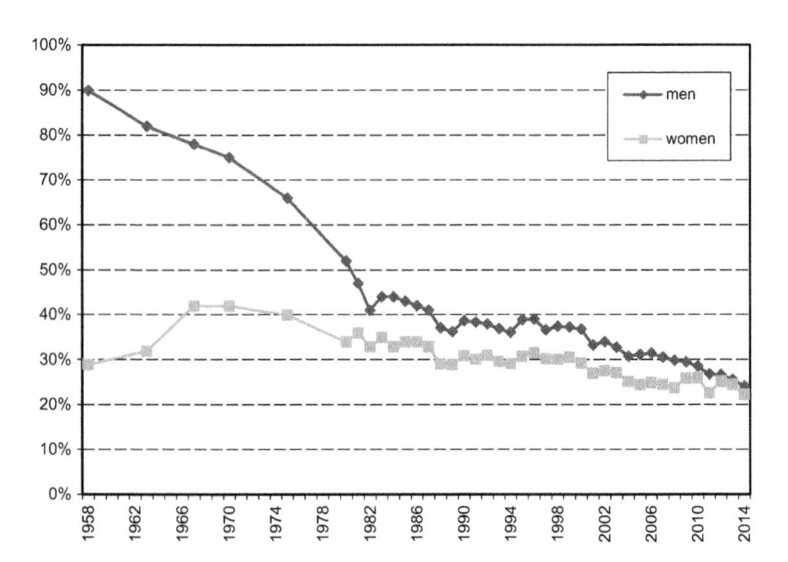

Fig. 4.2 Smoking prevalence in men and women since 1958. Sources: STIVORO (2012); Verdurmen, Monshouwer, and van Laar (2015). Note: whether one is a smoker or not is discerned by asking: "do you (ever) smoke or do you never smoke?"

decline from the 1980s onwards (OECD, 2014; Thun et al., 2012). In the Netherlands the percentage of women smoking peaked around 1970, followed by a reduction and convergence to male smoking levels in later decades. Internationally, the steep decline in smoking between 1960 and 1980 has been explained by widespread media attention to official governmental reports which showed that smoking causes death and disease (Farquhar, Magnus, & Maccoby, 1981; Reid et al., 1992). The Dutch public was confronted with similar messages in the media (see also Chap. 10) and many quit smoking despite the lack of governmental campaigns, while tobacco lost its aura of innocence and politicians called on the government to act.

In the 1980s smoking prevalence in the Netherlands was relatively high compared to other EU countries (European Commission, 1987). While the EU average was 37% in 1987, 44% of the Dutch population still smoked; only Denmark was higher with 46%. Although the decline in the general smoking rate followed roughly the same path in the Netherlands as in other developed countries (see Fig. 4.3 for a comparison with England and Canada), there was a noteworthy *increase* in the proportion of smokers between 1988 and 1996 (from 32% to 35%) in the Netherlands. Four years later, in 2000, the smoking rate was still higher than in 1988. In those years the Netherlands was very much a smoker's country. With 2951 cigarettes consumed per adult per year, the Netherlands ranked third highest in the EU for consumption, comparable to Russia and Greece and much higher than neighbours Belgium, Germany, and the United Kingdom (Gallus, Schiaffino, La Vecchia, Townsend, & Fernandez, 2006). The proportion of male smokers in 2002 was still slightly higher than the EU-25 average, while female smoking was among the five highest (Zatoński, Przewoźniak, Sulkowska, West, & Wojtyła, 2012).

Figure 4.3 shows how smoking rates declined in the Netherlands, the United Kingdom, and Canada. While smoking rates were about the same around 1988, in later years the United Kingdom and Canada did better. The long-term background rate fell by less than 0.5% per year between 1990 and 2010 in the Netherlands (Willemsen, 2010), while prevalence fell by around 0.75% in Canada and 0.7% in the United Kingdom (Royal College of Physicians, 2016).

Some other countries (the United Kingdom, Australia, Canada, and the United States) also witnessed a faltering in the decline of smoking in the beginning to mid-1990s (Wakefield & Chaloupka, 1998), but not as distinct nor as prolonged as in the Netherlands, where it continued until

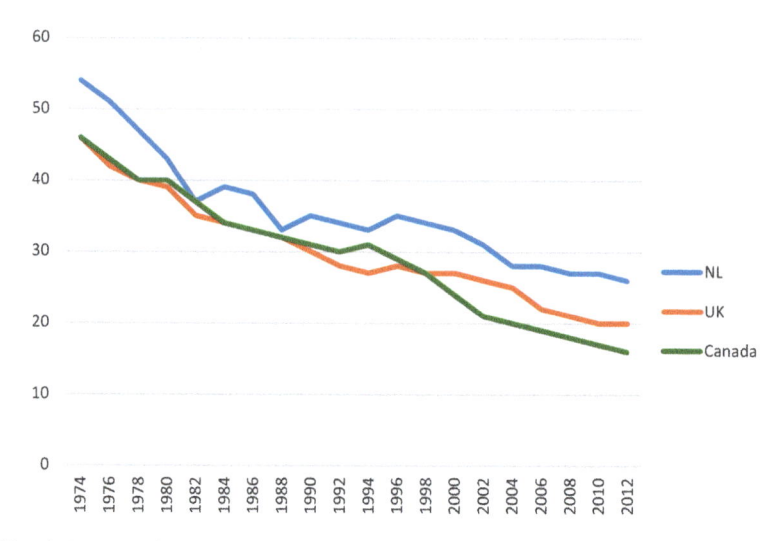

Fig. 4.3 Trends in adult smoking prevalence (men and women combined) in the Netherlands, the United Kingdom, and Canada. Sources: United Kingdom: General Lifestyle Survey; Canada: Canadian Tobacco Use Monitoring Survey (CTUMS); Netherlands: Dutch Continuous Survey of Smoking Habits (COR). Note: The way smoking prevalence is measured differs slightly between countries. In the United Kingdom, all aged 16+ were asked, "Do you smoke cigarettes at all nowadays?" while in the Netherlands all aged 15+ were asked the question, "Do you ever smoke or do you never smoke?" In Canada all 15+ aged were asked, "At the present time do you smoke cigarettes every day, occasionally, or not at all?" Smokers are daily smokers and non-daily smokers combined

2000. It is no coincidence that this 12-year period of standstill coincided with a period of virtually no tobacco control interventions that might have impacted on smoking rates, while tobacco industry influence was strong both behind the scenes and in the media (Willemsen, 2017). Tobacco industry tolerance campaigns re-normalised smoking (see Chap. 8). The tobacco control flywheel had clearly lost its energy. The period of stagnation ended when 800,000 smokers made a quit attempt during a large-scale mass media quit campaign at the turn of the millennium. The revised Tobacco Act in 2002 led to a further reduction of the smoking rate from 31% in 2002 to 28% in 2004, after which it continued to fall. The reduction in the Netherlands between 1999 and 2009 (−18.7%) was almost the same as the Organisation for Economic Co-operation and Development (OECD) average reduction (−17.9%) (Bruggink, 2013). After the "correction" initiated by Minister Borst, the Netherlands was on a trajectory towards a non-smoking society at about the same pace as most other developed countries, but in more recent years smoking rates have seemed to rise again, from 24.5% in 2012 to 26.3% in 2015 (Van Laar & Van Ooyen-Houben, 2016).

Between 1992 and 1996 youth smoking increased (Fig. 4.4), despite a shift from daily smoking to less frequent smoking in this period (Willemsen, 2005). Since 1996, youth smoking rates declined almost uninterruptedly. "Regular smoking" in youth (10- to 19-year-olds) is defined as having smoked at least once in the past month.

The reduction in adolescent smoking seems to follow the general trend seen earlier in the adult population, including a period of stagnation in the 1990s. When adult smoking rates go down, youth rates follow; when adult smoking goes up, youth smoking again follows. Some have noted this as the most likely explanation for reductions in youth smoking

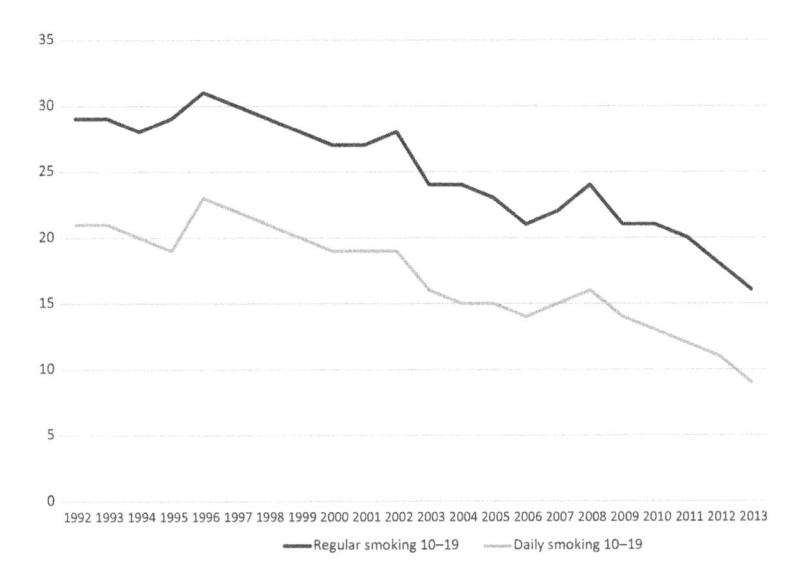

Fig. 4.4 Trends in youth smoking (10–19 year olds) between 1992 and 2013 in the Netherlands. Sources: STIVORO (2012); Verdurmen, Monshouwer, and Van Laar (2014)

(Chapman, 2007; Gielkens-Sijstermans et al., 2009; Hill, 1999). Young people are particularly sensitive to changes in what is regarded as "cool" in the wider society. Smoking has become less attractive since tobacco advertising was banned in 2002, and smokers were increasingly seen as social pariahs when smoking was banned in workplaces in that same year. Part of the explanation may also be that when parents quit smoking, fewer children are exposed to tobacco products at home and parents no longer are exemplars for smoking (Den Exter Blokland, Engels, Hale III, Meeus, & Willemsen, 2004).

Public Support for Tobacco Control

The flywheel model assumes that, at least in modern democracies, the adoption of policies reflects what the broader society wants. Tobacco policy generally reflects shifts in public opinion (Kagan & Nelson, 2001). Empirical evidence from US states has shown that when public opinion becomes more supportive of smoking bans, states are more likely to adopt them (Pacheco, 2012). Politicians know this and push for more stringent measures when they feel that society is ready. The battle is thus fought first in society, after which it moves to the political arena. When public opinion changes, politicians follow. As one former civil servant put it, "It is a very slow process to get societal support. Politics usually follow trends in society, because this assures that you remain in office and can come back again … it rarely happens that policy makers actively want to change public opinion."[5]

The need to have support from the general public is well known among Dutch politicians and policymakers. They routinely refer to public support when they defend or reject tobacco control policy proposals. For example, State Secretary for Health Joop van der Reijden (VVD) explicitly made decisions to intensify tobacco control contingent on the political discussion in parliament, which "shall made clear whether the climate is ripe for a really powerful policy" (WVC, 1986). In those days, the civil servants at the Ministry of Health who developed the first tobacco control policy measures complained that they did not feel supported by society or the medical sector.[6] Twenty years later, when Health Minister Borst defended her tobacco control bill in the senate, she said, "I believe that exceptions [to the ban] can only disappear when we have a totally different culture in the Netherlands, a culture in which nobody, exceptions granted, smokes. … We must not make things look nicer than they are. So we have to make exceptions for certain sectors."[7] In 2005 the government looked back and remarked that the 1999 revised Tobacco Act "attempted to catch up with the changes in how society regards smoking" (VWS, 2005). State Secretary Martin van Rijn said in 2014, "A basic assumption [of my policy making] is that I want to carry a consistent and effective policy that has support from society" (Van Rijn, 2014). Even Dutch parliamentarians who are vehemently in favour of stricter tobacco control cannot easily propagate policies that lack general support from the public. Carla Dik-Faber, parliamentarian for the Christian Union (CU), reacted to the idea of banning smoking on terraces: "This topic is very much debated in society. At the moment there is insufficient political support. I can imagine that at one point terraces will become smoke-free. However, it is still too early for this. Political decision making must follow developments in society" (Van der Laan, 2015).

In 1987, when most EU countries had not yet adopted major tobacco policy measures, the European Commission (EC) wanted to know how supportive Europeans were of tobacco control measures (European Commission, 1987). The Dutch population answered somewhat below average on all measures, with a relatively low level of support for an advertising ban. The low support for tobacco control in the Netherlands has become more pronounced in later years. A Eurobarometer poll from 2005 showed that the Dutch were not very supportive of a smoking ban in bars (TNS Opinion & Social, 2006): only 46% of the total population was "somewhat or totally in favour"— one of the lowest ever levels of support in the EU. In 2009 when the EC conducted another poll (TNS Opinion & Social, 2010), the Netherlands emerged as a country with little general support for tobacco control measures, scoring the absolute lowest on plain packaging and on banning the sale of tobacco via the internet. The poll was repeated in 2012 (TNS Opinion & Social, 2012) and showed little change in the Dutch position: the Netherlands still had the least support for plain packaging of all 27 EU countries.

What might explain such low levels of support? According to the flywheel model, public support reflects dominant social norms in society. Social norms depend on knowledge about the problems associated with smoking (particularly from passive smoking) and level of acceptance of these problems by the public. Given that the level of concern is relatively low in the Netherlands, as was shown previously, one would expect that support for tobacco control is also low. This is indeed the case. I already referred to the striking data from the ITC project about the relative lack of concern among Dutch smokers about tobacco and health. I found a strong correlation in Dutch national survey data between believing that passive smoking is harmful and support for smoking bans (Willemsen, 2006). This association was consistent among both highly educated and lower educated groups—an association also found in other countries. With some colleagues I analysed Eurobarometer data from 2009, and what stood out was that smokers who lived in countries with comprehensive tobacco policies were more likely to support tobacco control measures, and such support was greater when they were more concerned about whether their smoking harms non-smokers (Willemsen, Kiselinova, et al., 2012). In an older study we had found that Dutch non-smoking employees were more likely to ask co-workers not to smoke when they had more negative beliefs about the health consequences of passive smoking (Willemsen & De Vries, 1996). Compliance with smoking bans is higher if smokers are more supportive of them and if they are more aware of the health consequences of passive smoking (G. E. Nagelhout, de Vries, et al., 2012).

Conclusion

Smoking rates have declined following patterns similar to those in other developed countries, typified by a fast decline in the 1960s and 1970s and a slower decline from the 1980s onwards. However, during the 1990s smoking rates stagnated then rose again. In these years the Netherlands was a smoker's country, with more cigarettes consumed than in almost every other EU country. Smoking was socially well accepted, which might be partially attributed to the success of tobacco industry's tolerance campaigns from 1970 until the end of the 1990s (see Chap. 8 for details about industry tolerance campaigns). These were exceptionally well received in the Netherlands, since the Dutch cherished the collective idea of being a tolerant people. There was a 12-year standstill in smoking rates (1988–2000), which coincided with virtually no action from the government to regulate tobacco. Only after the revised Tobacco Act was implemented in 2002 did people start to quit again. Smoking rates have continued to go down since then, and smoking among youth followed the example of the adults and also has gone down.

Societal support for most tobacco control measures has been relatively low compared with other EU countries. Support was lowest for confrontational tobacco control elements, which might be explained by "feminine" cooperative value orientations in Dutch national culture. The smoking bans implemented in 2004 were more smoker-friendly than those in other countries, reflecting such values. The Dutch government has been reluctant to run health awareness media campaigns, which are seen as ineffective, costly, and paternalistic. The lack of health awareness campaigns contributed to the relatively low levels of concern about smoking and the less than optimal support for tobacco control in even today's society.

Notes

1. Translation of Dutch song text. Top 40 hit by Fluitsma and Van Tijn in 1996.
2. Parliamentary Papers II, 1999–2000, 26472, nr. 6, pp. 4–5.
3. Proceedings II, 1999–2000, 26472, nr. 6, p. 4.
4. Known in Dutch as *Continu Onderzoek Rookgewoonten* (COR), the surveys have been conducted since the 1970s by TNS-NIPO on behalf of STIVORO. They are available until 2014.
5. Interview, 6 October 2015.
6. Interview, 1 February 2017.
7. Proceedings I, 26 March 2002, 24, 1273.

References

Alamar, B., & Glantz, S. (2006). Effect of increased social unacceptability of cigarette smoking on reduction in cigarette consumption. *American Journal of Public Health, 97*, 1359–1362.

Baha, M., & Le Faou, A. L. (2010). Smokers' reasons for quitting in an antismoking social context. *Public Health, 124*(4), 225–231. https://doi.org/10.1016/j.puhe.2010.02.011

Beernink, J. F., & Plokker, J. H. (1975). Maatregelen tot beperking van het roken. Advies van de Gezondheidsraad. *Verslagen, Adviezen, Rapporten* (Vol. 23). Leidschendam: Ministerie van Volksgezondheid en Milieuhygiëne.

Best, A., Clark, P., Leichow, S. J., & Trochim, W. M. K. (2007). *Greater than the sum: Systems thinking in tobacco control.* Tobacco control monograph. Bethesda, MD: U.S. Department of Health and Human Services, National Institutes of Health, National Cancer Institute.

Betzner, A. E., Boyle, R. G., Luxenberg, M. G., Schillo, B. A., Keller, P. A., Rainey, J., ... Saul, J. E. (2012). Experience of smokers and recent quitters with smoke-free regulations and quitting. *American Journal of Preventive Medicine, 43*, S163–S170. https://doi.org/10.1016/j.amepre.2012.08.005

Biener, L., Hamilton, W. L., Siegel, M., & Sullivan, E. M. (2010). Individual, social-normative, and policy predictors of smoking cessation: A multilevel longitudinal analysis. *American Journal of Public Health, 100*, 547–554. https://doi.org/10.2105/ajph.2008

Biener, L., Reimer, R., Wakefield, M., Szczypka, G., Rigotti, N. A., & Connolly, G. (2006). Impact of smoking cessation aids and mass media among recent quitters. *American Journal of Preventive Medicine, 30*, 217–224.

Borland, R., & Balmford, J. (2003). Understanding how mass media campaigns impact on smokers. *Tobacco Control, 12*(Suppl 2), ii45–ii52. https://doi.org/10.1136/tc.12.suppl_2.ii45

Bosdriesz, J. R., Kunst, A., Muntaner, C., Willemsen, M. C., & O'Campo, P. (2017). The effect of tobacco tax and price increases on smoking cessation or reduction—A scoping realist review. *Article submitted.*

Bruggink, J.-W. (2013). Ontwikkelingen in het aandeel rokers in Nederland sinds 1989. *Tijdschrift voor Gezondheidswetenschappen, 91*(4), 234–240.

Burson-Marstellar. (1990). An accommodation strategy in EEMA: A strategic brief. *Philip Morris Collection*, Bates No. 2021181862–2021181887. Retrieved from https://www.industrydocumentslibrary.ucsf.edu/tobacco/docs/nppf0117

Chaiton, M. O., Cohen, J. E., & Frank, J. (2003). Population health and the hardcore smoker: Geoffrey Rose revisited. *Journal of Public Health, 307*, 429–432.

Chapman, S. (2007). *Public health advocacy and tobacco control: Making smoking history.* Oxford: Blackwell Publishing.

Clairmonte, F. F. (1983, December). The transnational tobacco and alcohol conglomerates: A world oligolopy. *New York State Journal of Medicine, 83*, 1322–1323.

Dechesne, F., Dignum, V., & Tan, Y.-H. (2011). Understanding compliance differences between legal and social norms: The case of smoking ban. In F. Dechesne, H. Hattori, A. Ter Mors, J. M. Such, D. Weyns, & F. Dignum (Eds.), *Advanced agent technology. AAMAS 2011. Lecture Notes in Computer Science* (Vol. 7068). Berlin: Springer.

Dechesne, F., Di Tosto, G., Dignum, V., & Dignum, F. (2013). No smoking here: Values, norms and culture in multi-agent systems. *Artificial Intelligence and Law, 21*, 79. https://doi.org/10.1007/s10506-012-9128-5

Den Exter Blokland, E. A. W., Engels, R. C. M. E., Hale, W. W., III, Meeus, W., & Willemsen, M. C. (2004). Lifetime parental smoking history and cessation and early adolescent smoking behavior. *Preventive Medicine, 38*(3), 359–368. https://doi.org/10.1016/j.ypmed.2003.11.008

Durkin, S., Brennan, E., & Wakefield, M. (2012). Mass media campaigns to promote smoking cessation among adults: An integrative review. *Tobacco Control, 21*(2), 127–138. https://doi.org/10.1136/tobaccocontrol-2011-050345

European Commission. (1987). *Survey: Europeans and the prevention of cancer. A working document of the services of the European Commission.* Brussels: European Commission.

Farquhar, J. W., Magnus, P. F., & Maccoby, N. (1981). The role of public information and education in cigarette smoking controls. *Canadian Journal of Public Health, 72*(6), 412–420.

Gallus, S., Schiaffino, A., La Vecchia, C., Townsend, J., & Fernandez, E. (2006). Price and cigarette consumption in Europe. *Tobacco Control, 15*(2), 114–119. https://doi.org/10.1136/tc.2005.012468

GfK Great Britain. (1998). ETS world report Philip Morris 1998. *Philip Morris Records*, Bates No. 2065221475–2065221544. Retrieved from http://legacy.library.ucsf.edu/tid/fnq90g00/pdf

Gielkens-Sijstermans, C. M., Mommers, M. A., Hoogenveen, R. T., Feenstra, T. L., Vreede, J. d., Bovens, F. M., & Schayck, O. C. v. (2009). Reduction of smoking in Dutch adolescents over the past decade and its health gains: A repeated cross-sectional study. *European Journal of Public Health, 20*(3), 146–150.

Goldberg, H. (1999). International accommodation programs. *Philip Morris Collection*, Bates No. 2074399542–2074399568. Retrieved from http://legacy.library.ucsf.edu/tid/thp11h00

Gravely, S., Giovino, G. A., Craig, L., Commar, A., Déspaignet, E. T., Schotte, K., & Fong, G. T. (2017). Implementation of key demand-reduction measures of the WHO Framework Convention on Tobacco Control and change in smoking prevalence in 126 countries: An association study. *The Lancet, 2*, e166–e174. https://doi.org/10.1016/S2468-2667(17)30045-2

Hammond, D., Fong, G. T., Zanna, M. P., Thrasher, J. F., & Borland, R. (2006). Tobacco denormalization and industry beliefs among smokers from four countries. *American Journal of Preventive Medicine, 31*(3), 225–232. https://doi.org/10.1016/j.amepre.2006.04.004

Helweg-Larsen, M., & Nielsen, G. A. (2009). Smoking cross-culturally: Risk perceptions among young adults in Denmark and the United States. *Psychology & Health, 24*(1), 81–93. https://doi.org/10.1080/08870440801932656

Hill, D. (1999). Why we should tackle adult smoking first. *Tobacco Control, 8*, 333–335.

Hofstede Centre. (2015). The Netherlands. Retrieved May 4, 2015, from http://geert-hofstede.com/netherlands.html

Hofstede, G. J. (1980). *Culture's consequences. International differences in work-related values.* Beverly Hills, CA: Sage.

Hosking, W., Borland, R., Yong, H. H., Fong, G., Zanna, M., Laux, F., ... Omar, M. (2009). The effects of smoking norms and attitudes on quitting intentions in Malaysia, Thailand and four western nations: A cross-cultural comparison. *Psychology & Health, 24*, 95–107. https://doi.org/10.1080/08870440802385854

ITC Project. (2015). *ITC Netherlands National Report. Findings from the Wave 1 to 8 Surveys (2008–2014)*. Waterloo, ON, Canada: University of Waterloo.

Kagan, R. A., & Nelson, W. P. (2001). The politics of tobacco regulation in the United States. In R. Rabin & S. Sugarman (Eds.), *Regulating tobacco* (pp. 11–38). New York: Oxford University Press.

Kim, S.-H., & Shanahan, J. (2003). Stigmatizing smokers: Public sentiment toward cigarette smoking and its relationship to smoking behaviors. *Journal of Health Communication, 8*, 343–367. https://doi.org/10.1080/10810730305723

Lopez, A. D., Collishaw, N. E., & Piha, T. (1994). A descriptive model of the cigarette epidemic in developed countries. *Tobacco Control, 3*(3), 242. https://doi.org/10.1136/tc.3.3.242

Martinez-Sanchez, J. M., Fernandez, E., Fu, M., Gallus, S., Martinez, C., Sureda, X., ... Clancy, L. (2010). Smoking behaviour, involuntary smoking, attitudes towards smoke-free legislations, and tobacco control activities in the European Union. *PLoS One, 5*(11), e13881. https://doi.org/10.1371/journal.pone.0013881

McCaul, K. D., Hockemeyer, J. R., Johnson, R. J., Zetocha, K., Quinlan, K., & Glasgow, R. E. (2006). Motivation to quit using cigarettes: A review. *Addictive Behaviours, 31*(1), 42–56. https://doi.org/10.1016/j.addbeh.2005.04.004

Nagelhout, G. E., de Vries, H., Fong, G. T., Candel, M. J., Thrasher, J. F., van den Putte, B., ... Willemsen, M. C. (2012). Pathways of change explaining the effect of smoke-free legislation on smoking cessation in The Netherlands. An application of the international tobacco control conceptual model. *Nicotine & Tobacco Research, 14*(12), 1474–1482. https://doi.org/10.1093/ntr/nts081

Nagelhout, G. E., Mons, U., Allwright, S., Guignard, R., Beck, F., Fong, G. T., ... Willemsen, M. C. (2011). Prevalence and predictors of smoking in "smoke-free" bars. Findings from the International Tobacco Control (ITC) Europe Surveys. *Social Science & Medicine, 72*(10), 1643–1651. https://doi.org/10.1016/j.socscimed.2011.03.018

National Cancer Institute. (2008). *The role of the media in promoting and reducing tobacco use*. NCI tobacco control monograph series (Vol. 19).

Ngo, A., Cheng, K.-W., Chaloupka, F. J., & Shang, C. (2017). The effect of MPOWER scores on cigarette smoking prevalence and consumption. *Preventive Medicine*. Retrieved from May 11, 2017. https://doi.org/10.1016/j.ypmed.2017.05.006

OECD. (2014). *Health at a glance: Europe 2014*. Brussels: Organisation for Economic Co-operation and Development (OECD).

Pacheco, J. (2012). The social contagion model: Exploring the role of public opinion on the diffusion of anti-smoking legislation across the American States. *Journal of Politics, 74*(1), 187–202.

Pasick, R. J., Onofrio, C. N., & Otero-Sabogal, R. (1996). Similarities and differences across cultures: Questions to inform a third generation of health promotion research. *Health Promotion Quarterly, 23*(Suppl 1), S142–S161.

Philip Morris. (1996). Corporate Affairs 1996/1997 The Netherlands. *Philip Morris Records*, Bates No. 2501076006–2501076023. Retrieved from https://www.industrydocumentslibrary.ucsf.edu/tobacco/docs/nzjl0112

Reid, D. J., Killoran, A. J., McNeill, A. D., & Chambers, J. S. (1992). Choosing the most effective health promotion options for reducing a nation's smoking prevalence. *Tobacco Control, 1*(3), 185. https://doi.org/10.1136/tc.1.3.185

Rennen, E., Nagelhout, G. E., Van den Putte, B., Janssen, E., Mons, U., Guignard, R., ... Willemsen, M. C. (2014). Associations between tobacco control policy awareness, social acceptability of smoking and smoking cessation. Findings from the International Tobacco Control (ITC) Europe Surveys. *Health Education Research, 29*(1), 72–82. https://doi.org/10.1093/her/cyt073

Roemer, R. (1982). *Legislative action to combat the world smoking epidemic.* Geneva: WHO.

Rose, G. (1992). *The strategy of preventive medicine.* Oxford: Oxford University Press.

Royal College of Physicians. (2016). *Nicotine without smoke: Tobacco harm reduction.* London: Royal College of Physicians.

Schwartz, S. (2006). A theory of cultural value orientations: Explication and applications. *Comparative Sociology, 5*(2), 137–182. https://doi.org/10.1163/156913306778667357

STIVORO. (2012). *Hoe ontmoediging verdween uit het tabaksontmoedigingsbeleid [Year Report 2011].* Den Haag: STIVORO.

Thun, M., Peto, R., Boreham, J., & Lopez, A. D. (2012). Stages of the cigarette epidemic on entering its second century. *Tobacco Control, 21*(2), 96–101. https://doi.org/10.1136/tobaccocontrol-2011-050294

Timmers, R., & Van der Wijst, P. (2007). Images as anti-smoking fear appeals: The effects of emotion on the persuasion process. *Information Design Journal, 15*, 21–36.

TNS Opinion & Social. (2006). *Special Eurobarometer 239: Attitudes of Europeans towards tobacco.* Brussels: European Commission.

TNS Opinion & Social. (2010). *Special Eurobarometer 332: Tobacco.* Brussels: European Commission.

TNS Opinion & Social. (2012). *Special Eurobarometer 385: Attitudes of Europeans towards tobacco.* Brussels: European Commission.

Unger, J. B., Cruz, T., Baezconde-Garbanati, L., Shakib, S., Palmer, P., Johnson, C. A., ... Gritz, E. (2003). Exploring the cultural context of tobacco use: A transdisciplinary framework. *Nicotine & Tobacco Research*, 5(Suppl 1), S101–S117. https://doi.org/10.1080/14622200310001625546

Unknown (Philip Morris). (1979). *Smoking & health—Five year plan*, Bates No 2501020542-2501020686. Truth Tobacco Industry Documents.

Van der Laan, S. (2015). Politiek ziet rookverbod op terras (nog) niet zitten. Retrieved October 14, 2015, from http://www.elsevier.nl/Nederland/achtergrond/2015/9/Politiek-ziet-rookvrij-terras-nog-niet-zitten-2679393W/?masterpageid=158493

Van Laar, M. W., & Van Ooyen-Houben, M. M. J. (2016). *Nationale Drug Monitor*. Utrecht: Trimbos-Institute.

Van Rijn, M. (2014). Onderzoeken naar effecten verkooppunten en leeftijdverificatiesystemen tabaksproducten. *Kamerbrief 626288-122861-VGP*.

Verdurmen, J., Monshouwer, K., & Van Laar, M. (2014). *Roken Jeugd Monitor 2013*. Utrecht: Trimbos-instituut.

Vogel, D., Kagan, R. A., & Kessler, T. (1993). Political culture and tobacco control: An international comparison. *Tobacco Control*, 2(4), 317–326.

VWS. (2005). *Evaluatie Tabaksontmoediging*. Den Haag: Ministerie van VWS.

Wakefield, M. A., & Chaloupka, F. J. (1998). Improving the measurement and use of tobacco control "inputs". *Tobacco Control*, 7(4), 333–335. https://doi.org/10.1136/tc.7.4.333

Wakefield, M. A., Durkin, S., Spittal, M. J., Siahpush, M., Scollo, M., Simpson, J. A., ... Hill, D. (2008). Impact of tobacco control policies and mass media campaigns on monthly adult smoking prevalence. *American Journal of Public Health*, 98(8), 1443–1450. https://doi.org/10.2105/ajph.2007.128991

Wakefield, M. A., Loken, B., & Hornik, R. C. (2010). Use of mass media campaigns to change health behaviour. *The Lancet*, 376, 1261–1271.

Willemsen, M. C. (2005). Tabaksgebruik: trends bij de Nederlandse bevolking. In L. Knol, C. Hilvering, D. J. T. Wagener, & M. C. Willemsen (Eds.), *Tabaksgebruik: Gevolgen en bestrijding*. Utrecht: Lemma.

Willemsen, M. C. (2006). *Rokers onder vuur? Invloed van de gewijzigde Tabakswet op rokers, met speciale aandacht voor verschillen tussen sociaal-economische klassen*. Den Haag: STIVORO.

Willemsen, M. C. (2010). Tabaksverslaving: de impact van gezondheidsvoorlichting en hulpverlening op de totale populatie rokers. *Psychologie en Gezondheid*, 38, 119–130.

Willemsen, M. C. (2011). *Roken in Nederland: De keerzijde van tolerantie [inaugural lecture]*. Maastricht: Maastricht University.

Willemsen, M. C. (2017). Het Nederlandse tabaksontmoedigingsbeleid: Mijlpalen in het verleden en een blik op de toekomst. *Nederlands Tijdschrift voor Geneeskunde*, 161, D949.

Willemsen, M. C., & De Vries, H. (1996). Saying "no" to environmental tobacco smoke: Determinants of assertiveness among nonsmoking employees. *Preventive Medicine*, 25(5), 575–582. https://doi.org/10.1006/pmed.1996.0092

Willemsen, M. C., Kiselinova, M., Nagelhout, G. E., Joossens, L., & Knibbe, R. A. (2012). Concern about passive smoking and tobacco control policies in European countries: An ecological study. *BMC Public Health, 12*, 876. https://doi.org/10.1186/1471-2458-12-876

WVC. (1984). Volksgezondheid bij beperkte middelen. *Kamerstuk 18108, nrs 1–2.*

WVC. (1986). Over de ontwikkeling van gezondheidsbeleid: feiten, beschouwingen en beleidsvoornemens (Nota 2000). *Handelingen II, 1985–1986, 19500, nr 1–2.*

Zatoński, W., Przewoźniak, K., Sulkowska, U., West, R., & Wojtyła, A. (2012). Tobacco smoking in countries of the European Union. *Annals of Agricultutal Environmental Medicine, 19*, 181–192.

Open Access This chapter is licensed under the terms of the Creative Commons Attribution 4.0 International License (http://creativecommons.org/licenses/by/4.0/), which permits use, sharing, adaptation, distribution and reproduction in any medium or format, as long as you give appropriate credit to the original author(s) and the source, provide a link to the Creative Commons license and indicate if changes were made.

The images or other third party material in this chapter are included in the chapter's Creative Commons license, unless indicated otherwise in a credit line to the material. If material is not included in the chapter's Creative Commons license and your intended use is not permitted by statutory regulation or exceeds the permitted use, you will need to obtain permission directly from the copyright holder.

CHAPTER 5

Making Tobacco Control Policy Work: Rules of the Game

Tobacco policy is made by actors who operate in an institutional environment with specific characteristics (Scharpf, 1997), and differences in these characteristics can explain much of the variation in tobacco control between countries. Governments and parliaments, and their bureaucracies, have formal and informal "rules of the game." Informal rules include conventions, unwritten procedures, and expectations. Formal rules are official and legal procedures. While the contextual factors discussed in Chap. 4 are relatively dynamic and amenable to change by tobacco control interest groups, the rules of the game that are the subject of the current chapter are more static. In terms of the Advocacy Coalition Framework, they are the constitutional structural factors (Breton, Richard, Gagnon, Jacques, & Bergeron, 2008; Sabatier, 2007) which determine how countries differ from each other—less about how countries change over time, although institutional factors and conditions can gradually change. Knowledge of these factors is not only key to understanding why tobacco policymaking is most of the time a tedious and slow process; it also helps to understand how tobacco interest groups may influence policymaking and why some groups are more successful at this than others.

Groups of countries that are politically and culturally similar and have comparable institutional arrangements are sometimes referred to as "families of nations". Policies in countries that are similar with respect to culture, institutional make-up, and economic development tend to converge

(Lenschow, Liefferink, & Veenman, 2005). Convergence between countries within the same family has been shown to occur for tobacco control, with similar countries choosing similar policies and adopting policies at roughly the same tempo (Studlar, 2007). The Netherlands is considered part of the continental (Western European) family, consisting of countries like Belgium, Germany, and Austria (Castles & Obinger, 2008; Obinger & Wagschal, 2001). Other families are an Anglo-Saxon (English-speaking) group (Australia, Canada, New Zealand, the United Kingdom, the United States), a cluster of Scandinavian countries, and a peripheral group of European countries (Italy, Spain, Portugal, Greece). The continental family, to which the Netherlands belongs, is characterised by the central position of Christian Democrats, a "politics of the middle way" (combining social democratic and liberal principles), and political cultures that are oriented towards bargaining and compromise seeking. This chapter describes this system. It starts with a discussion of the two most important aspects of Dutch policymaking: corporatism (pressure groups incorporated into the policymaking process) and the continuous need to seek consensus in a multi-party political system. The reader's attention is directed to the tension between party ideology and tobacco control policymaking. Separate sections deal with the process of drafting new legislation and the opportunities available for advocates to influence this process through lobbying, either directly (targeting civil servants of the ministry), or through parliament. Finally, our attention turns to two long-term processes that gradually undermined the position of the central government as the main producer of tobacco control: deregulation and decentralisation.

Corporatism

Dutch pragmatic policymaking is sometimes called interactive governance, but most often it is referred to as corporatism (Van Tulder, 1999). The Netherlands has a conservative-corporatist model of the welfare state (Fenger, 2007) and is a prime example of a corporatist country, where policymakers incorporate interests of legitimate stakeholders into the decision-making process. In a review of 23 studies that assessed the level of corporatism in developed countries, the Netherlands ranked fourth on corporatism after Austria, Norway, and Sweden (Siaroff, 1999).

Corporatism has been defined as "institutionalized and privileged integration of organized interests in the preparation and/or implementation of public policies" (Christiansen et al., 2010). In a corporatist structure, government and interest groups cooperate rather than compete (Andeweg & Irwin, 2009). Pressure groups do not need to influence the government from the outside since they are incorporated in the policymaking process—hence the name "corporatism." If the government formulates a new policy, parties such as trade unions, business representative organisations, and societal organisations—with an obvious interest in the policy—are routinely invited into the policymaking process. Some groups obtain a privileged monopoly over a policy topic, and these chosen few enjoy close relationships with state representatives. The government bargains and seeks compromise with these groups, trusting that this will result in "better" policy outcomes—more equal, flexible, or more effective. In corporatist systems a government is most likely to consult the tobacco industry on new tobacco control initiatives. This contrasts with pluralistic democracies, where interest groups freely interact with each other and compete for power (a "may the strongest party win" approach) and influence policy from the outside. Sometimes the term "lobbyism" is used for pluralist systems (Rommetvedt, Thesen, Christiansen, & Nørgaard, 2012). Outsider anti-tobacco lobbying groups thrive best in open and competitive pluralist environments (Studlar, 2007). Countries with strong pluralistic characteristics are New Zealand, Australia, the United Kingdom, Italy, Ireland, Canada, and the United States (Siaroff, 1999).

A feature of the corporatist system is that interest groups are more or less routinely invited by the government to comment on policy proposals. In the Netherlands, involvement of stakeholders is historically organised in an informal manner. Consultation is confidential and open only to invited stakeholders. This practice has benefitted the tobacco industry tremendously in the past (see Chap. 8 for examples), but is currently changing. In 2011, the cabinet announced that it wanted to use open internet consultation rounds more often, in addition to the traditional practice of invitation-only consultation—although the ministries are still only committed to submit 10% of their regulatory proposals for internet consultation. Recent consultations on tobacco covered the implementation of the European Union (EU) tobacco product directive, adaptations of tobacco taxation, and an intended ban on the display of tobacco products.[1]

In the Netherlands corporatism is grounded in Christian Democratic values and associated political principles, two of which are particularly relevant. The first is subsidiarity: the principle that decision-making should take place at the lowest possible (administrative) level. It means that regulation by the state is only appropriate if it is not possible to solve matters at regional or local levels. The second principle is the idea that *het maatschappelijke middenveld* (civil society) is needed for political support and to have effective policies (Andeweg & Irwin, 2009, pp. 177–178). This goes back to the nineteenth-century Calvinist doctrine of *soevereiniteit in eigen kring* (sovereignty in one's own circle), the idea that organisations determine their own fate independent of government. Christian Democrats believe that organisations such as churches, unions, welfare institutions, and voluntary organisations must not become too dependent on government support but must retain responsibility and have their own decision-making powers, and that this will benefit social cohesion. These historical principles were re-introduced by Prime Minister Balkenende—an influential ideologist in the Christian Democratic Party's think tank—. His idea that government must work together in partnership with business and society was a guiding principle in the 2002–2010 cabinets. In 2007 Health Minister Ab Klink, former director of the think tank of the Christian Democratic Party and co-author with Balkenende on CDA position papers, introduced it as the cornerstone of his prevention policy. During the debate on the Tobacco Act on 31 May 2001, Siem Buijs of the Christian Democratic Party (CDA) debated with Rob Oudkerk (Labour Party) on the need for an advertising ban instead of continued self-regulation. Oudkerk attacked Buijs for hiding behind self-regulation and being naïve about the real intentions of the industry: "Keep on dreaming, CDA, this is not how it works," Buijs replied:

> You keep on dreaming, Mister Oudkerk, that we can influence behaviour in this country through laws and regulations. Forget it! We see this in many places. This is not what the CDA wants with shared responsibility. ... We want behaviour to be influenced from the bottom up. It should not be controlled from the top down through laws, after which you can relax because everything is settled. I believe that is a sham. ... I want to say this to you: "I have a dream." It is a nice dream and I want to make it true. It assumes behavioural change and attitude change and not an iron rod and a stick.

In corporatist arrangements, if an interest group is not recognised by the government as a legitimate negotiation partner, it can be a voice in the wilderness. This is what happened to the Cancer Society's director Dr Meinsma in the 1970s, and explains why the confrontational, more aggressive lobbying strategy that was adopted around 2008 by the Dutch tobacco control coalition was ultimately ineffective and eventually contributed to the downfall of STIVORO (see Chap. 9). The national corporatist character explains why the Netherlands does not have a strong tradition of the type of grass roots activist movements that were crucial to advancing smoke-free legislation in the United States and Australia. This is not to say that civil lawsuits and citizens' initiatives play a marginal role in the Dutch system. They have an important role in voicing societal concerns and may occasionally succeed in putting tobacco on the political agenda, especially when they use the weapon of legal action (see the section on venue shopping, later in this chapter).

Consensus Seeking

The Netherlands has long been one of the purest examples of a consensus democracy (Lijphart, 1999). This means that the political landscape is so fragmented that no single party is likely to achieve a majority position in parliament. This sets the Netherlands apart from majoritarian democracies such as the United Kingdom and the United States, where governments can impose policy in a top-down manner as they do not need to obtain consensus from rival political parties (although this has changed somewhat in the United Kingdom in more recent years). The fragmented Dutch political landscape has its origins dating back to times when the Netherlands was divided into the four religious or ideological "pillars": Catholics, Protestant-Christians, Socialists, and liberals or neutrals. Because no group was large enough for a majority, they needed to cooperate to maintain a stable and viable society. This was done by a process of consultation between spokespersons from the four groups. Specific but mainly informal "rules of the game" were developed and abided by to safeguard democratic stability (Lijphart, 1999).

The four pillars no longer exist, but the political landscape is still fragmented. After the Second World War the lower chamber of parliament consisted of six political parties roughly conforming to the traditional pillars, but the number of parties had increased to 13 by 2017. Since governments prefer to have a majority in both chambers of parliament, they usually need two or three parties, sometimes even four, to form a government.

Minority cabinets are rare in the Netherlands. Coalitions are constructed in such a way that the government has an obedient majority and a relatively powerless minority in parliament. This can work in two ways. If the government presents a coalition agreement that includes a strong tobacco control paragraph, parliament can only delay its passage as the paragraph is accepted by the parties that make up the majority. Parliament cannot vote against it without risking the fall of the cabinet. On average, less than one government bill is defeated by parliament per year (Andeweg & Irwin, 2009). However, if a strong tobacco control paragraph is missing from the coalition agreement and the government is unwilling to advance tobacco control, the power of the parliament to push for tobacco control is extremely limited because it has little chance to obtain sufficient votes to reach a majority.

Because of its multi-party nature, the cabinet must seek approval from a coalition of parties for important decisions, especially about sensitive matters. Because of the continuous need to secure support from parties that have different ideologies and interests, yes or no decisions are avoided and politicians go to great lengths to avoid having identifiable winners and losers, since this could create resentment and would cause problems for future decisions where one might need support from the opponents of the day (Koopmans, 2011). The Dutch version of consensus-based policy-making became widely known as the *polder* model during the late 1990s, when employer organisations, trade unions, and the government made compromises regarding wages and social security, and the astonishing positive effect on the national economy attracted international attention. Nowadays *polderen* is used more broadly, referring to the process of finding compromises between political parties or between government and civil society. The first policy reflex to a new social problem is still to find a solution that does right by as many stakeholders as possible.

The Christian Democratic ideals of subsidiarity and the reliance on support from civil society and the associated tradition of *polderen* mean that informal self-restraint and self-regulatory agreements with industry and other interested parties are preferred. The government feels most comfortable with voluntary agreements by the sector as the first policy option, before eventually proposing and trying legislation. This has happened time and again in tobacco control policy making, and continues to be the first reflex of Dutch politicians, many of whom believe it has advantages. These were summarised in 1996 by the minister of economic affairs in a debate in parliament over tobacco policy:

> Self-regulation certainly has advantages: it makes it possible to have tailor-made solutions for each sector, it creates flexibility, and changes in agreements can be made relatively quickly because it is not necessary to come to formal changes in law. A disadvantage is that the legal status of agreements often is unclear.[2]

In a parliamentary debate in 2001 about the Tobacco Act, Minister of Health Els Borst called self-regulation "the royal way" for government.[3] The preference for self-regulation is held by political parties in the centre and on the right flank of the Dutch parliament (who usually hold the majority of seats), while parties from the left question it as they are more suspicious of the intentions of businesses.

Consensus Seeking in the Cabinet

Dutch ministers wear two hats, one as a minister who has tasks, responsibilities, and challenges unique to his or her department, the other ideological, resulting from representing a political party. After the breakdown of the ideal of pillars, consensus seeking became concentrated more and more within the cabinet itself, where departmental ministers compete and negotiate with their ministerial colleagues and political ideologies are taken into consideration. From the 1960s on, the cabinet became increasingly politicised (Andeweg & Irwin, 2009, pp. 142–145). A state secretary and a minister in the same department are often from different political parties, so that the coalition parties are represented in a balanced manner in the cabinet. Health ministers were most often from liberal or Christian parties (Table 5.1). Few have had a background in health: from 1967, this has been the case in only 6 of 15 instances, and none has had a medical profile since 2002 (Table 5.1). Another point to note is that until 1994 tobacco control was handled by state secretaries (junior ministers). This gave tobacco control a none too strong negotiating position, because state secretaries are not present at the weekly cabinet meetings and do not have the right to vote. They attend only when a topic in their area is being discussed.

The cabinet is further politicised through the practice of holding party meetings of political parties' ministers and state secretaries with their leaders and party chairpersons in the second and first chamber the day before each weekly cabinet meeting to prepare for next day's agenda. Party discipline may be enforced so that ministers vote along party lines.

COALITION AGREEMENTS

After an election, the political leaders of the parties of a new ruling coalition draft a set of policy intentions. As in other multi-party countries, such coalition agreements are the result of a sometimes long and difficult negotiation between party leaders and are subject to extensive lobbying from

Table 5.1 Members of cabinet who have held the tobacco policy portfolio

Period	Name	Position in Ministry of Health	Political party	Academic background
1967–1971	Roelof Kruisinga	State secretary	CHU[a]	Medical doctor
1971–1973	Louis Stuyt	Minister[b]	KVP[c]	Medical doctor
1973–1977	Jo Hendriks	State secretary	KVP	No academic background, manager of a sickness fund
1977–1981	Els Veder-Smit	State secretary	VVD	Law
1981–1982	Ineke Lambers	State secretary	D66	Law
1982–1986	Joop van der Reijden	State secretary	CDA	Economy, affinity to the health sector
1986–1989	Dick Dees	State secretary	VVD	Pharmacist
1989–1994	Hans Simons	State secretary	PvdA	Political sciences and sociology
1994–2002	Els Borst	Minister	D66	Medical doctor
2002–2002	Eduard Bomhoff	Minister	LPF	Economy, long-time affiliation with the Labour party (PVDA) before entering cabinet as member of populist party LPF
2002–2003	Clémence Ross-van Dorp	State secretary (interim)	CDA	English teacher, Sinologue
2003–2007	Hans Hoogervorst	Minister	VVD	Historian, worked at Ministry of Finance, was Minister of Finance in 2002–2003
2007–2010	Ab Klink	Minister	CDA	Sociology, worked at Ministry of Justice and at the scientific bureau of the CDA
2010–2012	Edith Schippers	Minister	VVD	Political sciences, worked at VNO-NCW (employer lobby organisation)
2012–2017	Martin Van Rijn	State secretary	PvdA	Economy, career civil servant at Ministry of Health, Ministry of Interior Affairs, and Ministry of Public Housing

[a]KVP = *Katholieke Volkspartij* (Catholic People's Party)
[b]There was no state secretary at the Ministry of Health in 1971–1973
[c]CHU = *Christelijk-Historische Unie* (Christian Historical Union)

interests groups. The outcome is "a register of policies that coalition parties wish ministers to implement" (Moury, 2011). About two-thirds of pledges formulated in Dutch coalition agreements are transferred into government decisions, according to one study that examined this for two cabinets (Lubbers III, 1989–1994; Kok II, 1998–2002) (Moury, 2011). Coalition partners tend to negotiate policy intentions for the next four years at a rather high level of detail so that there is little room for the new government to decide on new policy except for unexpected issues and responses to crises. If we disregard decisions about things such as crises, Dutch ministers make less than 20% of policy decisions spontaneously. They must promise to adhere to the coalition agreement before they are sworn in, and they sometimes refer to it as their "Holy Bible" (Andeweg & Irwin, 2009).[4] Jeroen Dijsselbloem, Labour Party politician and former Minister of Finance, described such a coalition agreement as "a sad thing. It lists many far-reaching policy intentions, intentions that are devised and negotiated by a small group of political insiders behind closed doors. Civil society and science are not taken into consideration, so that it has no non-political checks and balances" (Slob & Staman, 2012).

Tobacco control was mentioned three times in the coalition agreements of the 15 cabinets since 1972 (Elsevier, 2010; Van den Braak & Van den Berg, 2017). The first was in the second cabinet of Labour Party Prime Minister Kok (1998–2002). Tobacco policy was called a priority: tobacco control was to be intensified and it was announced that when the code of conduct regarding tobacco advertising ended (in May 1999), the European directive on tobacco advertising would be implemented. This gave Health Minister Els Borst a strong mandate to realise her Tobacco Act, since it meant that the Liberal–Conservative *Volkspartij voor Vrijheid en Democratie* (People's Party for Freedom and Democracy) (VVD), part of the ruling coalition, was committed to the agreement and could not put up much of a fight. The second time that tobacco was mentioned was in the fourth cabinet of Christian Democratic Prime Minister Balkenende (2007–2010), in which the Labour Party also participated. The tobacco control lobby succeeded in getting a sentence about a smoke-free hospitality sector in the coalition agreement that said that, in collaboration with the hospitality sector, the government would work towards a smoke-free hospitality sector. The next coalition between VVD and CDA (Rutte I) announced in 2010 in its coalition agreement that the smoking ban for bars would be relaxed because "in many small pubs, where there is no personnel employed, there is no need for a smoking ban." Rutte explained it in his public statement about the coalition agreement: "We give responsibility back to the people in this country. No patronising, no untenable smoking bans in small cafés, and furthermore no unnecessary regulations" (Elsevier, 2010, p. 176). This was the outcome of a deal between the VVD and the CDA. The CDA would give up its wish for smoke-free bars in exchange for an assurance that it would be compensated in other dossiers.[5]

Securing Long-Term Tobacco Control Policy

Dutch tobacco control policymaking is a drawn-out process. The Ministry of Health pushes for a stricter and more effective tobacco policy, supported by tobacco control organisations. This is most effective when there is sufficient collective memory and capacity within the bureaucracy to support long-term policymaking, independent of the whim of the day and the ever-changing ideologies of Dutch governments. However, this capacity is restricted. In the past, institutional policy continuity was supported by the fact that high-level officials remained at their posts when governments changed, so that policy knowledge was preserved. However, since the emergence of the *Algemene Bestuursdienst* (senior civil service) at the end of the 1990s, top-level bureaucrats (secretaries-general, directors-general, and inspectors-general) are supposed to change position every four or five years in order to reduce compartmentalisation. This has led to the emergence of career civil servants: managers with little affinity for the subject matter. According to one person, "that's the big story of these top levels who rotate faster and faster so there's less and less collective memory. This plays into the hands of the industry."[6] In more recent years, institutional memory within the tobacco control unit of the Ministry of Health has been further hampered when civil servants from lower levels also changed positions. Between 2008 and 2013 there was much turnover, with civil servants "doing" tobacco control for short periods of time.[7]

One way of overcoming problems of such institutional amnesia is to rely on organisations and individuals outside the governmental bureaucracy to provide continuity and the preservation of knowledge (Smith, 2013). In the Netherlands, STIVORO traditionally fulfilled this role, and new civil servants in the Ministry of Health could quickly become familiar with the tobacco control "dossier" after a few meetings with experts from this organisation.[8]

One mechanism that supports policy continuity from one administration to the next is the practice of introductory dossiers, presented to a new minister on the first day in office. They are written by high-level civil servants and are a list of policy intentions, unresolved issues, and pressing matters that need to be solved in the short- and mid-term. Introductory dossiers are also an attempt by the bureaucratic system to assure that a minister stays as close as possible to mid- and long-term policy issues.

Compromises Between Ministries

While tobacco control policy is subject to compromises between political parties and between the government and interest groups, compromises are also sought between different ministries: particularly between the Ministry of Economic Affairs, which protects business interests, and the Ministry of Health, which protects public health. Until the mid-1990s tobacco policy was jointly determined by these two departments, after which it became the prime responsibility of the Ministry of Health. Health Minister Borst's tobacco policy document in 1996 was the last one co-signed by both ministers. This signified an important transformation from an economic to a public health-dominated perspective on the tobacco problem. A similar handing over of responsibilities from trade to health has occurred in other high-income countries (Cairney, Studlar, & Mamudu, 2012): in the United Kingdom, for instance, such a shift took place in 2003 (Cairney et al., 2012), six years later than in the Netherlands. In the Netherlands, despite this shift in formal responsibilities, the trade ministry continues to have a say in tobacco control policy (see Chap. 8). For one thing, the health minister, like every other minister, has to have support for plans and budget proposals from the full cabinet.

Proposals for new tobacco policy are usually made after frequent consultation between civil servants from the Ministry of Health and their counterparts from the Ministry of Economic Affairs, but may also involve the Ministry of Social Affairs (in the case of smoking bans), the Ministry of Education (e.g., regarding youth prevention programmes and smoke-free schools), and the Ministry of Finance (for taxation of tobacco and requests for a larger budget). Tobacco taxation, which is the most effective tobacco control measure, is still firmly in the hands of the Ministry of Finance. Ministers do not want issues to be discussed in the cabinet while they are in their infancy, so civil servants from ministries negotiate with each other until a compromise is reached. By the time an issue is brought to the cabinet meeting for approval, it has been thoroughly discussed and reworked by the bureaucracy.

Disputes that cannot be solved by civil servants at the highest level are negotiated in cabinet meetings. The practice of consultation with other ministries encourages slow decision-making and compromises. Minister Els Borst reflected on the long time it took to realise a new tobacco policy:

> There are 15 different ministers in this cabinet, with different opinions, often based on personal beliefs about tobacco and alcohol policy. They further have a specific political stance and these three political parties [which form the government] have different views on the matter. It is not the case that the minister of health and the minister of economic affairs can decide on tobacco policy quickly on their own. These discussions on tobacco control policy (...) have taken much time within the full cabinet.[9]

When debating in parliament, the minister is supposed to speak on behalf of the cabinet. Ministers mask disputes with colleague ministers. When Borst was trying to get her proposal for revision of the Tobacco Act adopted, she was in constant conflict with Minister of Economic Affairs Annemarie Jorritsma, who vigorously defended tobacco industry interests and sent Borst so-called blue letters[10] urging her to tone down her policy intentions. In 2000 MP Jan Marijnissen (Socialist Party) initiated a debate in a fruitless attempt to get to the bottom of this.[11]

Lobbying the Bureaucracy of the Ministry

After a minister or state secretary has instructed the bureaucracy to draft a bill, civil servants go to work on it. The start of the creation of new legislation "is the most relevant part of decision-making, where most influence can be exerted" (Scheltema Beduin & Ter Weele, 2015). The process usually involves talks with stakeholders. Lobbying at this stage, before any formal public consultation may be organised, is regarded as the most important and opportune moment to influence decision-making, and this lobby is completely unchecked in the Netherlands (Scheltema Beduin & Ter Weele, 2015)—although this improved for tobacco control since the implementation of Article 5.3 of the FCTC (more on this in Chap. 6). As one Dutch tobacco industry lobbyist put it, "You need to sit with the person who has the white paper sheet in front of him" (Van der Poel & Gutter, 2011). In 2000 Socialist Party parliamentarian Jan Marijnissen questioned the fact that civil servants from the Ministry of Economic

Affairs gave suggestions about the wording and content of the proposal for the new Tobacco Act after being prepared by officials from the Ministry of Health—that had led to textual changes.[12] Marijnissen suggested that the tobacco industry had influenced the policymaking process through the trade ministry. The health minister replied that "there are constantly contacts about tobacco prevention policy between the Ministry of Health, Economic Affairs, sometimes Finance and sometimes Social Affairs. (...) These are normal, common contacts." However, it is clear that these interdepartmental contacts gave the tobacco industry ample opportunity to influence tobacco control policy via contacts with civil servants.

Approval from other ministries is also sought at this stage. When the civil servants have written a draft legislation, it gets "in the line" for approval and amendments by ever higher echelons of bureaucracy until it receives a paragraph of approval from the minister. It is then discussed in a small committee with the involved ministers. After that, it is discussed in the cabinet before being sent for advice to the Council of State and to a commission that checks whether the proposal imposes administrative burdens to society and businesses. Only when it has passed these hurdles is it sent to the second chamber of parliament. It is then discussed in an expert committee of the parliament with the minister, after which it is subject to a plenary debate in parliament. Only then does the bill become public. The parliament can, and most often does, propose further amendments. Amendments need a simple majority vote. This process of amending and rewriting may take several years in the case of politically controversial issues such as tobacco policy, after which it is sent back to the second chamber for a final vote. After approval it is sent for scrutiny to the first chamber (the senate).

In the Netherlands about 250 bills are introduced each year, and they take on average 14 months to reach the adoption stage in the senate, but there have been cases where the process took more than 20 years (Andeweg & Irwin, 2009). The first Tobacco Act took four years (1984–1988) from presentation of the first draft to the second chamber and approval by the first chamber, but the preparatory work had started already around 1981. The second (amended) Tobacco Act took two years (1999–2001), but the political and bureaucratic process had already started in 1996 when the government presented its tobacco control policy intentions for scrutiny and debate in parliament.

It is a peculiarity of the Dutch legislative process that bills do not die with a change of government, as is the case in some countries. Despite the fact that drafting a piece of legislation does not stop when a cabinet resigns, ministers are keen to complete the legislation process while they are still in power, since the survival of a bill is uncertain when a new majority coalition takes over. It was crucial to the realisation of the second Tobacco Act that Minister of Health Els Borst remained in office for two full cabinet periods (1994–2002). In the last year she and her bureaucracy put much pressure on the process, supported by the tobacco control network, and she managed to get the act through the senate just before the cabinet resigned.

After legislation has been approved, the government can issue regulations for the implementation phase. Governmental decrees (orders-in-council)[13] and ministerial decrees[14] are part of a higher-order legislative act, and are used for fine-tuning legislation during implementation. Formal approval by vote from the parliament is not necessary. This so-called delegated legislation was extensively used while working on the Tobacco Act and postponed the most controversial elements of the legislation to a later date. Decrees are often used since they make legislation possible while at the same time functioning as a big stick to put pressure on self-regulatory trajectories, for example, with the various temporary exceptions to the workplace smoking ban under the revised Tobacco Act.

Lobbying Parliament

The drafting of legislation is the joint constitutional responsibility of government and parliament. The second chamber of parliament (lower house, house of representatives) may take the initiative to draft a law and has the right to amend pieces of legislation that are proposed by the government, while the first chamber (upper house, senate) can only adopt or block proposals. It does not have the right to amend laws, although it can force the minister to reconsider a law, withdraw it, or send a revised version to the senate. In practice, the second chamber of parliament rarely uses its right of initiative (Van Outeren & Pergrim, 2015). New legislation stems mainly from the governmental bureaucracy, but this may be, to various degrees, adjusted and amended in parliament.

There is a strict party discipline in parliament. Votes on a proposal are by show of hands. Normally only the hands of the leaders of the parliamentary factions are counted, since it is assumed that party members vote uniformly. A recent count revealed that in a period of four years (2008–2012), there were 11,000 cases where parliamentarians had to vote (Okhuijsen, 2012). Only in 64 cases was there a roll-call vote, where individuals were counted, and in only 25 of the 11,000 cases did members of parliament cross the floor. In tobacco control policymaking, only once was there a situation where a member of parliament went against party discipline: when the lower house voted on the amendments to the Tobacco Act in 2002 by show of hands. Erica Terpstra broke VVD ranks and voted in favour of the bill.

Despite its relatively weak power position, opposition in the parliament has influenced tobacco control policy considerably. The main way parliament may influence legislation is to adopt resolutions (motions) during debates. In order to be tabled, draft resolutions have to be seconded by at least four other MP's. The purpose is to urge a minister to act or to change intended legislation, for example, to come up with a new or additional proposal. Resolutions are not binding, but when a parliamentary majority approves them, ministers are expected to carry them out. Most resolutions introduced in the Dutch parliament to strengthen tobacco legislation have been defeated because of majority support for the government's position. However, in some cases, resolutions received backing from both ruling and opposing parties, and were influential. For example, parliament strengthened tobacco control by including the worksite smoking ban in the amended Tobacco Act. On the other hand, it diluted or delayed tobacco control by opting for an age key system instead of a ban on tobacco vending machines, by setting the age limit for the sale of tobacco at 16 instead of 18 years, by demanding exemptions to the smoking ban and by rejecting new policy ideas such as graphic health warnings in 2006 (discussed in Chap. 2). Box 5.1 presents more examples of resolutions that influenced tobacco control, illustrating how the parliament is an important lobbying venue for both sides of tobacco control. On balance, the industry lobby seems to have been most successful.

Box 5.1 Important pro- and anti-tobacco control parliamentary resolutions

In 1996 Marijnissen (Socialist Party) received a majority vote with backing from the Christian Democrats.[15] The resolution requested that the government come up with a plan to restrict the sale of tobacco to specialty shops. To this day the government has not executed the motion, but it is still occasionally referred to and in that manner continues to plague the government such as in 2013 when State Secretary Martin van Rijn was challenged by parliament to come up with a proposal to reduce the number of points of sale.[16]

> In 1997 the VVD (with support from D66 and CDA) was successful in weakening the advertising and promotion ban by exempting the brand names or trademarks of tobacco product already in use for non-tobacco merchandise before the law went into effect.[17] The industry could continue circumventing the ban by promoting its brand through clothes, shoes, and the like.
>
> In 2001 the Labour Party, together with the Socialist Party, managed to round up a majority for a resolution demanding that the government make effective smoking cessation support eligible for financial reimbursement through the national health insurance plan.[18] This eventually contributed to the adoption of the current reimbursement system, although it took ten years to be implemented.
>
> In 2002 CDA Senator Werner received full support for a resolution that requested that the government find the necessary budget for media campaigns to help smokers quit smoking as an accompaniment to the workplace smoking ban.[19] It was contingent on this condition that the senate was prepared to approve the Tobacco Act.
>
> In 2005 conservative parties, with support from the Socialist and the Green-left parties, forced the government to consider ventilation as an alternative to smoking bans.[20]

As in other democracies, Dutch parliamentarians have the right to ask oral or written questions to ministers, who are obliged to answer within three weeks to written questions. Questioning is therefore an important additional means for parliamentarians to control government and, through friendly members of parliament, for lobbyists to put pressure on the government. See Chap. 10 for a further discussion of parliamentary questions.

Parliamentarians: Targets for Lobbyists

In the Netherlands lobbying is part of day-to-day politics. It is less regulated than in many other countries in Europe (Scheltema Beduin & Ter Weele, 2015). At best, Dutch parliamentarians have only one personal staff member to help them with their complex tasks. They are among the least equipped parliamentarians in Europe, making them particularly vulnerable to lobbyists (Korteweg & Huisman, 2016, p. 17). Parliamentarians often rely on interest groups to help them control the government or draft initiative laws, as they lack both the specialised knowledge and the time to gather all the facts and figures they need. How they process information they receive from lobbyists is at their own discretion—they do not have to declare or make this public.

There is increasing demand for lobbying transparency in Dutch society and the media. In 2012 the *Algemene Rekenkamer* (Court of Audit) noted that the information possessed by the tobacco sector is better than that of specialised parliamentarians (Algemene Rekenkamer, 2012).[21] When former Health Minister Elco Brinkman became a lobbyist for Philip Morris and in this capacity contacted the state secretary for finance about a European taxation matter, this was exposed in the media. Soon afterwards Lea Bouwmeester, a Labour Party parliamentarian, announced that she was preparing a bill that would make it mandatory for the government to include a "lobbyists paragraph" in each proposal for new legislation.[22] Such a paragraph would require disclosure of lobbying contacts that occurred in the drafting process of laws and give details about who, on behalf of which organisation, visited which policymaker, with what intentions; similar requirements exist in other jurisdictions, including the United States, England, and the European Union. Three years later the initiative law had still not been introduced. According to Bouwmeester, "writing such a proposal is complicated and the parliament has too little support for it" (Meeus, 2015).

In 2016 journalists revealed that one quarter of ex-politicians (ministers and parliamentarians) had become lobbyists (Huisman, Kooistra, & Korteweg, 2016). In 2017 the cabinet responded for the first time to calls from the Labour Party for more transparency, and decided that there would be a restriction on ex-ministers and state secretaries accepting lobbying positions in their field of expertise for two years after leaving office. It has also become more difficult for tobacco industry lobbyists to contact government officials directly due to a stricter adherence by the government to Article 5.3 FCTC (more on this in Chap. 6).

Lobbying Through Different Venues

The Netherlands is not a federal state like Canada, Australia, or the United States. Federal states offer interest groups ample opportunity to place tobacco control on the political agenda. In Australia, it has been noted that "Australian states are like dominos, and when one state takes the first step, the others will likely follow shortly after" (Bryan-Jones & Chapman,

2008). In the United States when tobacco control activists have no success at the central federal level, they simply turn their attention to local and state policymakers. The advantage of such "venue shopping" has been suggested as a reason why the United States has stronger tobacco control than Denmark, which has a single-venue system like that of the Netherlands (Albæk, Green-Pedersen, & Nielsen, 2007). While there seems some truth in the single/multiple venue explanation, it is overly simplistic, since counter-examples can be found easily. Germany has a federal system but is a tobacco control laggard, while a leader like New Zealand is a single-venue country. The next chapter will explore the increasing importance of European and global legislation for tobacco control and lobbying opportunities for venue shopping in an international context.

A special "shopping venue" is the judicial system. This has frequently been used by both sides (pro- and anti-tobacco advocacy groups) in the Netherlands, and has forced breakthroughs when policymaking was slow. A case that received much media exposure was the Nanny Nooijen case of 2000: an employee of the Dutch postal office won a court case against her employer, who had failed to protect her from exposure to second-hand smoke from her colleagues. A few more court cases were needed before the workplace smoking ban finally made the legal route redundant, and one of these was in 2003, where the court forced Isala Clinics to financially compensate an employee with asthma for health damage as a consequence of exposure to tobacco smoke.[23] In March 2002, during the debate in the senate about the Tobacco Act, senator Ruers (SP) said, "I want to point out that the only real breakthrough in the Netherlands regarding the smoke-free workplace was the court case the previous year. An employee had the courage to start a lawsuit, which she won. This caused a tremendous change in the Netherlands. (...) A civilian accomplished more for society than all [other] measures taken together."[24] Another example of the importance of the legal system involved the non-smokers' rights group Clean Air Netherlands (CAN), which won an important court case against the state in 2014. CAN successfully pleaded that small bars must not be exempted from the workplace smoking ban, referring to Article 8 of the Framework Convention on Tobacco Control (FCTC) treaty. But not only did the health network successfully use the legal venue: four years before the CAN ruling, small bar owners, with help from the industry, won court cases where local judges ruled that small bars without personnel had to be exempted. Chapter 8 gives some further examples of the tobacco manufacturers' use of the court system to frustrate tobacco control or intimidate tobacco control organisations.

The Story of Deregulation

This chapter about institutional factors has to include a discussion of the process of deregulation, which started in the 1980s. Later Dutch cabinets followed a neo-liberalist agenda that aimed at less government, less bureaucracy, and more free market. This section discusses the consequences for Dutch tobacco control.

The first Lubbers Cabinet (1982–1986), which consisted of CDA and the liberal–conservative VVD, wanted to reduce administrative burdens on businesses and initiated a regulatory "reform" programme, informed by similar deregulation initiatives in the United States and the United Kingdom. An important motive for this so-called deregulation operation was to overcome the economic crisis by improving business competitiveness, but it also had ideological motives. Deregulation was one of six elements in a substantial programme aimed at reducing high unemployment rates and central budget deficits. Other elements were reconsideration of the role of the government (making it smaller), decentralisation, reorganisation of the governmental bureaucracy, reduction of the number of civil servants, and extensive privatisation (Van der Voet, 2005).

Proposals for new laws had to be submitted to a deregulation commission. This "Commission Van der Grinten" advised on whether regulation was necessary and, if so, how it could be simplified. Not all proposals were sent to this commission: the cabinet decided on a selection. Among these was the proposal for a Tobacco Act, and the involvement of this commission was one of the reasons why the process of drafting the initial act took four years.[25] The commission's advice was not to impose smoking bans but to leave this to industry self-regulation.[26] Cabinet ignored the advice, but adopted the commissions' wish not to ban the sale of cigarettes to minors (16-year-olds) nor to ban cigarette sales through vending machines and self-service outlets. The draft Tobacco Act was adjusted to reflect these amendments before it was sent to parliament.

Commission Van der Grinten was active until 1995, when a new form of regulatory impact assessment, called the *Marktwerking, Deregulering en Wetgevingskwaliteit Operatie* (market competition, deregulation, and quality of legislation) (MDW Operation), replaced it. This was the new answer to the government's continued desire for a simplified regulatory environment offering fewer hurdles to businesses. Formal top-down interventions had to be constrained, and self-regulation by industry and citizens was the default. MDW was operative until 2003, when the second Balkenende cabinet (VVD, CDA, D66), which had as a motto "more participation, more work and less regulation," introduced its own version under the heading "B4."[27] Tobacco industry lobbyists regularly referred to the cabinet's wish to minimise bureaucracy and reduce administrative burdens for business, which had been estimated at €16.4 billion per year.

Since 1998 new regulation has been subject to scrutiny from ACTAL.[28] This independent advisory board assesses whether new legislation is suitable for decision-making in the cabinet (Hoppe, Woldendorp, & Bandelow, 2015) and requires policymakers to provide specifications of the exact administrative burden it will impose on businesses. In order to do this, civil servants may contact industries for information about the expected costs of new legislation to their sector. Only after a stamp of approval from ACTAL can a proposal for new legislation be sent to the cabinet.

The Dutch experience with deregulation for businesses has been considered an example to other nations making attempts to reduce bureaucracy in the EU (see Box 5.2). The tobacco industry, with support from other multinational corporations such as the oil industry, pharmaceutical companies, and the food and alcohol industry, lobbied successfully to introduce such business-friendly adaptations of legislation making in the Brussels bureaucracy, making it more difficult to pass legislation that protects public health (Smith et al., 2010; Smith, Fooks, Gilmore, Collin, & Weishaar, 2015).

Box 5.2 Dutch inspiration for a business-friendly policy agenda in Europe

Around 1994 British American Tobacco (BAT) started to lobby for regulatory reforms in the EU similar to what was common practice in the United Kingdom and the Netherlands (Smith et al., 2010). The Netherlands was one of the strongest supporters of "better regulation" in the EU, after Germany, the United Kingdom, and Ireland. When the Dutch assumed the EU presidency in 1997, BAT recognised an opportunity as "The Dutch appear even more committed to the principles of cost-benefit analysis and risk assessment ... and would support a treaty amendment to achieve this objective" (BAT, 1996). BAT, with support from other multinationals, promoted the idea that the EU would be more competitive when legislation was simplified and when proposals for new legislation, including those that protect health, were subject to rigorous cost-benefit analyses and impact assessments. As a consequence of BAT's lobbying efforts, a "better regulation" agenda that included a mandatory impact assessment of new legislation and requirements to consult industry at an early stage of the policymaking process was implemented as part of the Treaty of Amsterdam (1997) (Smith et al., 2010). This achievement was heralded by BAT as "an important victory" for the company (BAT, n.d.). It helped the industry prevent the introduction of EU-wide public smoking restrictions and delay tobacco advertising restrictions.

Decentralisation

Governments choose the path of decentralisation for ideological and financial reasons (De Vries, 2000). Since the 1980s the Dutch government has decentralised a great number of tasks, including health promotion, to local governments and the private sector assuming that this will improve operational efficiency and that in this way central government can downsize and reverse its growth (De Vries, 2000). This had direct consequences for how government approached national tobacco control policy making, since responsibility was increasingly given to the local level.

Decentralisation of public health policy began in 1986 with *Nota 2000*, a 600-page memorandum on public health (Dekker & Saan, 1990). It outlined new ambitions in the field of public health and a political commitment to WHO's global strategy, "Health for All by the year 2000" (WVC, 1986). WHO called on governments to improve health through a strategy encompassing not only individuals but also their environment, all levels of society, and all sectors that might influence health. The new idea of an intersectoral approach and organising health promotion at the lowest level caught on. Health policy and prevention was to be restructured as part of a broader administrative reform of retreating government and liberalisation of public tasks, initiated by the Lubbers cabinets (1982–1994) (WVC, 1991). The idea was that the Ministry of Health would continue to coordinate, set targets, and monitor, but that execution would devolve to the local level. The Netherlands is not unique in this: many EU countries decentralised in the 1990s and later (Marks & Hooghe, 2003).

With the *Wet Collectieve Preventie Volksgezondheid* (Public Health Collective Prevention Act) (WCPV) of 1990, prevention of disease became a responsibility that the national government shared with municipalities.

According to law, every four years all municipalities (there were 393 in 2015) have to develop a public health policy document in which they outline priorities for the next four years. Local policymakers are free to choose priorities and targets based on regional epidemiological data and are expected to make use of evidence-based interventions—although this is not mandatory. Municipalities have to finance health promotion from the general municipality budget, which shrank over the years due to budget cuts by the central government, and are thus required to look for additional financial means, such as applying for competitive grants or initiating private–public partnerships with insurance companies or commercial businesses. Municipalities increasingly take the lead in public health at the local and regional level, and receive support from *Gemeentelijke Gezondheidsdienst* (Regional Public Health Services) (GGD) with this task. Officials of the *Inspectie voor de Gezondheidszorg* (Inspectorate for Health Care) (IGZ) visit the GGDs every year to assess the execution of their duties within the law.

In 2003 an amendment to the Public Health Collective Prevention Act made local governments' periodic status reports on disease prevention mandatory by law. Local municipalities were also required to play a specific role in what became known as the "prevention cycle" (VWS, 2011b). In 2008 the WCPV was integrated in a new public health act (*Wet Publieke Gezondheidszorg* (WPG)), another step towards strengthening the prevention cycle and handing responsibility to the local level. According to a recent national health policy document, health promotion is now a decentralised task and the joint responsibility of local government and health insurers (VWS, 2011a). Although the formal responsibility for tobacco policy remains with the cabinet, because Article 22 of the national constitution stipulates that the government has a legal obligation to protect and promote public health, municipalities are expected to coordinate tobacco control activities at the municipal level and by doing so contribute to the reduction of national smoking rates.

Tobacco Control Lost Between the National and the Local Level?

The responsibility for municipalities in the field of public health is daunting, for there are great complexities and small budgets. Many municipalities are not sufficiently equipped to develop and implement prevention strategies. On 25 March 2010, IGZ reported on the lack of effectiveness. The day of publication was chosen carefully, because on the same day the *Rijksinstituut voor Volksgezondheid en Milieu* (National Institute for Public

Health and the Environment) (RIVM) published its new *Volksgezondheid Toekomst Verkenning* (Public Health Status and Foresight) (VTV) report (see Chap. 10 for more about the RIVM and VTV reports). Both reports came to the devastating conclusion that the prevention cycle was not functioning and that local health promotion policies do not contribute to reductions of obesity, smoking, alcohol abuse, or depression at the national level (Inspectie van de Gezondheidszorg, 2010). The message was that the central government must take back control. At an unusually frank press conference, Marc Sprenger, director-general of the RIVM, commented to the press that "the government must have the courage to firmly and normatively take up its role. It is one thing to distribute nice folders in schools, but that is not enough. One must also be prepared to take tough measures … that support local programmes" (NRC, 2010).

The government may promote decentralisation and citizen participation when it simply wants to cut spending. At such times Dutch tobacco policy risks getting lost between the national and the local level: the national government may delegate responsibility to lower levels and emphasise citizens' own responsibility, while municipalities evade responsibility and point back to the government. The potential advantages of decentralisation, such as tailoring policies to local circumstances, encouraging citizen participation, and being more efficient, are questionable if they are not adequately facilitated by the central government. The current attempt by the Dutch government to stimulate local initiatives in public health through the National Prevention Program (NPP) is not supported by the necessary budget. Instead, the government assumes that societal and commercial organisations will pay for the health promotion programmes themselves. This may work for some issues, but is problematic for tobacco control. Municipal councillors have many other more pressing concerns than tobacco, and tobacco prevention is not a topic that will earn them credit from the public (see Box 5.3). In addition, they have to overcome resistance from local functionaries who feel uncomfortable interfering in a private habit such as smoking (Van der Meer, Spruijt, & De Beer, 2012).

These problems have been recognised by *the Raad voor de Volksgezondheid en Zorg* (Council for Public Health and Health Care) (RVZ), an independent advisory body. It urged the government to take a stronger lead, to set quantifiable targets, and to resume coordination and control (RVZ, 2010). In one report RVZ concluded that national public health tasks can only be effectively administered by municipalities if they are supported by a complementary central policy, and if the minister has voiced a clear normative standpoint (RVZ, 2011). The advice echoes the call for action from the director-general of the RIVM, Mark Sprenger, the year before. RVZ recognised that "there are political–ideological arguments against applying the most effective interventions (especially supply side restrictions). ... These have to do with the prime responsibility that a citizen has for the choices it makes, an opinion that seems to have more supporters in the Netherlands than elsewhere." The council was critical about the government's weak prevention policy and its inertness, and recommended that the shift towards local health policy be accompanied by strong measures such as higher tobacco taxes and a larger budget for prevention.

> **Box 5.3 Municipalities and national tobacco control goals**
> A 2011 study among health policy officers of 151 municipalities revealed that 39% had not included tobacco control in their policy intentions (Huijsman, van der Meer, de Beer, van Emst, & Willemsen, 2013). Of those who did, only 41% indicated that they had a distinct tobacco reduction programme. In most cases this was part of a broader addiction or lifestyle programme. The concrete activities were related to education, mostly smoking prevention programmes in schools, and occasional organised cessation support for smokers wanting to quit. The main reason for not implementing local tobacco control policy was that it is too labour intensive (especially for smaller municipalities) and that they felt that tobacco policy could best be tackled at the national level. One officer was quoted saying: "With the restricted means and time that we have, we want to make a choice in what to do in our health policy. It is better to do a few topics well, than many badly. Because tobacco control can be done much more effectively at the national level (smoking bans, smoking cessation support through national health insurance) we choose to do other topics [than tobacco]." In 2013, the low priority given to tobacco control by local authorities was confirmed in an inventory by the national organisation of community health services. This showed that one-third of the municipalities did not tackle smoking (GGD Nederland, 2013). Alcohol prevention was given more priority. A more recent study found that tobacco control is still virtually non-existent at the local level. Local decision makers see few advantages, because they "are not familiar with the possibilities they have to control smoking. Smoking is such a small issue for them that they do not take the time to get to grips with it" (Mulder, Bommelé, Branderhorst, & Hasselt, 2016).

Conclusion

Several aspects of the Dutch policy environment work against expeditious adoption of tobacco control. For many years Christian Democratic principles of subsidiarity, coupled with the corporatist tradition of policymaking and consensus seeking, combined to make it "logical" for policymakers to invite representatives of the tobacco industry to present their views on tobacco control, with business-friendly solutions (self-regulation instead of legislation) as the outcome. Dutch policymakers tried to avoid polarisation and conflicts between groups, and informal stakeholder consultation became a popular strategy to this end—which presented ample opportunity to the tobacco industry to influence and delay tobacco control. This was facilitated by calls to reduce the administrative burden to businesses during periods of economic recession, resulting in extensive deregulation operations in the 1980s and later. Another aspect of the policy environment not conducive to tobacco control was the neo-liberalist agenda of most cabinets, which preferred a limited role by the government.

Given the multiple-party nature of Dutch politics, the drafting of new policies must follow the specifics laid out in a coalition agreement, which is the end result of intense negotiations between the co-ruling political parties. The tobacco control coalition has only been successful twice in getting tobacco control proposals into coalition agreements.

In the Dutch system, where ministers are politically appointed and rarely have a background in health or medicine, the chance that ministers will become tobacco control champions is small. The political make-up of the cabinet is crucial, but the political orientation of the majority in parliament is also important. Parliament will usually support the government, but its opposition may amend or delay government proposals and influence the political agenda through the presentation of resolutions and parliamentary questions. Parliament is an important venue for lobbyists from both sides, but the industry has been most successful, since delaying or adapting policy intentions is easier than getting new legislation on the agenda in the first place. The inside lobby for many years has been unchecked and barely accountable in the Netherlands, and less regulated than in many other democracies, although this is now improving. Dutch parliamentarians are understaffed and depend on lobbyists for information and support with drafting bills and motions. For years the industry has had an advantage as their lobbyists stayed at their posts for decades, while both the civil servants who specialised in tobacco control experienced regular turnover.

A long and gradual process of decentralisation of public health tasks away from the central government to the municipal level increased the risk that tobacco control will be lost between the national and local levels, as it made it easier to escape responsibilities. Municipalities have little means and lack the motivation to take on national tobacco control tasks. The judicial system has become increasingly important as the corporatist elements of Dutch policymaking diminish, and the court has been responsible for important breakthroughs, especially regarding smoking bans.

Notes

1. https://www.internetconsultatie.nl/zoeken/resultaat?Trefwoorden=tabak&TrefwoordenSearchScope=TitelEnTekst
2. Proceedings II, 1996–1997, 24743, nr. 12, p. 7.
3. Proceedings II, 31 May 2001, 82–5234.
4. Dutch decision makers feel equally constrained by coalition agreements as their colleagues in Belgium, but somewhat more than in Germany and much more than in Italy (Moury & Timmermans, 2013).
5. Proceedings II, 2010–2011, 32,011, nr. 15.
6. Interview, 6 November 2015.
7. This is in contrast with the industry sector, where lobbyists such as Jan-Willem Roelofs for the SSI, Jan Willem Burgering for NSO, Alexander van Voorst Vader for VNK, Niek Jan van Kesteren for VNO–NCW, Ton Wurtz for SRB, and Robert Wassenaar voor for Philip Morris were more or less permanent factors of influence for decades.
8. With the termination of STIVORO in 2013, the continuity of historical knowledge and expertise was affected, although much of it was taken over by the Trimbos Institute.
9. Proceedings II, 1999–2000, 12 October 2000, 834–847.
10. Blue letters are letters or notes between two ministers, not open to public scrutiny.
11. Proceedings II, 1999–2000, 12 October 2000, 834–847.
12. Proceedings II, 1999–2000, TK12, 12 Oktober 2000, pp. 834–847.
13. In Dutch: Algemene Maatregel van Bestuur (AMvB).
14. Examples are decisions regarding how many grammes of tobacco should be in a pack of cigarettes or roll-your-own tobacco, or yearly adaptations of tobacco taxation levels.
15. Motie Marijnissen, 1996, nr. 5 (24743).
16. Motie Dik-Faber, 2015, nr. 38 (32011).
17. Motie Kamp, 1997, nr. 28 (21501–21519).
18. Motie Oudkerk, Kant, 2001, nr. 19 (26472).

19. Motie Werner, Stekelenburg, Van Schijndel, Van den Berg, Ruers, Hessing en Van de Beeten, 2002, nr. 59ᵉ (26472).
20. Motie Schippers, Buijs, Van der Ham, Hermans, Kant, 2005, nr. 109 (29800-XVI).
21. Not only parliament, but government also can have information disadvantages compared to the industry. For example, officials from the Ministry of Finance rely on information on tobacco market prices and effects of tax increases provided by the industry.
22. Bouwmeester had already declared in 2009 that she wanted to develop a code of practice for lobbyists after she had learned that the group of small bar owners who fought against a smoking ban in small pubs and bars was financed and supported by the tobacco industry.
23. http://www.cer-leuven.be/passiefroken/rechtszaken/zaakriphagen.htm
24. Proceedings I, Tabakswet 26 maart 2002, 24–1253.
25. Parliamentary Papers II, 1985–1986, 18749, nr. 6, p. 6.
26. Parliamentary Papers II, 1984–1985, 17931, nr. 61.
27. B4 = "Beter Bestuur voor Burger en Bedrijf" (better governance for citizen and enterprise).
28. ACTAL = "Adviescollege Toesting Administratieve Lasten" (Advisory Board on Administrative Burden Reduction).

References

Albæk, E., Green-Pedersen, C., & Nielsen, L. B. (2007). Making tobacco consumption a political issue in the United States and Denmark: The dynamics of issue expansion in comparative perspective. *Journal of Comparative Policy Analysis: Research and Practice, 9*, 1–20.

Algemene Rekenkamer. (2012). *Bestrijding van accijnsfraude bij alcohol en tabak. EU-beleid: naleving en effecten.* Den Haag: Sdu Uitgevers.

Andeweg, R. B., & Irwin, G. A. (2009). *Governance and politics of the Netherlands* (3rd ed.). Hampshire: Palgrave Macmillan.

BAT. (1996). EU issues. *British American Tobacco Records*, Bates No. 322122073–322122107. Retrieved from https://www.industrydocumentslibrary.ucsf.edu/tobacco/docs/rkyb0207

BAT. (n.d.). Shaping the regulatory environment: Advertising and public smoking. *British American Tobacco Records*, Bates No. 322121140–322121143. Retrieved from https://www.industrydocumentslibrary.ucsf.edu/tobacco/docs/jpcd0211

Breton, E., Richard, L., Gagnon, F., Jacques, M., & Bergeron, P. (2008). Health promotion research and practice require sound policy analysis models: The case of Quebec's tobacco act. *Social Sciences & Medicine, 67*(11), 1679–1689. https://doi.org/10.1016/j.socscimed.2008.07.028

Bryan-Jones, K., & Chapman, S. (2008). Political dynamics promoting the incremental regulation of secondhand smoke: A case study of New South Wales, Australia. *BMC Public Health, 6*, 192.

Cairney, P. (2012). *Understanding public policy: Theories and issues.* Basingstoke: Palgrave Macmillan.

Cairney, P., Studlar, D. T., & Mamudu, H. M. (2012). *Global tobacco control: Power, policy, governance and transfer.* New York: Palgrave Macmillan.

Castles, F. G., & Obinger, H. (2008). Worlds, families, regimes: Country clusters in European and OECD area public policy. *West European Politics, 31*, 321–344. https://doi.org/10.1080/01402380701835140

Christiansen, P. M., Norgaard, A. S., Rommetvedt, H., Svensson, T., Thesen, G., & Oberg, P. (2010). Varieties of democracy: Interest groups and corporatist committees in Scandinavian policy making. *Voluntas, 21*(1), 22–40. https://doi.org/10.1007/s11266-009-9105-0

De Vries, M. S. (2000). The rise and fall of decentralization: A comparative analysis of arguments and practices in European countries. *European Journal of Political Research, 38*, 193–224.

Dekker, E., & Saan, H. (1990). Policy papers, papers or policies: HFA under uncertain political conditions. *Health Promotion International, 5*, 279–290.

Elsevier. (2010). *Wacht op onze daden: Alle regeringsverklaringen van Lubbers tot en met Rutte.* Amsterdam: Elsevier Boeken.

Fenger, F. (2007). Welfare regimes in Central and Eastern Europe: Incorporating post-communist countries in a welfare regime typology. *Contemporary Issues and Ideas in Social Sciences, 3*(2), 1–30.

GGD Nederland. (2013). *Gezondheidsbeleid in de groei.* Utrecht: GGD Nederland.

Hoppe, R., Woldendorp, J., & Bandelow, N. (2015). *2015 Netherlands report.* Gütersloh: Bertelsmann Stiftung.

Huijsman, F., van der Meer, R. M., de Beer, M. A. M., van Emst, A. J., & Willemsen, M. C. (2013). Decentralisation of tobacco control: Smoking policy falls through the cracks. *Tijdschrift voor Gezondheidswetenschappen, 91*, 52–59.

Hummel, K., Willemsen, M. C., Monshouwer, K., De Vries, H., & Nagelhout, G. E. (2016). Social acceptance of smoking restrictions during 10 years of policy implementation, reversal, and reenactment in the Netherlands: Findings from a national population survey. *Nicotine & Tobacco Research, 19*, 1–8. https://doi.org/10.1093/ntr/ntw169

Inspectie van de Gezondheidszorg. (2010). *De staat van de gezondheidszorg: Meer effect mogelijk van publieke gezondheidszorg.* Utrecht: IGZ.

Koopmans, F. S. L. (2011). Going Dutch: Recent drug policy developments in the Netherlands. *Journal of Global Drug Policy and Practice, 5*(3), 1–9.

Korteweg, A., & Huisman, E. (2016). *Lobbyland: De geheime krachten in Den Haag.* Amsterdam: De Geus.

Lenschow, A., Liefferink, D., & Veenman, S. (2005). When the birds sing. A framework for analysing domestic factors behind policy convergence. *Journal of European Public Policy, 12*(5), 797–816. https://doi.org/10.1080/13501760500161373

Lijphart, A. (1999). *Patterns of democracy: Government forms and performance in thirty-six countries.* New Haven, CT: Yale University Press.

Marks, G., & Hooghe, L. (2003). Contrasting visions of multi-level governance. In I. Bache & M. Flinders (Eds.), *Multi-level governance* (pp. 15–30). Oxford: Oxford University Press.

Meeus, T.-J. (2015, November 7/8). Bericht uit Den Haag: Burger, u bent nog lang niet boos genoeg. *NRC Handelsblad*, 17.

Moury, C. (2011). Coalition agreement and party mandate: How coalition agreements constrain the ministers. *Party Politics, 17*(3), 385–404. https://doi.org/10.1177/1354068810372099

Moury, C., & Timmermans, A. (2013). Case study three: The Netherlands. In *Coalition government and party mandate: How coalition agreements constrain ministerial action.* New York: Routledge.

Mulder, J., Bommelé, J., Branderhorst, D., & Hasselt, N. v. (2016). *De Rookvrije Generatie als kans voor gemeenten. Een needs-assessment onder gemeentelijke beleidsmakers en GGD-adviseurs.* Utrecht: Trimbos-instituut.

NRC. (2010). Onderzoek: overheid faalt bij projecten gezondheid. *NRC Handelsblad.* Retrieved from https://www.nrc.nl/nieuws/2010/03/25/overheid-faalt-bij-projecten-gezondheid-11868351-a282303

Obinger, H., & Wagschal, U. (2001). Families of nations and public policy. *West European Politics, 24*(1), 99–114. https://doi.org/10.1080/01402380108425419

Okhuijsen, S. (2012). Fractiediscipline tweede kamer op 99,998%. Retrieved March 8, 2016, from http://sargasso.nl/fractiediscipline-tweede-kamer-op-99999/

Rommetvedt, H., Thesen, G., Christiansen, P. M., & Nørgaard, A. S. (2012). Coping with corporatism in decline and the revival of parliament: Interest group lobbyism in Denmark and Norway, 1980–2005. *Comparative Political Studies, 46*, 457–485.

RVZ. (2010). *Perspectief op gezondheid 20/20.* Den Haag: Raad voor de Volksgezondheid en Zorg.

RVZ. (2011). *Preventie van welvaartsziekten. Effectief en efficiënt georganiseerd.* Den Haag: Raad voor de Volksgezondheid en Zorg (RVZ).

Sabatier, P. A. (2007). *Theories of the policy process* (2nd ed.). Cambridge, MA: Westview Press.

Scharpf, F. W. (1997). *Games real actors play: Actor-centred institutionalism in policy research.* Oxford: Westview Press.

Scheltema Beduin, A., & Ter Weele, W. (2015). *Lifting the lid on lobbying: Enhancing trust in public decisionmaking in the Netherlands*. Amsterdam: Transparency International Nederland.

Siaroff, A. (1999). Corporatism in 24 industrial democracies: Meaning and measurement. *European Journal of Political Research, 36*, 175–205.

Slob, M., & Staman, J. (2012). *Beleid en het bewijsbeest: Een verkenning van verwachtingen en praktijken rond evidence based policy*. Den Haag: Rathenau Instituut.

Smith, K. E. (2013). Understanding the influence of evidence in public health policy: What can we learn from the 'Tobacco Wars'? *Social Policy & Administration, 47*(4), 382–398. https://doi.org/10.1111/spol.12025

Smith, K. E., Fooks, G., Collin, J., Weishaar, H., Mandal, S., & Gilmore, A. B. (2010). "Working the System"—British American Tobacco's influence on the European Union treaty and its implications for policy: An analysis of internal tobacco industry documents. *PLoS Medicine, 7*(1), e1000202. https://doi.org/10.1371/journal.pmed.1000202

Smith, K. E., Fooks, G., Gilmore, A. B., Collin, J., & Weishaar, H. (2015). Corporate coalitions and policy making in the European Union: How and why British American Tobacco promoted "Better Regulation". *Journal of Health Politics, Policy and Law, 40*(2), 325–372. https://doi.org/10.1215/03616878-2882231

Studlar, D. T. (2007). *What explains policy change in tobacco control policy in advanced industrial democracies?* Paper presented at the European Consortium of Political Research, Helsinki.

Van den Braak, B. H., & Van den Berg, J. T. J. (2017). Kabinetsformatie sinds 1945. *Parlement & Politiek*. Retrieved August 23, 2017, from http://www.parlement.com/id/vh8lnhrsr2z2/kabinetsformaties_sinds_1945

Van der Meer, R., Spruijt, R., & De Beer, M. (2012). *Zoeken naar Nieuwe Kansen voor Lokaal Gezondheidsbeleid en Roken Project Structureel Aanbod Gemeenten Tabakspreventie Eindrapportage 2011*. The Hague: STIVORO.

Van der Poel, T., & Gutter, A. (2011). Transcripten interviews. *Dutch Tobacco Industry Collection*, Bates No. JB0561. Retrieved from https://www.industrydocumentslibrary.ucsf.edu/tobacco/results/#q=transcripten%20interviews&col=%5B%22Dutch%20Tobacco%20Industry%20Collection%22%5D&h=%7B%22hideDuplicates%22%3Atrue%2C%22hideFolders%22%3Atrue%7D&subsite=tobacco&cache=true&count=3

Van der Voet, G. W. (2005). *De kwaliteit van de WMCZ als medezeggenschapswet*. Den Haag: Boom Juridische Uitgevers.

Van Outeren, E., & Pergrim, C. (2015, November 11). Weer zet de denaat er een streep door. *NRC Handelsblad*, 9.

Van Tulder, R. (1999). Small, smart and sustainable? Policy challenges to the Dutch model of governance (together) with multinationals. In R. Narula & R. van Hoesel (Eds.), *Multinational enterprises from the Netherlands*. London: Routledge.

VWS. (2011a). *Gezondheid dichtbij. Landelijke nota gezondheidsbeleid*. Den Haag: Ministerie van VWS.

VWS. (2011b). *Wet publieke gezondheid: De preventiecyclus*. Den Haag: Ministerie van VWS.

WVC. (1986). Over de ontwikkeling van gezondheidsbeleid: feiten, beschouwingen en beleidsvoornemens (Nota 2000). *Handelingen II, 1985–1986, 19500, nr 1–2*.

WVC. (1991). Gezondheid met beleid. *Handelingen II, 1991–1992, 22459, nr 2*.

Open Access This chapter is licensed under the terms of the Creative Commons Attribution 4.0 International License (http://creativecommons.org/licenses/by/4.0/), which permits use, sharing, adaptation, distribution and reproduction in any medium or format, as long as you give appropriate credit to the original author(s) and the source, provide a link to the Creative Commons license and indicate if changes were made.

The images or other third party material in this chapter are included in the chapter's Creative Commons license, unless indicated otherwise in a credit line to the material. If material is not included in the chapter's Creative Commons license and your intended use is not permitted by statutory regulation or exceeds the permitted use, you will need to obtain permission directly from the copyright holder.

CHAPTER 6

The International Context: EU and WHO

Since the 1960s, governments around the world have been developing policies to control tobacco. Countries have employed different combinations of measures (World Bank, 1999), taking national circumstances into account. For example, the United Kingdom attached importance to building a national infrastructure of smoking cessation support in combination with having the highest cigarette prices in Europe, while Australia invested in mass media campaigns and was at the forefront of pictorial health warnings and plain packaging, in addition to high tobacco taxes. In contrast, the United States combined strong smoking bans to protect non-smokers, with restrictions on the sale of tobacco to youth and a long history of litigation against the tobacco industry, but has relatively low cigarette taxes, modest health warnings on cigarette packs, and weak advertising restrictions (Kagan & Nelson, 2001). Despite such differences, there is an increasing convergence of strategies across countries (Studlar, 2006). There are two aspects to this. The first is the process of governments and tobacco control coalitions becoming inspired by countries that lead the way, facilitated by increased levels of corporation and coordination of tobacco control advocacy at the international level. The second is the emergence of "hard" international law to which national governments need to abide. This is facilitated by supranational legislation from the EU and WHO forcing countries to adopt similar policies. In Europe these processes add two extra layers of governance above the national and sub-national levels, and as a result tobacco control policymaking has become the outcome of a continuous negotiation among nested governments at several tiers, a process which has been described as multi-level governance (Asare, Cairney, & Studlar, 2009; Marks & Hooghe, 2003).

The previous chapter discussed the division of responsibilities between the national and the local levels. The current chapter examines the relationship between the national and international levels. I start with EU policymaking, followed by an account of the emergence of WHO's Framework Convention on Tobacco Control (FCTC) and what this meant for Dutch national policymaking. A key part of FCTC is Article 5.3, which was included to assure that the tobacco industry is kept away from the process of making tobacco control policy.

European Tobacco Control Policy

The EU developed several mechanisms to coordinate and develop policy-making across EU countries.[1] Nowadays tobacco control laws are part of the EU *acquis communautaire*, the body of laws by which countries that join the EU must abide.

During the first decades of tobacco control, no supranational coordination or legislation existed. The formulation of an EU tobacco control policy began in 1984, when tobacco control was mentioned for the first time as a potential EU task, next to drug addiction and prevention of infectious diseases (European Commission, 1984). The EU regarded it as its task to coordinate the various programmes and actions that individual member states were already taking against tobacco. In 1985 the European Council of Health Ministers announced a programme against cancer, in an attempt to bring the European project closer to the real concerns of Europeans—for cancer was a great concern to many. Smoking was given high priority within this programme, and the Europe Against Cancer programme became a catalyst for EU-initiated tobacco control (Gilmore & McKee, 2004).

The EU developed various ways of controlling tobacco, and it is important to understand the differences. Directives, Decisions, and Regulations are legally binding, while Recommendations and Resolutions are not. Directives must first be transposed into national law and be adjusted to member states' particular circumstances, while Regulations have the immediate force of law. For tobacco control, Directives have been most important. The European Commission (EC) enforces Directives by sending notifications, then issuing warnings, and finally referring to the European Court of Justice when member states do not implement them in their national legislation (Asare et al., 2009). Non-compliance is punished by financial sanctions ("hard law"). Other tobacco control measures such as protection of non-smokers, education, and smoking cessation support are dealt with in Recommendations and Resolutions, which are not legally binding ("soft law"). In addition to hard and soft laws, the EU initiated and funded various tobacco control capacity building activities, such as the European Network of Smoking Prevention (ENSP) and media campaigns to discourage smoking in youth. The Europe Against Cancer programme consisted mainly of educational measures like media campaigns, but it inspired the EC to develop and adopt no less than six Directives, one Regulation, and one Resolution between 1989 and 1992.

The swift adoption at the beginning of the 1990s of so many binding EU measures to control tobacco was possible because the tobacco industry had not yet developed a strong lobbying position in Brussels (Gilmore & McKee, 2004) and the proposed measures were no real threat to individual EU countries since most had already implemented them—such as bans on tobacco advertising on television and text warnings on cigarette packs. In the course of the 1990s the tobacco lobby became more organised. It had some success in delaying or watering down EU initiatives, including tobacco advertising Directives and tobacco product Directives (Costa, Gilmore, Peeters, McKee, & Stuckler, 2014; Hastings & Angus, 2004; Peeters, Costa, Stuckler, McKee, & Gilmore, 2016). However, its effectiveness should not be overrated. For example, in the case of the first Tobacco Product Directive (TPD-1), the industry was unable to prevent the directive from coming into force nor did it manage to dilute it, despite intensive lobbying (Mandal et al., 2009).

The EU's Competence in Tobacco Control

The 1986 Single European Act recognised, albeit in vague terms, health as a factor to take into account when strengthening European economic integration and building a single market, but the EU has never acquired a mandate to issue regulations solely for the sake of public health (Duina & Kurzer, 2004). The EU's public health competence is laid down in article 152 EC (formerly Article 129), which requires that public health be protected in all EU policies and activities. However, the article excludes harmonisation of hard laws and Regulations and therefore cannot serve as a legal basis for tobacco control laws (Boessen & Maarse, 2008; Mandal et al., 2009; Verschuuren, 2011). In the absence of a legal base to regulate smoking, the EU had to fall back on the creative use of other EU treaties (Boessen & Maarse, 2008). After much debate it finally based its competence on tobacco control through EU jurisdiction concerning the internal market (Article 95 EC, formerly Article 100a). All EU tobacco legislation regarding labelling, advertising, and product regulation are founded on the EU's jurisdiction to ensure the free movement of goods and services throughout the EU (Verschuuren, 2011). This is not a clear-cut matter, since it requires the EC to show that tobacco control interventions, which in essence restrict markets, have at least an element that improves internal markets (Boessen & Maarse, 2008). The EC argued that a uniform EU-wide tobacco advertising ban was necessary to end distortion of competition across borders, which might be the result if one country gave advertising agencies more freedom to promote tobacco in magazines and newspapers than did another.

EU's legal competence to control tobacco has frequently been disputed by the tobacco industry, and by some governments. The most notorious example was when the German government challenged the EU's jurisdiction to enforce tobacco advertising restrictions, resulting in an annulment by the European Court of Justice of the advertising Directive, after which the EC was forced to be content with a less comprehensive advertising ban (Mandal et al., 2009). The ban was proposed in 1989 and supported by several countries, notably Italy and France, for whom such a ban would confirm existing national legislation, while the United Kingdom, Denmark, Germany, and the Netherlands opposed and successfully vetoed proposals (Bitton, Neuman, & Glantz, 2002) (see Box 6.1). Duina and Kurzer (2004) argue that these four countries shared "national traditions of libertarianism characterised by minimal state intrusion in the private sphere of consumption," (p. 65) and that the tobacco industry had a strong influence on these governments throughout the 1990s.

Box 6.1 The Dutch blockade of the EU tobacco advertising ban
In 1990 Philip Morris intensified its lobbying efforts against the European advertising Directive (Dollisson, 1990) and very soon "the largest and best financed lobbying campaign ever mounted by tobacco and advertising companies" descended on the members of the European Parliament (Boessen, 2008, p. 77). Because the ban would be based on the EU's jurisdiction over the internal market (Article 95 EC), it was subject to qualified majority voting. For a minority to veto the ban, 26 or more votes were required. The minority at the time consisted of Denmark (3 votes), Germany (10), Greece (5), the Netherlands (5), and the United Kingdom (10). The Netherlands blocked the EU advertising ban for many years, for economic reasons and because it preferred self-regulation, but formally on the grounds that the EC had no legal competence in the field of public health (Boessen & Maarse, 2008). According to a German civil servant, "most legal arguments, especially those regarding competence, were just smoke screens for countries who wanted to block the ban" (Boessen & Maarse, 2008). Philip Morris tried to preserve Dutch opposition through "contacts with the trade ministry to keep the health minister from undermining the Dutch position" and planned to "continue lobbying all country EC ambassadors and health attachés" (Philip Morris, 1993a). In 1993 the Dutch government decided it would reconsider its blocking position only in the event that the Dutch vote became decisive.

A few months after the inauguration of the new Purple cabinet in August 1994, a resolution of the Ninth World Conference on Tobacco or Health in Paris condemned the Netherlands and two other countries for blocking EU advertising legislation (Slama, 1995). Blocking the implementation of the directive was "an international scandal and is detrimental to the health of all citizens of the European Union, and by example of the citizens in all developing regions of the world who look to the European Union for leadership in public health policy" (Tubiana, 1994).

In November 1995 the official position of the Dutch government was still that as long as an EU decision on advertising ban did not depend solely on the Dutch vote, the Dutch national policy was to continue to trust the industry that it could restrain its advertising and promotion efforts without needing direct governmental intrusion.[2] This changed in 1997 after Tony Blair's landslide election victory in the United Kingdom. The new UK Labour government decided to support the ban. Without the United Kingdom in the blocking group, the Dutch vote was no longer crucial. In November 1997 Health Minister Borst joined the United Kingdom in support of the EU proposal. The next month, at the EU Health Ministers' Council meeting, a majority of countries supported the advertising ban, paving the way for the EU to proceed. However, the industry managed to have the advertising Directive annulled by the European Court of Justice, after which a watered down version was adopted in 2003, resulting in Directive 98/43/EC. Denmark, the United Kingdom, France, and the Netherlands choose to use the original, more comprehensive, version of the advertising Directive as the basis for its national tobacco advertising and promotion ban (VWS, 2005).

Impact of the EU on Tobacco Control

The importance of the EU for tobacco control should not be undervalued. Very influential were the second Tobacco Advertising Directive (Directive 2003/33/EC or TAD-2), and the two Tobacco Product Directives (2001/37/EC (TPD-1) and 2014/40/EU (TPD-2)). Nowadays cross-border advertising and promotion of tobacco products is banned throughout the EU. TPD-2 mandated pictorial health warnings, which are now implemented throughout the EU. Other Directives harmonised tobacco taxes across the EU by setting minimum taxation levels, which led to higher prices in southern European countries and in those EU member states that joined in 2004 (ASPECT Consortium, 2004).

Implementation of Directives

Transposition of EU tobacco regulation into national law is more or less a formality, since EU law supersedes national law. However, the tobacco industry may influence the interpretation of an EU law. Since both chambers of the parliament need to approve changes in existing national laws, this offers possibilities for lobbying. In the case of TPD-1, there were lengthy discussions in both houses of parliament about interpretations of the text, fuelled by claims from the industry that the Dutch interpretation was more far-reaching than strictly necessary. One issue was whether the black border around the new health warnings should be included or excluded from the warning space (Lie, Willemsen, De Vries, & Fooks, 2016). Ultimately the Dutch government agreed to the industry's interpretation, against the advice of the EC. Other issues were the requirement for tobacco manufacturers to hand over lists of ingredients, and a ban on misleading wordings on cigarette packs such as "light" and "mild." There were long debates between both houses of parliament and the cabinet in 2002, the result of intensive lobbying by the tobacco industry network through the *Volkspartij voor Vrijheid en Democratie* (People's Party for Freedom and Democracy) (VVD) and *Christen-Democratisch Appèl* (Christian Democratic Party) (CDA). Member of parliament Geert Wilders (then still with the VVD) questioned the government's interpretation that the ban on misleading descriptors such as "light" and "mild" implied that colouring associated with lightness and mildness must also be restricted, so that light shades would be prohibited.[3] He argued that this did not directly follow from the English text of the EU directive, although it might be derived from a strict choice of words in the Dutch translation. Health Minister Bomhoff agreed with Wilders that the Netherlands had no ambition to be a pioneer in Europe, since other countries did not seem to follow the more strict Dutch interpretation. The government asked the EC if they could "correct" the Dutch official translation, confirmed that the English text was leading and that differences in colours within the same brand were thus allowed.

EU Recommendations

EU's Recommendations are less committal than Directives, and are therefore perceived as less important by national policymakers. The EC has issued two Recommendations on tobacco control. The first, in 2003 (Recommendation 2003/54/EC), urged EU countries to develop comprehensive approaches to tobacco control, including measures to prevent tobacco sales to children, restricting access to vending machines, removing tobacco products from self-service displays, prohibiting alternative forms of tobacco promotion not covered by Directive 2003/33/EC, and implementing tax measures to discourage consumption. Since the Netherlands had just implemented its revised Tobacco Act, the EU

Recommendation was hardly noted. The second Recommendation was about the protection of non-smokers and smoking cessation (in line with FCTC article 8), and dated from 2009 (2009/C296/02). It asked member states to optimise protection from exposure to tobacco smoke in workplaces, public places, and public transport. It also called on governments to provide smokers with adequate treatment for tobacco dependence, and to consider plain packaging of tobacco products. This latter idea was particularly threatening to the industry, which lobbied intensively to tone it down. Dutch civil servants were targeted as well (see Box 8.3 in Chap. 8 for a detailed account of how the industry tried to get plain packaging out of the Recommendation).

The Principle of Subsidiarity

In 1992 the EU introduced the criterion of subsidiarity, which means that the EU may only intervene by means of a Regulation or Directive if it can act more effectively than individual member states are able to. This principle made it harder to implement EU-wide tobacco control regulation and was explicitly used in industry argumentation. According to Philip Morris, "in order to delay EU action we shall dialogue with supportive governments (the United Kingdom, Germany, Holland and Denmark) to encourage their opposition to EU legislation on the grounds of subsidiarity" (Philip Morris, 1993b). This strategy was indeed frequently applied in the Netherlands, where it resonated well with Christian Democratic principles. Already, in the beginning of the 1990s, the Dutch government had rejected the proposal for a tobacco advertising Directive on the grounds that this could better be resolved at a national level.[4] Box 6.1 talked about the Dutch government's opposition to the EU advertising ban. An internal industry document emphasised that "the United Kingdom and the Netherlands are the two member states which are the most opposed to the proposal, on the grounds of subsidiarity and proportionality. They believe that the means are too strong to achieve the objectives, and that the member states should regulate the situation themselves" (BAT, 1996). The same reasoning was heard in 2007 when the government replied to consultation from the EC about the best policy to protect Europeans from tobacco smoke (the green paper *Towards a Europe free from tobacco smoke: Policy options at EU level* (European Commission, 2007)). The advice of the government was to leave it to member states to decide on smoking bans, a decision motivated by increased negative public opinion of the

Brussels bureaucracy in the Netherlands (De Goeij, 2007). Since 2006 not only the government but also both chambers of parliament have tested new EU regulations by conducting a "subsidiarity check," in response to increased calls from society to reduce the power of Brussels.

Coordination of Tobacco Control Policy Across the EU

In 2001, across country coordination between national- and EU-level tobacco control was strengthened by the establishment of a regulatory committee for tobacco control, under Article 10 of Directive 2001/37/EC. Once a year officials from the European national health ministries met in this committee, coordinated by the EC's Health Directorate. They discussed the progress of implementation of EU regulations in the various countries and were informed by the EC of the next steps towards EU tobacco control. The Netherlands was a steadfast participant at these meetings, which were also attended by the *Rijksinstituut voor Volksgezondheid en Milieu* (National Institute for Public Health and the Environment) (RIVM) and sometimes by the *Nederlandse Voedsel en Waren Autoriteit* (Netherlands Food and Consumer Product Safety Authority) (NVWA) (European Commission, 2017b). In 2014 the committee was replaced by an "expert group"; it has basically the same civil servants, but meets about four times per year (European Commission, 2017a). There are subgroups on issues such as tobacco ingredients and electronic cigarettes. This is an important network for civil servants who work on tobacco control, because this is where they exchange experiences and can support each other over practical and legal problems related to the implementation of EU tobacco control regulations. It is also a platform where country representatives discuss measures that member states may take that go beyond minimum EU requirements, such as tobacco product display bans, higher age limits for sales, and plain packaging. According to a Dutch participant in these meetings, "international cooperation increases our knowledge and offers new insights to reduce tobacco use further" (Mackay, 2017). Tobacco control has also been an important topic during most of the meetings of the European health ministers, who convene about twice a year in Brussels. The influence of the European Health Council thus goes beyond the adoption of new regulations or recommendations: the ministers exchange ideas and may learn from colleagues how to advance tobacco control at the national level (ASPECT Consortium, 2004, p. 115).

The World Health Organization

WHO is a specialised agency of the United Nations concerned with international public health. It is the main driving force for global tobacco control (Mamudu, Cairney, & Studlar, 2015). National tobacco control initiatives are increasingly developed in response to WHO recommendations and, after the FCTC treaty was adopted in 2015, following FCTC requirements. The FCTC treaty was the end station of a long process by experts and WHO officials working towards a global tobacco control treaty (Mamudu, Gonzalez, & Glantz, 2011). According to WHO, the main pillars of a comprehensive tobacco control approach include measures that reduce the supply of tobacco (bans on tobacco advertising and promotion, and the use of taxation to increase tobacco prices), the demand for tobacco (mass media awareness campaigns and providing effective smoking cessation support to quitters), and the protection of non-smokers through smoking bans. These elements were already well known in the Netherlands in the 1980s (Baan, 1986) and are reminiscent of the recommendations from the earlier Health Council's report (Beernink & Plokker, 1975). In this respect, the FCTC treaty did not offer novel ideas about how to tackle smoking for Dutch tobacco control advocates and Dutch government officials.

In 1994, the World Health Assembly adopted the "International Strategy for Tobacco Control" resolution, which finally, after a long process of negotiation between individual states, led to the FCTC. The treaty came into force in 2005, after the required 40 countries had ratified it. Since then the number of ratifying countries has risen to 180, covering 89% of the world's population (Framework Convention Alliance, 2017). WHO initiated a process of negotiation between participating countries through a series of Conferences of the Parties (COPs) in which guidelines were developed with details on how FCTC articles should be interpreted and implemented.

The Netherlands was among the countries in the EU (others were supposedly Germany, the Czech Republic, Austria, and Slovakia) that were reluctant to sign the FCTC treaty.[5] Only because Dutch civil servants downplayed the consequences for the national tobacco policy, emphasising that WHO had no sanctioning power and that the treaty did not contain strict obligations for the state, and by treating it as a low-key topic, was it possible to get it through the Dutch bureaucracy. The government presented the treaty for tacit approval to both chambers of parliament in

December 2004.[6] It did not go completely unnoticed, for CDA, VVD, and LPF raised concerns about how the treaty would affect the national cigar manufacturing industry.[7] Furthermore, the Dutch Antilles and Aruba did not want to be subject to the treaty, because they were afraid that it could not be implemented and enforced in their part of the kingdom.[8] Nevertheless, on 27 January 2005 the Netherlands ratified FCTC and the treaty came into force one month later.

Importance of WHO's FCTC Treaty for the Netherlands

The FCTC did not play a significant role in the Netherlands in the first years after ratification, although there was a passing reference to it in the National Tobacco Control Plan 2006–2010 (STIVORO, 2005; VWS, 2006) and the Partnership Stop Smoking[9] identified FCTC as setting "minimum norms for an effective policy to reduce the harm from tobacco" (Partnership Stop met Roken, 2004). It seldom surfaced during the regular talks between the *Stichting Volksgezondheid en Roken* (Dutch Smoking or Health Foundation) (STIVORO) and civil servants from the Ministry of Health, where mutual tobacco control campaigns and activities were discussed. Officials from the ministry were content that they had succeeded in having the Netherlands sign and ratify the FCTC, without opposition from parliament. They avoided discussions about whether the Netherlands was sufficiently compliant. Dutch officials, including the Council of State, had taken a close look at the text of the treaty and concluded that, strictly speaking, the Netherlands was already complying with the main FCTC requirements. They felt they could argue that the government was compliant, although they knew that there were many areas where the FCTC text went further than the Tobacco Act—certainly in its spirit.[10] One ex-civil servant commented: "We felt that we had already accomplished a lot at the time: the smoke-free workplaces and advertising bans. We had the feeling that it [FCTC] was too late and superfluous."[11] There also was an understanding among bureaucrats that FCTC was mostly relevant to third-world countries, who could use the treaty as leverage to improve tobacco policy, but that it was less relevant in the Dutch context.

Around 2010 the FCTC was finally given more consideration, after the first Rutte cabinet announced that finance for tobacco control would be cut and tobacco control measures were to be reversed. STIVORO responded by emphasising the government's neglect of its FCTC requirements. STIVORO became a member of the international lobbying organisation Framework Convention Alliance (FCA), set up in 1999 by the United Kingdom's Action on Smoking and Health (ASH) with support from WHO as a central coordinating network of tobacco control advocates during FCTC negotiations and to push governments to implement the FCTC (Gneiting & Schmitz, 2016; Mamudu & Glantz, 2009).

Implementation of the FCTC Treaty

By signing and ratifying the FCTC, a country commits to implementing the policies that are part of the treaty. Many elements in the FCTC are mandatory and even legally binding under international law. Governments are required periodically to report to WHO about progress in implementing the FCTC. Every two years, governments meet at a Conference of the Parties (COP)[12] where details of guidelines for implementation and interpretation of the treaty are discussed and established. COPs are opportunities for extensive lobbying, both on the part of the tobacco control community (organised by the Framework Convention Alliance), and the tobacco industry lobby (Kalra, Bansal, Wilson, & Lasseter, 2017). Before and during COP meetings, governments try to come to agreement over the final text of new guidelines, which often requires compromises. This creates difficult situations in cases where the subject matter of the guideline is also on a national policy agenda, and government representatives may abstain from voting, in order not to undermine the (oftentimes more important) negotiations at the national parliament.

The Role of NGO's

Although FCTC is legally binding upon governments, just like in other UN treaties there are no effective enforcement mechanisms. It is therefore left to civil society to make governments accountable, and even challenge them in court in the case of non-compliance. In some countries, tobacco control non-governmental organisations (NGOs) published "shadow reports" that told a more critical story than the periodic implementation progress reports that governments have to send to the WHO. Inspired by a shadow report from Canada (Global Tobacco Control Forum, 2010), STIVORO published an FCTC shadow report in March 2011 on behalf of the Cancer Society, the Heart Foundation, and the Lung Foundation (Rennen & Willemsen, 2012). The report gave a detailed account of shortcomings regarding the Dutch government's FCTC obligations. Member of parliament Esmé Wiegman (Christian Union party) questioned the health minister on the issue and tabled a motion that the government should develop a comprehensive tobacco control policy in line with FCTC.[13] The *Alliantie Nederland Rookvrij* (Dutch Alliance for a smoke-free society) (ANR) presented a second shadow report in January 2015, which again pointed to the huge gap between current tobacco control policy in the Netherlands and full implementation of the FCTC treaty, although it acknowledged that the government was getting back on track (Heijndijk & Willemsen, 2015).

The correct implementation of one of the FCTC Articles (8.2) was put to the test in a court case by Clean Air Netherlands (CAN) against the Dutch State. In October 2014 the Supreme Court ruled that the Dutch government's decision to exempt small cafes from the smoking ban ran contrary to FCTC Article 8.2, which states that countries shall adopt legislation in order to protect citizens from exposure to tobacco smoke in indoor workplaces and other public places, and should therefore be considered binding. The government responded by reinforcing the smoking ban in all cafes. This was the first time anywhere in the world that a national court decided that an FCTC requirement outranked a contradictory national law (Campaign for smoke-free kids, 2014).

FCTC's Article 5.3: Excluding the Industry from Tobacco Control Policymaking

A key element in the FCTC treaty is Article 5.3, which aims to exclude tobacco industry lobbyists from the policymaking process. WHO FCTC Article 5.3 states: "In setting and implementing their public health policies with respect to tobacco control, Parties shall act to protect these policies from commercial and other vested interests of the tobacco industry in accordance with national law"(WHO, 2003). In 2008 at the third Conference of the Parties in Durham, South Africa, further guidelines for the implementation of Article 5.3 were approved (WHO, 2008). A few weeks later in a personal meeting in December, Dutch Health Minister Klink talked with the *Stichting Sigaretten Industrie* (Dutch Cigarette Manufacturers Association) (SSI) and *Vereniging Nederlandse Kerftabakindustrie* (Dutch Fine Cut Tobacco Industry Association) (VNK) about the consequences of the outcomes of the COP. Klink confirmed that the Netherlands had expressed reservations about the implementation of the guidelines, declaring that because the sale of tobacco is a legal economic activity, it must remain possible to have contacts with all stakeholders, including the tobacco industry. According to a summary of the meeting written by the industry, Klink referred to the principle of subsidiarity, a central element in CDA ideology and central in EU regulation: "The Netherlands (…) should not have to implement FCTC guidelines if it already has a good prevention policy in place" (SSI & VNK, 2009). Klink affirmed that he was happy to continue talking with the industry and hearing their side of the argument regarding tobacco control policy proposals.

Following frequent media attention and parliamentary questions about contacts between the government and the tobacco industry at the end of 2011 and the beginning of 2012, the *Stichting Rookpreventie Jeugd* (Youth Smoking Prevention Foundation) (SRJ) took the State to court for violating Article 5.3. Under the Dutch Freedom of Information Act, it had obtained hundreds of documents revealing contacts between Dutch government officials and the tobacco industry over the period 2009–2014. Although the case was lost in court, the government did set up rules to clarify Article 5.3 requirements (Youth Smoking Prevention Foundation, 2015). This was facilitated by a report commissioned by ANR, which outlined to the government how it should implement the article (Oude Gracht Groep, 2015), and technical instructions from WHO on implementation of Article 5.3 (WHO, 2012). In September 2015 State Secretary van Rijn sent a letter to both chambers of parliament outlining the government's policy regarding contacts with the tobacco industry,[14] and in March 2016 a protocol was published and sent to all levels of government (ministries, provinces, municipalities) (VWS, 2016). Government officials were required to be restrained in their contacts with the tobacco industry "to prevent the industry from having influence on policy. That is why contacts (…) must be restricted to matters of technical execution." Regular meetings were no longer allowed, contacts had to be transparent, and notes of meetings were to be published on the internet, including letters and email contacts.[15] Cooperation with the industry as part of corporate social responsibility activities was regarded as subject to Article 5.3 as well. Since then, it has become substantially more difficult for industry representatives and lobbyists to get an appointment with a government official (Scheltema Beduin & Ter Weele, 2015, pp. 65–66; Van der Lugt, 2016).

Conclusion

Tobacco policy is no longer the exclusive domain of the national government. Sovereignty is shared with supranational legislative bodies, especially the EU and WHO. The EU has a notoriously weak tobacco control regime, with restricted jurisdiction (only binding regulation if it contributes to free movement of goods and services across the EU), a slow policy formation process subject to intensive industry lobby, and a tendency to adopt policies after they have been implemented at the national level by most member states. The Dutch government is generally critical of EU interference with national tobacco control policy, and weighs EU proposals against subsidiarity criteria. However, once an EU directive is adopted by the European parliament, the government must transpose it into national law and implement it. In this way, EU regulation has become an important aspect of national tobacco control policy. Most important are EU requirements regarding tobacco packaging and the product itself (tobacco product Directives). In addition to such "hard law," the European tobacco control community has become important as an inspiration and example for national policy efforts, facilitated by coordination from Brussels-based tobacco control advocacy organisations such as the ENSP and the Smoke Free Partnership (SFP), and the fact that government officials (including ministers) frequently confer with colleagues from other EU countries.

It took some time before WHO's FCTC Treaty, which was ratified by the Dutch government in 2005, became influential in the Netherlands. In the first five years after ratification, the treaty had no impact whatever, mainly because it was not recognised by health organisations as a powerful advocacy tool. Since WHO has no mechanism to enforce through sanctions, the main value of the FCTC is that national advocacy organisations can use it to put moral or legal pressure on the government to do more. Only when the Dutch government reversed tobacco control in 2010, and it became clear that the government was on a path of weakening its FCTC commitments, did the FCTC become the benchmark for tobacco control advocacy groups in the Netherlands.

Notes

1. See Lelieveldt and Princen (2011) for an introduction.
2. Parliamentary Papers, 1995–1996, 24126, nr. 7, p. 2.

3. Proceedings II, 26 September 2002, 6, 344.
4. Parliamentary Papers, 1991–1992, 22300 KVI, nr. 36, p. 9.
5. Interview, 6 October 2015.
6. Parliamentary papers II, 2004–2005, 29927, nr. 1.
7. Parliamentary papers II, 2004–2005, 29927, nr. 3.
8. Parliamentary papers II, 2004–2005, 29927, nr. 2.
9. See Chap. 9 for a description of the Partnership.
10. Interview, 6 November 2015.
11. Interview, 20 October 2015.
12. The COP is the governing body of the WHO's FCTC and is comprised of all parties to the Convention.
13. Proceedings II, 2011–2012, 32,793, nr. 43; Motion nr. 41 (32,793).
14. Parliamentary Papers II, 2015–2016, 32,011, nr. 47.
15. They can be found on: https://www.rijksoverheid.nl/onderwerpen/roken/transparant-over-contact-tabaksindustrie

References

Asare, B., Cairney, P., & Studlar, D. T. (2009). Federalism and multilevel governance in tobacco policy: The European Union, the United Kingdom, and devolved UK institutions. *Journal of Public Policy, 29*, 79. https://doi.org/10.1017/s0143814x09000993

ASPECT Consortium. (2004). *Tobacco or health in the European Union: Past, present and future*. Luxembourg: European Commission.

Baan, B. (1986). Strategieen ter bevordering van het niet-roken. *Nederlands Tijdschrift voor Geneeskunde, 130*, 1232–1139.

BAT. (1996). EU issues. *British American Tobacco Records*, Bates No. 322122073–322122107. Retrieved from https://www.industrydocumentslibrary.ucsf.edu/tobacco/docs/rkyb0207

Beernink, J. F., & Plokker, J. H. (1975). Maatregelen tot beperking van het roken. Advies van de Gezondheidsraad. *Verslagen, Adviezen, Rapporten* (Vol. 23). Leidschendam: Ministerie van Volksgezondheid en Milieuhygiëne.

Bitton, A., Neuman, M. D., & Glantz, S. A. (2002). *Tobacco industry attempts to subvert European Union tobacco advertising legislation*. San Francisco, CA: Center for Tobacco Control Research and Education University of California.

Boessen, S. (2008). *The politics of European health policy-making: An actor-centred institutionalist analysis* (Doctoral dissertation), Maastricht University, Maastricht.

Boessen, S., & Maarse, H. (2008). The impact of the treaty basis on health policy legislation in the European Union: A case study on the tobacco advertising directive. [20]. *BMC Health Services Research, 8*, 77. https://doi.org/10.1186/1472-6963-8-77

Campaign for smoke-free kids. (2014). Dutch Association of CAN v. Netherlands. Retrieved October 30, 2013, from http://www.tobaccocontrollaws.org/litigation/decisions/nl-20141010-dutch-association-of-can-v.-ne

Costa, H., Gilmore, A. B., Peeters, S., McKee, M., & Stuckler, D. (2014). Quantifying the influence of the tobacco industry on EU governance: Automated content analysis of the EU Tobacco Products Directive. *Tobacco Control, 23*(6), 473–478. https://doi.org/10.1136/tobaccocontrol-2014-051822

De Goeij, J. I. M. (2007). Kabinetsreactie Groenboek rookvrij Europa. *Dutch Tobacco Industry Collection*, Bates No. JB0441. Retrieved from https://www.industrydocumentslibrary.ucsf.edu/tobacco/docs/tthb0191

Dollisson, J. (1990). EEC advertising directive. *Philip Morris Records*, Bates No. 2024671385–2024671388. Retrieved from http://legacy.library.ucsf.edu/tid/box36e00/pdf?search=%222024671385%201388%22

Duina, F., & Kurzer, P. (2004). Smoke in your eyes: The struggle over tobacco control in the European Union. *Journal of European Public Policy, 1*, 57–77. https://doi.org/10.1080/1350176042000164307

European Commission. (1984). *Cooperation at community level on health related problems. Communication from the Commission to the Council*. Brussels: European Commission.

European Commission. (2007). *Green paper towards a Europe free from tobacco smoke: Policy options at EU level*. Brussels: European Commission, Directorate C—Public Health and Risk Assessment.

European Commission. (2017a). Register of communication expert groups and other similar entities: Group of experts on tobacco policy (E03150). Retrieved April 14, 2017, from http://ec.europa.eu/transparency/regexpert/index.cfm?do=groupDetail.groupDetail&groupID=3150

European Commission. (2017b). Tobacco: All events. Retrieved July 7, 2017, from http://ec.europa.eu/health/tobacco/events/index_en.htm#anchor6

Framework Convention Alliance. (2017). Latest ratifications of the WHO FCTC. Retrieved July 7, 2017, from http://www.fctc.org/about-fca/tobacco-control-treaty/latest-ratifications

Gilmore, A., & McKee, M. (2004). Tobacco-control policy in the European Union. In E. A. Feldman & R. Bayer (Eds.), *Unfiltered: Conflicts over tobacco policy and public health* (pp. 219–245). London: Harvard University Press.

Global Tobacco Control Forum. (2010). *Canada's implementation of the Framework Convention on Tobacco Control: A civil society 'shadow report'*. Ottawa: Global Tobacco Control Forum (GTCF).

Gneiting, U., & Schmitz, H. P. (2016). Comparing global alcohol and tobacco control efforts: Network formation and evolution in international health governance. *Health Policy Plan, 31*(Suppl 1), i98–i109. https://doi.org/10.1093/heapol/czv125

Hastings, G., & Angus, K. (2004). The influence of the tobacco industry on European tobacco-control policy. In The ASPECT Consortium (Ed.), *Tobacco or health in the European Union: Past, present and future*. Luxembourg: European Commission.

Heijndijk, S. M., & Willemsen, M. C. (2015). *Dutch tobacco control: Moving towards the right track?* FCTC Shadow Report 2014. Den Haag: Alliantie Nederland Rookvrij.

Kagan, R. A., & Nelson, W. P. (2001). The politics of tobacco regulation in the United States. In R. Rabin & S. Sugarman (Eds.), *Regulating tobacco* (pp. 11–38). New York: Oxford University Press.

Kalra, A., Bansal, P., Wilson, D., & Lasseter, T. (2017). Inside Philip Morris' campaign to subvert the global anti-smoking treaty. Retrieved July 15, 2017, from https://www.reuters.com/investigates/special-report/pmi-who-fctc/

Lelieveldt, H., & Princen, S. (2011). *The politics of the European Union*. Cambridge: Cambridge University Press.

Lie, J., Willemsen, M. C., De Vries, N. K., & Fooks, G. (2016). The devil is in the detail: Tobacco industry political influence in the Dutch implementation of the 2001 EU Tobacco Products Directive. *Tobacco Control, 25*, 545–550. https://doi.org/10.1136/tobaccocontrol-2015-052302

Mackay, C. (2017). Internationale samenwerking tegen tabak. *Columns NET*. Retrieved April 14, 2017, from http://columns-net.trimbos.nl/column-03-2017

Mamudu, H., & Glantz, S. A. (2009). Civil society and the negotiation of the Framework Convention on Tobacco Control. *Global Public Health, 4*(2), 150–168. https://doi.org/10.1080/17441690802095355

Mamudu, H., Gonzalez, M., & Glantz, S. (2011). The nature, scope, and development of the global tobacco control epistemic community. *American Journal of Public Health, 101*(11), 2044–2054. https://doi.org/10.2105/AJPH.2011.300303

Mamudu, H. M., Cairney, P., & Studlar, D. T. (2015). Global public policy: Does the new venue for transnational tobacco control challenge the old way of doing things? *Public Administration, 93*(4), 856–873. https://doi.org/10.1111/padm.12143

Mandal, S., Gilmore, A. B., Collin, J., Weishaar, H., Smith, K., & McKee, M. (2009). *Block, amend, delay: Tobacco industry efforts to influence the European Union's Tobacco Products Directive (2001/37/EC)*. Bath: University of Bath, School for Health.

Marks, G., & Hooghe, L. (2003). Contrasting visions of multi-level governance. In I. Bache & M. Flinders (Eds.), *Multi-level governance* (pp. 15–30). Oxford: Oxford University Press.

Oude Gracht Groep. (2015). *Onderzoeks- en adviesrapportage m.b.t. de uitvoering van 'Artikel 5.3 van het WHO-Kaderverdrag inzake tabaksontmoediging (FCTC)' in Nederland*.

Partnership Stop met Roken. (2004). *Beleidsaanbevelingen voor de behandeling van tabaksverslaving*. Den Haag: Partnership Stop met Roken.
Peeters, S., Costa, H., Stuckler, D., McKee, M., & Gilmore, A. B. (2016). The revision of the 2014 European tobacco products directive: An analysis of the tobacco industry's attempts to 'break the health silo'. *Tobacco Control, 25*(1), 108–117. https://doi.org/10.1136/tobaccocontrol-2014-051919
Philip Morris. (1993a). Marketing freedoms. *Philip Morris Records*, Bates No. 2501021740-2501021746. Retrieved from http://legacy.library.ucsf.edu/tid/wet19e00
Philip Morris. (1993b). Smoking restrictions 3 year plan. *Philip Morris Records*, Bates No. 2025497291–2025497303. Retrieved from http://legacy.library.ucsf.edu/tid/vlz88e00
Rennen, E., & Willemsen, M. C. (2012). *Dutch tobacco control: Out of control? FCTC shadow report 2011*. Amsterdam: KWF Kankerbestrijding.
Scheltema Beduin, A., & Ter Weele, W. (2015). *Lifting the lid on lobbying: Enhancing trust in public decisionmaking in the Netherlands*. Amsterdam: Transparency International Nederland.
Slama, K. (1995). Resolutions of the Ninth World Conference on Tobacco and Health. In K. Slama (Ed.), *Tobacco and Health* (pp. 1017–1018). New York: Springer.
SSI & VNK. (2009). [Letter to Klink concerning talks about WHO FCTC draft guidelines on December 11]. *Dutch Tobacco Industry Collection*, Bates No. JB0413. Retrieved from https://www.industrydocumentslibrary.ucsf.edu/tobacco/docs/hshb0191
STIVORO. (2005). *Nationaal Programma Tabaksontmoediging 2006–2010*. Den Haag: STIVORO.
Studlar, D. T. (2006). Tobacco control policy instruments in a shrinking world: How much policy learning? *International Journal of Public Administration, 29*, 367–396. https://doi.org/10.1080/01900690500437006
Tubiana, M. (1994). [Letter from Tubiana to Borst-Eilers and Prime Minister Kok]. *Dutch Tobacco Industry Collection*, Bates No. JB2584. Retrieved from https://www.industrydocumentslibrary.ucsf.edu/tobacco/docs/hphp0219
Van der Lugt, P. (Producer). (2016, May 20). Nieuwe tabaksregels dwingen industrie tot bezinning. [Written article]. Retrieved from https://www.ftm.nl/artikelen/nieuwe-sigarettenpakjes-doen-harde-tabakslobby-veranderen
Verschuuren, M. (2011). *International policy overview: Smoking*. Bilthoven: RIVM.
VWS. (2005). *Tobacco Act: Tobacco control in the Netherlands* (International Publication Series Health, Welfare and Sport no. 22). The Hague.
VWS. (2006). *Nationaal Programma Tabaksontmoediging*. Den Haag: Ministerie van VWS.
VWS. (2016). *Protocol over de wijze van omgang met de tabaksindustrie*. Den Haag: Ministerie van VWS.

WHO. (2003). *WHO framework convention on tobacco control*. Geneva: World Health Organization.

WHO. (2008). Elaboration of guidelines for implementation of Article 5.3 of the Convention *Conference of the Parties to the WHO Framework Convention on Tobacco Control Third session Durban, South Africa, 17–22 November 2008*. Geneva: World Health Organisation.

WHO. (2012). *Technical Resource for Country Implementation of WHO FCTC Article 5.3*. Geneva: World Health Organization.

World Bank. (1999). *Curbing the epidemic: Governments and the economics of tobacco control*. Washington: The World Bank.

Youth Smoking Prevention Foundation. (2015). Huge progress made thanks to court case against Dutch State Retrieved May 26, 2017, from http://www.stichtingrookpreventiejeugd.nl/over-rookpreventie-jeugd/english/item/67-huge-progress-made-thanks-to-court-case-against-dutch-state

Open Access This chapter is licensed under the terms of the Creative Commons Attribution 4.0 International License (http://creativecommons.org/licenses/by/4.0/), which permits use, sharing, adaptation, distribution and reproduction in any medium or format, as long as you give appropriate credit to the original author(s) and the source, provide a link to the Creative Commons license and indicate if changes were made.

The images or other third party material in this chapter are included in the chapter's Creative Commons license, unless indicated otherwise in a credit line to the material. If material is not included in the chapter's Creative Commons license and your intended use is not permitted by statutory regulation or exceeds the permitted use, you will need to obtain permission directly from the copyright holder.

CHAPTER 7

Scientific Evidence and Policy Learning

Scientific evidence plays an important role in the policymaking process. Facts about the seriousness of a problem need to be accepted before a problem will be fully addressed, and evidence needs to be available for policymakers to decide about solutions. The Netherlands is among those countries where an evidence-based public health policy is best developed (CHRODIS, 2015; Smith, 2013, p. 4). When the evidence-based movement in public policy reached its apotheosis in the United Kingdom in 1997, with the new Labour government declaring "what matters is what works" (Davies, Nutley, & Smith, 2000), this was already common in the Netherlands. However, sometimes the call for more evidence may paralyse the policy process. There are also limits to the power of evidence. While a prerequisite for current policymaking in the field of public health is that important policy choices are "evidence based," in practice this often means that policy is at best "evidence informed" (Slob & Staman, 2012).

Political scientists make a distinction between ambiguity and uncertainty (Cairney & Oliver, 2017; Cairney, Oliver, & Wellstead, 2016; Majone, 1992; Zahariadis, 2007, pp. 66–67). When considering policy options, ambiguity refers to a state of ambivalence: there are various ways of thinking about an issue (efficacious, moral, ideological, economic) leading to confusion about what to do. This is different from uncertainty. Uncertainty refers to inadequate knowledge and precision to determine whether something is likely to work or not, or about what the exact

© The Author(s) 2018
M. C. Willemsen, *Tobacco Control Policy in the Netherlands*,
Palgrave Studies in Public Health Policy Research,
https://doi.org/10.1007/978-3-319-72368-6_7

magnitude of a problem is. Scientists and research institutes regard their role primarily as a source of uncertainty reduction, producing evidence about the size of a problem and the effectiveness and cost-effectiveness of policy options. Collecting more data will reduce uncertainty but not necessarily ambiguity. Ambiguity is resolved by argument. The process of agenda setting (discussed in Chap. 10) is primarily about resolving ambiguity through issue framing: drawing attention to one specific way of perceiving the problem so that policymakers feel more comfortable with a solution. Even in the field of tobacco control, which is widely regarded as a field with abundant scientific evidence—and there are many examples where scientific evidence has played a key role in policy debates—merely producing evidence with scientific rigour is not enough. International experts ranked the availability of scientific evidence as "having had a 'substantial' impact on the adoption of clean indoor air policy, taxation and cessation treatment policy, and a 'modest' effect on all of the other policy areas" (Warner & Tam, 2012). Advocates need to find ways to combine the scientific evidence with effective messages that appeal to policymakers (American Cancer Society, 2003).

This chapter takes a closer look at how the Dutch government responded to scientific facts about the health risks associated with active and passive smoking. It describes how and when the health risk definitely became accepted as "scientific fact" by the government. This happened somewhat later in the Netherlands than in leading countries. Attention will be paid to the diffusion of ideas and knowledge, from the international tobacco control community to the national setting. Since tobacco control policy does not automatically follow best evidence, I also explore the mediating role of ideology on knowledge diffusion and emulation.[1]

Evidence About the Risks of Smoking

The Dutch Health Council noted already in 1957 that lung cancer rates had increased to an alarmingly high level and that this was associated with smoking (Wester, 1957). However, the members of the council could not reach consensus about whether the association was causal, and "from a psychological standpoint, focusing too much on a possible causal relation between smoking and lung cancer has great disadvantages." Following advice from the council, the government made an official warning through the media to young people not to smoke, but phrased in a way that would not distress older, addicted smokers. The government responded to the

Health Council's advice by instructing a second Health Council committee to make a plan for *how* youth should be approached, and some general warnings through the media (Bouma, 2001). The passive Dutch governmental response was in contrast to the US government, which quickly mandated warning labels on cigarettes and initiated a ban on broadcasting cigarette advertisements.

When a new compelling report from the UK Royal College of Physicians came out in 1971, this was quickly translated and widely distributed in the Netherlands by the Dutch Cancer Society (Meinsma, 1972). However, while in the United Kingdom health warnings appeared on cigarette packs in 1971 and the government allowed their health education committee to run explicit media campaigns to confront the public with the devastating harm that smoking inflicts, the Dutch government needed more than ten years of further study and deliberation before cigarette packs were provided with health warnings.[2] Media awareness campaigns showing the health damage to smokers did not appear in the Netherlands.

Instead of taking action, State Secretary for Health Roelof Kruisinga commissioned the Health Council to write a new (the third one) report, this time on how to address the tobacco problem. The report (discussed in Chap. 2) called for an integrative set of policy measures (Beernink & Plokker, 1975). However, the report was not as outspoken about the gravity of the risks of smoking as US and UK reports. The council estimated that smoking causes about 12,000 deaths per year, but it did not elaborate on specific health damages (Beernink & Plokker, 1975). The section discussing the evidence about health consequences was barely more than four pages long. The subsequent report by the *Interdepartementale Commissie Beperking Tabaksgebruik* (Interdepartmental Committee for Reducing Tobacco Use) (ICBT) (discussed in Chap. 2), issued to formulate proposals for regulative measures, was even more vague: "the starting point for the commission has been that, based on scientific studies, it is certain that the use of tobacco products, particularly cigarettes and roll-your-own tobacco, has a harmful effect on the health of the user" (ICBT, 1981). Both the ICBT report and the Health Council report noted that the effects depended on factors such as number of cigarettes smoked per day, the choice of tobacco, use of filters, way of smoking, and number of years of smoking. Mainstream thinking about smoking in these years, even among Dutch academics, was that it was possible to smoke "sensibly," (Drogendijk, 1978). In an interview in 1999, Borst said that the Health

Council should have sent out a more powerful message about the health risks of smoking between 1956 and 1975 (Bouma, 1999). With some understatement, she remarked about the late introduction of the health warnings that "a little late might ... be defendable, but much later is not very nice."

Debates About Second-Hand Smoke

At the end of the 1970s the government contemplated the need to protect non-smokers from exposure to tobacco smoke. The main motive was to accommodate the wishes of non-smokers; health concerns did not yet play a role.[3] There was considerable disagreement about the seriousness of health risks for non-smokers. Dutch Cancer Society's director Lenze Meinsma, the main health activist at the time, did not believe that the risks of environmental tobacco smoke (ETS) were important enough for government interference. In the 1980s the government regarded passive smoking as problematic because it caused hindrance and discomfort. Complaining non-smokers could suffer social isolation or conflict at work, while vulnerable groups like babies and asthma patients might suffer from direct exposure.[4]

The year 1986 is generally regarded as the year that the public perception of second-hand smoke risks changed worldwide. Two reports from the United States presented comprehensive and authoritative scientific accounts of the health risks (National Research Council, 1986; US Surgeon General, 1986). In addition, the WHO-affiliated International Agency for Research on Cancer concluded that "passive smoking gives rise to some risk of cancer" (IARC, 1986). In an effort to estimate the health risks for the Dutch population, State Secretary for Health Dick Dees ordered the Health Council in 1989 to critically examine the existing international scientific evidence, taking the international reports as their starting point. The Dutch Health Council reviewed the reports and concluded that it was very likely that prolonged exposure to ETS increased the risk of lung cancer (Gezondheidsraad, 1990). However, the report was more restrained than the US reports. The Surgeon General Report's major conclusion that "involuntary smoking is a cause of disease, including lung cancer, in healthy non-smokers" (US Surgeon General, 1986) was re-formulated by the Dutch Health Council as "it is likely that long-term exposure to tobacco smoke may increase the lung cancer risk of non-smokers," emphasising that the increase "could be partly due to flaws in the design of the epidemiological studies." Although the US National

Research Council experts did recognise misclassification problems and methodological difficulties in estimating the number of cancer cases, they felt confident enough to conclude from the evidence that about 21% of the lung cancers in non-smoking women and 20% in non-smoking men were attributable to exposure to tobacco smoke (National Research Council, 1986). The Dutch Health Council was more cautious and concluded that a quantitative estimation of the risk was not possible.

In the 1980s the evidence about the health consequences of prolonged exposure to second-hand smoke were thus less definitive in the Netherlands than in the United States. The Dutch tobacco control health network realised that the issue of involuntary smoking was key to getting public and political support for stronger tobacco control. The *Stichting Volksgezondheid en Roken* (Dutch Smoking or Health Foundation) (STIVORO), on behalf of the three charities which sat on their board and with support from the ministry, started campaigns to educate the public about the risks. This brought STIVORO into direct conflict with the industry, which continued to cast doubt on the established scientific knowledge (see Chap. 9).

In 1992, a report from the US Environmental Protection Agency declared tobacco smoke a human carcinogen, and concluded that second-hand smoke is a cause of lung cancer in non-smoking adults (EPA, 1992). Epidemiologists from the Dutch Cancer Institute estimated, based on the US Environmental Protection Agency (EPA) report, that in the Netherlands each year between 110 and 270 people died because of exposure to ETS (Jansen, Van Barneveld, & Van Leeuwen, 1993). When the EPA's conclusions about the causal effect of exposure to ETS and lung cancer were attacked by the tobacco industry through a high-profile advertising and public relations campaign (Oreskes & Conway, 2010), the EPA quickly set the record straight with a decisive rebuttal (EPA, 1994). Despite the endorsement of the EPA for the conclusions of the Dutch scientists, it took another ten years before the Dutch Health Council felt confident enough to quantify the risk.

Involuntary smoking continued to be the subject of debate, ignited by tobacco industry think tanks, smokers' rights groups, and industry-sponsored scientists. Surveys among Dutch employees in 1993 found that only 49% of non-smokers and 25% of smokers believed that non-smokers had more chance of getting cancer because of exposure to tobacco smoke in the workplace (Willemsen, De Vries, & Genders, 1996). In the United Kingdom the matter was more or less settled in 1998 with a meta-analysis of the evidence by the Scientific Committee on Tobacco and Health (SCOTH, 1998). In 1996 researchers commissioned by Philip Morris reviewed the available evidence from industry-led studies worldwide about public perceptions of the risks of environmental tobacco smoke. They reported that the belief that ETS was "a serious health risk" was lowest in the Netherlands (21% agreed), compared with other European countries surveyed (e.g., Germany 30%, Ireland 30%, the United Kingdom 42%, France 52%, and Italy 53%) (Philip Morris, 1996).

The Dutch Health Council finally concluded in 2003 that exposure to ETS increased the risk of lung cancer by 20%, resulting in "several hundreds of lung cancer deaths" per year and an additional "several thousands" of deaths as a result of heart disease (Gezondheidsraad, 2003). This was more than 15 years after US reports had come to similar conclusions.

THE EVIDENCE BASE FOR TOBACCO CONTROL POLICY

Nowadays international scientific knowledge about what works best to reduce smoking, and *how* it works, is immense. Hoffman and Toan (2015), in a review of reviews, identified 59 systematic reviews covering 1150 primary studies of the likely population impact of measures that are part of the Framework Convention of Tobacco Control (FCTC). Evidence was most robust for the effect of smoking bans (they improve population health outcomes through reduced exposure to tobacco smoke, and reduced smoking) and raising tobacco prices (they decrease cigarette consumption, stimulate smoking cessation, and lower population smoking rates). Increasing the price of tobacco was by far the most effective policy instrument to reduce tobacco consumption (Chaloupka, Straif, & Leon, 2011; Chaloupka, Yurekli, & Fong, 2012; IARC, 2011). Positive results were also found for health warnings on cigarette packs and mass media campaigns, which are most effective as part of larger multicomponent programmes (Hoffman & Toan, 2015). Far more studies have been done on the effects of anti-tobacco media campaigns than on any other health-related topic, so that the evidence base is exceptionally strong (Wakefield, Loken, & Hornik, 2010). The US National Cancer Institute made an extensive review of the scientific literature and identified no less than 25 controlled field experiments with youth media campaigns, 40 with adult targeted campaigns, and 57 population-based state/national mass media campaigns (National Cancer Institute, 2008). Carefully planned and sustained mass media campaigns can change smoking behaviour across large populations (Bala, Strzeszynski, Topor-Madry, & Cahill, 2013; Sims et al., 2014; Wakefield et al., 2010), provided they are adequately budgeted (Durkin, Brennan, & Wakefield, 2012). However, the Dutch government did not invest in national media campaigns to raise awareness of the health consequences of smoking (see Box 7.1). Evidence for advertising bans is less conclusive, but strong enough to conclude that they remain important.

WHO officials and experts who collaborated in drafting the FCTC took as their starting point that the treaty must be evidence-based and follow best practices from leading countries (WHO, 2003; World Bank, 1999). Most of the treaty's articles are grounded on a well-developed evidence base (Warner & Tam, 2012). The main tobacco control building blocks for the global treaty were already laid out in a report from a WHO expert committee in 1979 (WHO, 1979) and were fine-tuned in subsequent WHO reports (Roemer, 1982; WHO, 1998, 2004a, 2004b), substantiated by scientific evidence collated in reports from the US government (CDC, 1999; IOM (Institute of Medicine), 2007; U.S. Department of Health and Human Services, 2000).

WHO understood very early that governments need support and encouragement to implement FCTC measures. One of the strategies was the promotion of "MPOWER," a user-friendly way to single out and bring the six most important "proven policies" to the attention of policymakers (WHO, 2008). These are monitoring smoking and prevention policies (M), protecting people from second-hand smoke (P), offering help to people who want to quit (O), warning about the dangers of tobacco (W), enforcing bans on advertising (E), and raising taxes (R). The MPOWER package was brought to the attention of Dutch politicians and policymakers in 2010 (STIVORO, 2010).

Box 7.1 Confrontational media campaigns to deter smoking
For long, Dutch officials have been sceptical about the ability of media campaigns to influence health behaviour. Scepticism can be traced to a critical report from the Dutch Court of Audit in 1991 that concluded that most government media campaigns were conducted without proper evaluation so that effects were not demonstrable or

negligible (Algemene Rekenkamer, 1991). Parliament demanded immediate cuts in government spending on campaigns and a more critical reflection about their use to influence unhealthy lifestyle. Despite improvements in the general quality of campaign designs, the Health Council concluded 15 years later that mass media campaigns "have, at best, only a modest effect on behaviour," although it was acknowledged that they can be important as part of comprehensive approaches (Gezondheidsraad, 2006).

Tobacco risk awareness campaigns are seen by some as "fear mongering." Ten years ago, the Dutch Health Council advised that fear appeals were not an effective means to influence behaviour and should therefore be avoided (Gezondheidsraad, 2006). There was some debate among Dutch researchers from different scientific backgrounds about the usefulness of this type of campaign for tobacco control (Ruiter & Kok, 2006; Van der Kemp & Bekker, 2007; Zeeman, Willemsen, & van Gennip, 2007). Researchers from different scientific backgrounds may reach different but equally legitimate conclusions when they study the same phenomenon (Sarewitz, 2004), but when this happens, it makes it more difficult for policymakers to reach a decision.

THE INTERNATIONAL TOBACCO CONTROL EPISTEMIC COMMUNITY

The spread of knowledge from one country to another is facilitated and accelerated by "epistemic communities," "networks of professionals with recognised expertise and competence in a particular domain and an authoritative claim to policy relevant knowledge within that domain" (Stronks, van de Mheen, Looman, & Mackenbach, 1997). In the past 50 years, a worldwide tobacco control network has emerged. Its members share a common understanding of the science base for effective tobacco control, shaped after years of interaction and participation in scientific debates about the best way forward (Mamudu, Gonzalez, & Glantz, 2011). A study based on interviews with 181 members from 39 countries between 1999 and 2006 revealed that the international tobacco control network consists of four types of actors: scientists who are also advocates; pure advocates; pure scientists; and expert government officials (Mamudu et al., 2011). To a large extent, they share a "consensual knowledge" about what works best in tobacco control: for example, they view tobacco control as a public health issue, regard tobacco use as an addiction, recognise the strength of the tobacco industry lobby, and advocate a comprehensive approach to tobacco control. This epistemic community is linked through e-mail networks, social media, conferences, international research projects, and international non-governmental organisations, and is dominated by experts from the United States, Australia, and the United Kingdom. Dutch experts play a role, through collaborations with international research networks, such as through the International Tobacco Control (ITC) Policy Evaluation Project (ITC Project, 2015).

The Netherlands is an open country, with one of the highest levels of inhabitants speaking English as a second language. Dutch policymakers are more steered by international developments than politicians in large autarkic societies like the United States, the United Kingdom, Germany, and France. There are few barriers in the Netherlands to prevent the quick diffusion of new ideas and evidence from abroad to policymakers. The process of policies spreading from one government to another is known as "policy diffusion" (Graham, Shipan, & Volden, 2012): when a policy has been proven effective in one country, others learn from its success and adaptation may follow. Policy diffusion can be better understood if we again consider the concept of a "family of nations" (discussed in Chap. 5). The Netherlands belongs to a group of Western-European "continental" countries including Belgium, Germany, and Austria: countries that share similar cultural values and political arrangements. This means that Dutch politicians and policymakers are more likely to look at best practices from these countries and might be sceptical of examples from other families of nations. For example, Health Minister Klink was known to get ideas about tobacco control from German newspapers and magazines. Dutch government officials indeed seem most comfortable looking for best practices within Europe, since tobacco control has more and more become a European Union (EU) affair and the civil servants working in tobacco control meet frequently with their European colleagues (see Chap. 6). Civil servants from the Ministry of Health learn from their colleagues from other European countries at regular, sometimes monthly, meetings in Brussels where they prepare and discuss tobacco legislation. During meetings, European countries look up to countries that are most active during discussions and have most knowledge to share. The Netherlands is in this active group, as are the United Kingdom, France, Belgium, and Scandinavian countries.[5] While the government orients towards European tobacco control, national tobacco control advocacy organisations often look for wider inspiration, particularly to the English-speaking countries which dominate the global tobacco control epistemic community (the United Kingdom, Australia, the United States), sometimes ignoring the fact that these countries have different tobacco control environments and institutional arrangements and might not share the same cultural values.

A second important source for the government is through national knowledge "broker" organisations. These are governmental or semi-governmental expert centres and scientific advisory boards, tasked with producing scientific evidence on which to base policy. It has been shown that the existence of national organisations for scientific knowledge brokering facilitate the uptake of evidence by policymakers (Liverani, Hawkins, & Parkhurst, 2013). In the Netherlands, the *Rijksinstituut voor Volksgezondheid en Milieu* (National Institute for Public Health and the Environment) (RIVM) and the Netherlands Expertise Center for Tobacco Control (NET) at the Trimbos Institute are currently important knowledge brokers for the government on tobacco control policy. The RIVM provides expertise and advice on risks of existing and novel tobacco products, estimates the population impact of measures, and does cost-benefit analyses. The Trimbos Institute's NET reviews the effectiveness of tobacco control measures and monitors national smoking prevalence rates.

Nowadays the EU is an important driver of tobacco control policy convergence and a source of policy learning (see also Chap. 6). Policy learning between tobacco control advocacy groups within Europe takes place through various European tobacco control organisations. The most important ones are the SFP (Smoke Free Partnership), ENSP (European Network of Smoking Prevention), the EHN (European Heart Network), and the ECL (the Association of European Cancer Leagues). Over the years the three Dutch charities (Cancer Society, Heart Foundation, Lung Foundation) built lasting contacts with these groups and organisations. The absorption of tobacco control policy knowledge is further facilitated through the World Conferences on Tobacco or Health (WCToH) and their European equivalents (ECToH). STIVORO and Dutch civil servants from the Ministry of Health visited these international tobacco control conferences, but it is unusual for high-level Dutch government officials, let alone ministers, to attend. One exception occurred in 1983 when State Secretary for Health Joop van der Reijden made a personal visit to the fifth World Conference on Tobacco or Health in Winnipeg, Canada, accompanied by STIVORO's director.

SCIENCE AND IDEOLOGY

Rigorous science is crucial for the establishment of effective tobacco control policy. Simply put, policy that is based on incomplete, incorrect, or bad science is not likely to be effective. However, it is seldom that a new research finding directly alters the way policymakers approach a problem such as tobacco. Rather, according to some scholars, research findings influence policy through a slow process where knowledge eventually filters into policymakers' decisions, a process which has been called "knowledge creep" or "percolation" (Radaelli, 1995; Weiss, 1980). Research findings cumulatively build towards a solid knowledge base, which policymakers use to legitimise their decisions.

For policy change to come about, the science to support the policy must be available the moment that an issue is discussed as part of the policymaking agenda (Schwartz & Rosen, 2004). It is important to understand that evidence is more likely to be used when it informs policymakers about *how* to implement something, rather than whether they *should* (Schwartz & Rosen, 2004). The latter type of decision more likely reflects political preferences (Liverani et al., 2013; Warner & Tam, 2012). As one ex-civil servant explained to me, "Research can never replace policy."[6]

Ideological preferences are likely to determine what policy solutions are selected. Paul Huijts, director-general at the Ministry of Health, said:

> The Health Council does not consider the societal acceptance of a measure in her advice. Of course the ministry has to take that into account. When we expect much resistance against a measure, this can mean that we will not implement that measure—despite the fact that implementation would be scientifically rational. (Slob & Staman, 2012)

He added, "Sometimes a scientific standpoint can clash with the political responsibility that a minister feels."

Ideological differences in the Netherlands tend to centre around three issues. First, whether the government believes that it is able to make the best choices for its citizens—believe in a modifiable society versus regarding state interference as paternalism. Second, whether the government believes that it is always best to start from the notion of own responsibility, respecting citizens' freedom of choice. Thirdly, the importance the government attaches to solidarity between demographic groups. These preferences are explicitly mentioned in an influential Dutch advisory report as the appropriate starting point for the government when it must choose between policy instruments (Werkgroep IBO Gezonde leefstijl, 2016). The first step is to identify which measures have proven effectiveness; the second to select from those the ones that best satisfy the ideological preferences.

Sometimes bureaucrats use evidence for strategic purposes. Seeking advice from an official expertise centre or advisory board is a political act in itself: it signals that the issue at hand is under consideration. It is revealing that the last time the government asked for an official expert's advice about tobacco control was in 1998 (Roscam Abbing, 1998) and it was a report by the Netherlands School of Public Health (NSPH) which became the bedrock on which the revised Tobacco Act was built. Another strategic motive is that policymakers need evidence to show that they have selected the best policy solution. One study from the United Kingdom interviewed policymakers and found that many are sceptical about the importance of research such as systematic literature reviews, impact assessments and health impact modelling to inform policy selection (Stewart & Smith, 2015). Many regard the usefulness of research more for its symbolic value: as a sign of good decision-making, and as a tool to convince proponents and the public that the chosen policy is sensible and responsible.

The role of ideology was particularly evident during the first years that Minister Schippers (2010–2012) was responsible for tobacco control. She consistently used libertarian arguments to underscore that tobacco control is not an issue that the government should be concerned with. When ideological considerations dominate, fact-free politics is often the result. She said in her maiden speech to parliament in 2010, when talking about tobacco control policy, "We are politicians. We are no technocrats who say: this is a list of measures which work best, so this is what we will do automatically. You might then just as well leave it up to a computer."[7] Schippers decided against prevailing evidence and dismantled much of the tobacco control infrastructure.

Conclusion

From the start, Dutch tobacco control policy lacked strong governmental commitment and firm backing by scientific authorities. Reports by the Health Council were hesitant and vague about the dangers of active smoking, despite the availability of alarming authoritative reports from the United States and the United Kingdom, which were very explicit about health risks. The government left it to civil organisations such as the Dutch Cancer Society to communicate about health risks, but these organisations were not in a position to put the issue convincingly on the societal and political agenda, as the government would have been. This has probably contributed to the slow start of the process of tobacco control policy making, relative to other European countries, as concluded in Chap. 3, which examined the tempo of tobacco control efforts in the Netherlands.

Commissioned experts from the Health Council were slow in processing the international body of knowledge about the health risks of second-hand smoke and came to more cautious conclusions than US experts. Disbelief about the health risks of passive smoking was reinforced by targeted actions by the tobacco industry to cast doubt on the science behind the claim that passive smoking causes serious disease and death. This might have contributed to a delay in the adoption of smoking bans—but this was not unique to the Netherlands. The United States and the United Kingdom, where the most authoritative and influential reports were produced, also witnessed a substantial lag between the time that the scientific knowledge on second-hand smoke was "set in stone" at the beginning of the 1990s and the time that the first comprehensive smoking bans were implemented. This was 1995 in California and early to mid-2000s for most other US states, and 2007 in the United Kingdom (two years later than in the Netherlands). Years after the international scientific community had reached consensus, press coverage in most countries continued to proclaim that the research was controversial, quoting industry spokespersons who criticised the epidemiological methodology.

Being from an open country with English as a second language, Dutch tobacco control groups are well connected with the international tobacco control community, dominated by English-speaking countries, particularly the United States, the United Kingdom, and Australia. Dutch government officials tend to look for best practice examples in Europe, as tobacco control is increasingly decided in Brussels. The Dutch government has ample access to information on what works best, including data from semi-governmental expert centres such as the RIVM and the Trimbos Institute. The general level of knowledge about tobacco control policy options is high, but health ministers tend to base their policy choices on political considerations, sometimes disregarding evidence about what is most efficacious and cost-effective. Considerations of deregulation, decentralisation, and budget control are competing issues, and at times more important.

Notes

1. Emulation may be defined as "borrowing ideas and adapting policy approaches, tools or structures to local conditions" (Stone, 2001).
2. This happened in 1982.
3. Proceedings II, 1977–1978, 14,800, hoofdstuk XVII, nr. 34.
4. Proceedings II, Tabakswet 23 juni 1987, 90–4570.
5. Interview, 29 October 2015.
6. Interview, 1 February 2017.
7. Proceedings II, Preventieve gezondheidsprojecten 28 October 2010, 15–14.

References

Algemene Rekenkamer. (1991). *Voorlichtingscampagnes van het Rijk*. Den Haag: SDU.
American Cancer Society. (2003). *Tobacco control strategy planning guide #1. Strategy planning for tobacco control advocacy*. Atlanta, GA: American Cancer Society.
Bala, M. M., Strzeszynski, L., Topor-Madry, R., & Cahill, K. (2013). Mass media interventions for smoking cessation in adults. *Cochrane Database of Systematic Reviews, 6*, CD004704.
Beernink, J. F., & Plokker, J. H. (1975). Maatregelen tot beperking van het roken. Advies van de Gezondheidsraad. *Verslagen, Adviezen, Rapporten* (Vol. 23). Leidschendam: Ministerie van Volksgezondheid en Milieuhygiëne.
Bouma, J. (1999). De overheid werd te laat actief. *Trouw*.
Bouma, J. (2001). *Het rookgordijn: De macht van de Nederlandse tabaksindustrie*. Amsterdam: Veen.
Cairney, P., & Oliver, K. (2017). Evidence-based policymaking is not like evidence-based medicine, so how far should you go to bridge the divide between evidence and policy? *Health Research Policy and Systems, 15*, 35. https://doi.org/10.1186/s12961-017-0192-x

Cairney, P., Oliver, K., & Wellstead, A. (2016). To bridge the divide between evidence and policy: Reduce ambiguity as much as uncertainty. *Public Administration Review, 76*, 399–402.

CDC. (1999). *Best practices for comprehensive tobacco control programs*. Atlanta: U.S. Department of Health and Human Services, Centers for Disease Control and Prevention, National Center for Chronic Disease Prevention and Health Promotion, Office on Smoking and Health.

Chaloupka, F. J., Straif, K., & Leon, M. E. (2011). Effectiveness of tax and price policies in tobacco control. *Tobacco Control, 20*(3), 235–238. https://doi.org/10.1136/tc.2010.039982

Chaloupka, F. J., Yurekli, A., & Fong, G. T. (2012). Tobacco taxes as a tobacco control strategy. *Tobacco Control, 21*(2), 172–180. https://doi.org/10.1136/tobaccocontrol-2011-050417

CHRODIS. (2015). *Health promotion and primary prevention in 14 European countries: A comparative overview of key policies, approaches, gaps and needs*. Brussels: CHRODIS.

Davies, H. T. O., Nutley, S., & Smith, P. C. (Eds.). (2000). *What works? Evidence-based policy and practice in public services*. Bristol: The Policy Press.

Drogendijk, A. C. (1978). *Verstandig roken*. Amsterdam: Buijten & Schipperheijn.

Durkin, S., Brennan, E., & Wakefield, M. (2012). Mass media campaigns to promote smoking cessation among adults: An integrative review. *Tobacco Control, 21*(2), 127–138. https://doi.org/10.1136/tobaccocontrol-2011-050345

EPA. (1992). *Respiratory health effects of passive smoking (also known as exposure to secondhand smoke or Environmental Tobacco Smoke—ETS)*. Washington, DC: U.S. Environmental Protection Agency (EPA).

EPA. (1994). *Setting the record straight: Secondhand smoke is a preventable health risk*. Washington, DC: U.S. Environmental Protection Agency (EPA).

Gezondheidsraad. (1990). *Passief roken: Beoordeling van de schadelijkheid van omgevingstabaksrook voor de gezondheid*. Den Haag: Gezondheidsraad.

Gezondheidsraad. (2003). *Volksgezondheidsschade door passief roken*. Den Haag: Gezondheidsraad.

Gezondheidsraad. (2006). *Plan de campagne: Bevordering van gezond gedrag door massamediale voorlichting*. The Hague: Health Council of the Netherlands.

Graham, E. R., Shipan, C. R., & Volden, C. (2012). The diffusion of policy diffusion research in political science. *British Journal of Political Science, 43*(3), 673–701. https://doi.org/10.1017/S0007123412000415

Hoffman, S. J., & Toan, C. (2015). Overview of systematic reviews on the health-related effects of government tobacco control policies. *BMC Public Health, 15*, 744.

IARC. (1986). Tobacco smoking. IARC monographs on the evaluation of carcinogenic risks of chemicals to humans. In *IARC monographs no 38* (Vol. 38). Lyon: International Agency for Research on Cancer (IARC).

IARC. (2011). *Effectiveness of tax and price policies for tobacco control. IARC handbooks of cancer prevention: Tobacco control* (Vol. 14). Lyon: International Agency for Research on Cancer (IARC).

ICBT. (1981). *Advies inzake maatregelen ter beperking van het tabaksgebruik.* Den Haag: Interdepartementale Commissie Beperking Tabaksgebruik (ICBT), Ministerie van Volksgezondheid en Milieu.

IOM (Institute of Medicine). (2007). *Ending the tobacco problem: A blue-print for the nation.* Washington, DC: The National Academies Press.

ITC Project. (2015). ITC Netherlands National Report. Findings from the Wave 1 to 8 Surveys (2008–2014). Waterloo, ON, Canada: University of Waterloo.

Jansen, D. F., Van Barneveld, T. A., & Van Leeuwen, F. E. (1993). *Passief roken en longkanker: Het EPA rapport.* Amsterdam: Nederlands Kanker Instituut.

Liverani, M., Hawkins, B., & Parkhurst, J. O. (2013). Political and institutional influences on the use of evidence in Public Health Policy. A systematic review. *PLoS One, 8*(10), e77404. https://doi.org/10.1371/journal.pone.0077404

Majone, G. (1992). *Evidence, argument, and persuasion in the policy process.* New Haven, CT: Yale University Press.

Mamudu, H., Gonzalez, M., & Glantz, S. (2011). The nature, scope, and development of the global tobacco control epistemic community. *American Journal of Public Health, 101*(11), 2044–2054. https://doi.org/10.2105/AJPH.2011.300303

Meinsma, L. (1972). *Roken en gezondheid nu: Een nieuw rapport en samenvatting over het roken en de gevolgen daarvan voor de gezondheid van het Royal College of Physicians te London.* Naarden: Strengholt.

National Cancer Institute. (2008). *The role of the media in promoting and reducing tobacco use.* NCI tobacco control monograph series (Vol. 19).

National Research Council. (1986). *Environmental tobacco smoke: Measuring exposure and assessing health effects.* Washington, DC: National Academy Press.

Oreskes, N., & Conway, E. M. (2010). *Merchants of doubt: How a handful of scientists obscured the truth on issues from tobacco smoke to global warming.* New York: Bloomsbury Press.

Philip Morris. (1996). Corporate Affairs 1996/1997 The Netherlands. *Philip Morris Records*, Bates No. 2501076006–2501076023. Retrieved from https://www.industrydocumentslibrary.ucsf.edu/tobacco/docs/nzjl0112

Radaelli, C. M. (1995). The role of knowledge in the policy process. *Journal of European Public Policy, 2*, 159–183.

Roemer, R. (1982). *Legislative action to combat the world smoking epidemic.* Geneva: WHO.

Roscam Abbing, E. W. (1998). *Tabaksontmoedigingsbeleid: Gezondheidseffectrapportage.* Utrecht: Netherlands School of Public Health (NSPH).

Ruiter, R., & Kok, G. (2006). Response to Hammond et al. showing leads to doing, but doing what? The need for experimental pilot-testing. *European Journal of Public Health, 16*, 225. https://doi.org/10.1093/eurpub/ckl014

Sarewitz, D. (2004). How science makes environmental controversies worse. *Environmental Science and Policy, 7*, 385–403.
Schwartz, R., & Rosen, B. (2004). The politics of evidence-based health policymaking. *Public Money & Management, 24*(2), 121–127. https://doi.org/10.1111/j.1467-9302.2004.00404.x
SCOTH. (1998). *Report of the Scientific Committee on tobacco and health.* London: Department of Health.
Sims, M., Salway, R., Langley, T., Lewis, S., McNeill, A., Szatkowski, L., & Gilmore, A. B. (2014). Effectiveness of tobacco control television advertising in changing tobacco use in England: A population-based cross-sectional study. *Addiction, 109*(6), 986–994. https://doi.org/10.1111/add.12501
Slob, M., & Staman, J. (2012). *Beleid en het bewijsbeest: Een verkenning van verwachtingen en praktijken rond evidence based policy.* Den Haag: Rathenau Instituut.
Smith, K. (2013). *Beyond evidence-based policy in public health: The interplay of ideas.* London: Palgrave Macmillan.
Stewart, E., & Smith, K. (2015). 'Black magic' and 'gold dust': The epistemic and political uses of evidence tools in public health policy making. *Evidence & Policy, 11*, 415–437.
STIVORO. (2010). *Van onderop en van bovenaf: De toekomst van tabaksontmoediging in Nederland 2011–2020.* Den Haag: STIVORO.
Stone, D. (2001). Learning lessons, policy transfer and the international diffusion of policy ideas. *CSGR Working Paper No. 69/01.*
Stronks, K., van de Mheen, H. D., Looman, C. W. N., & Mackenbach, J. P. (1997). Cultural, material, and psychosocial correlates of the socioeconomic gradient in smoking behavior among adults. *Preventive Medicine, 26*(5), 754–766. https://doi.org/10.1006/pmed.1997.0174
U.S. Department of Health and Human Services. (2000). *Reducing tobacco use: A report of the Surgeon General.* Atlanta: U.S. Department of Health and Human Services, Centers for Disease Control and Prevention, National Center for Chronic Disease Prevention and Health Promotion, Office on Smoking and Health.
US Surgeon General. (1986). *The health consequences of involuntary smoking.* Rockville: USDHHS.
Van der Kemp, S., & Bekker, B. (2007). Wat is effectief? De kruistocht van Kok. *TSG, 85*, 236–238.
Wakefield, M. A., Loken, B., & Hornik, R. C. (2010). Use of mass media campaigns to change health behaviour. *The Lancet, 376*, 1261–1271.
Warner, K. E., & Tam, J. (2012). The impact of tobacco control research and policy: 20 years of progress. *Tobacco Control, 21*, 103–109.
Weiss, C. H. (1980). Knowledge creep and decision accretion. *Science Communication, 1*(3), 381–404. https://doi.org/10.1177/107554708000100303
Werkgroep IBO Gezonde leefstijl. (2016). *IBO Gezonde leefstijl Eindrapportage van de werkgroep "IBO Gezonde leefstijl".* Den Haag: Ministerie van Financiën.

Wester, J. (1957). Roken en gezondheid. Rapport van de Gezondheidsraad. *Nederlands Tijdschrift voor Geneeskunde, 107*, 459–464.

WHO. (1979). *Controlling the smoking epidemic: Report of the WHO Expert Committee on Smoking Control.* WHO technical report series no. 636. Geneva: World Health Organization.

WHO. (1998). *Guidelines for controlling and monitoring the tobacco epidemic.* Geneva: World Health Organization.

WHO. (2003). *WHO framework convention on tobacco control.* Geneva: World Health Organization.

WHO. (2004a). *Building blocks for tobacco control: A handbook.* Geneva: World Health Organization.

WHO. (2004b). *Tobacco control legislation: An introductory guide* (2nd ed.). Geneva: World Health Organization.

WHO. (2008). *MPOWER.* Geneva: World Health Organisation.

Willemsen, M. C., De Vries, H., & Genders, R. (1996). Annoyance from environmental tobacco smoke and support for no-smoking policies at eight large Dutch workplaces. *Tobacco Control, 5*(2), 132–138.

World Bank. (1999). *Curbing the epidemic: Governments and the economics of tobacco control.* Washington: The World Bank.

Zahariadis, N. (2007). The multiple streams framework: Structure, limitations, prospects. In P. Sabatier (Ed.), *Theories of the policy process* (2nd ed.). Boulder, CO: Westview Press.

Zeeman, G., Willemsen, M. C., & Van Gennip, L. (2007). Foto's op pakjes passen in overheidsbeleid om tabaksgebruik te denormaliseren. *Tijdschrift voor Gezondheidswetenschappen, 85*, 234. https://doi.org/10.1007/BF03078670

Open Access This chapter is licensed under the terms of the Creative Commons Attribution 4.0 International License (http://creativecommons.org/licenses/by/4.0/), which permits use, sharing, adaptation, distribution and reproduction in any medium or format, as long as you give appropriate credit to the original author(s) and the source, provide a link to the Creative Commons license and indicate if changes were made.

The images or other third party material in this chapter are included in the chapter's Creative Commons license, unless indicated otherwise in a credit line to the material. If material is not included in the chapter's Creative Commons license and your intended use is not permitted by statutory regulation or exceeds the permitted use, you will need to obtain permission directly from the copyright holder.

CHAPTER 8

Tobacco Industry Influence

The origins of the tobacco market can be traced back to the seventeenth century. The famous Dutch golden age was an era of prosperity for tobacco merchants. They traded not only in spices and slaves but also in tobacco, and made Dutch towns extremely wealthy and financed the famous grand houses lining the canals of Amsterdam today. The habit of smoking tobacco spread from the New World and from England to the Dutch harbours. The act of smoking can be seen on many Dutch paintings from the seventeenth century. According to historian Schama (1987, p. 189), in the Golden Age "the smell of the Dutch Republic was the smell of tobacco." He referred to accounts by visitors to the Netherlands who were struck by the omnipresence of tobacco smoke in inns and towing barges, and the common sight of men and women smoking in public. Dutch clay pipes became an important export product. In the first half of the seventeenth century, tobacco was imported from the Americas, processed in Amsterdam, and exported to Russia and the Baltic. Amsterdam was the biggest staple market for Virginia and Maryland tobacco. The Dutch tobacco trade received a further boost when merchants set up tobacco plantations on Dutch soil, especially in the middle of the country, around the city of Amersfoort, and in the province of Gelderland. Around the year 1700 the total volume of exported mixed tobacco to Denmark, Sweden, Russia, and the Baltic states was about 10–15 million pounds per year,

© The Author(s) 2018
M. C. Willemsen, *Tobacco Control Policy in the Netherlands*,
Palgrave Studies in Public Health Policy Research,
https://doi.org/10.1007/978-3-319-72368-6_8

much larger than the 1.2 million that England exported to the Nordic countries (Roessingh, 1976).

Tobacco was still a thriving local agricultural and manufacturing sector in the Netherlands in the nineteenth century, after which the country gradually became the playground of a few multinational companies in the twentieth century. By the 1980s the Dutch tobacco industry had become an oligopoly, with two companies (Imperial Tobacco and British American Tobacco) dominating the roll-your-own market and four companies (BAT, Imperial Tobacco, Japan Tobacco International, and Philip Morris) dominating the cigarette and cigar market. They had selected the Low Countries as an international stronghold, and the Netherlands became one of the largest tobacco exporting countries in the world. This made the industry difficult to regulate because it was relatively powerful: it did not stand alone in its fight against regulators, but was supported by a network of allies with a common interest in protecting the status quo concerning selling tobacco, or who shared a common libertarian ideology. In this chapter I describe how the tobacco industry organised its lobbying apparatus, followed by a discussion of tobacco industry media advocacy to sway public opinion about passive smoking and attempts at influencing tobacco control through the ministries and the parliament.

TOBACCO MANUFACTURERS JOIN FORCES

Organised national tobacco industry lobbies developed sooner than organised tobacco control lobbies. In 1952 the manufacturers of roll-your-own tobacco joined forces and founded the *Vereniging Nederlandse Kerftabakindustrie* (Dutch Fine Cut Tobacco Industry Association) (VNK). Three years later cigarette manufacturers followed their example and founded the *Stichting Sigaretten Industrie* (Dutch Cigarette Manufacturers Association) (SSI). VNK and SSI shared the same lobbying apparatus, including communal office space in The Hague. Both employed one lobbyist and one supporting staff member. In 2017, VNK and SSI merged into one organisation: the *Vereniging Nederlandse Sigaretten- en Kerftabakfabrikanten* (Association for Dutch Cigarette and Fine Cut Tobacco Manufacturers) (VSK). The interests of Dutch cigar manufacturers are represented by the *Nederlandse Vereniging voor de Sigarenindustrie* (Dutch Cigar Industry Association) (NVS), established in 1971. Important allies of the tobacco manufacturers who share an economic interest in tobacco are the retail, wholesale, and vending machine sectors. Tobacco lobbyists sometimes refer to their closest allies as belonging to "the tobacco family" (Philip Morris, 1979). For many years the tobacco retail sector had two interest groups: a general and a Catholic. They merged in 1974 into the Dutch tobacco retail organisation *Nederlandse Sigarenverkopers Organisatie* (Dutch Cigar Sale Organisation) (NSO). Since 1996, motivated by the threat of legal restrictions on the sale of tobacco, the tobacco distributers and exploiters of tobacco vending machines united in a separate lobbying group, *Landelijke Belangenvereniging van Tabaksdistributeurs Nederland* (National Association for Tobacco Distributors) (LBT) (Van Oosten, 1996). Around that time the tobacco retailers also set up an organisation to coordinate activities related to implementing age of sale restrictions (the PVT).

VNK, SSI, NVS, and NSO were (and still are) natural allies when it came to the wish to normalise smoking and to prevent government regulation, but they were also competitors, driven by material self-interest. The VNK wanted to retain low taxation levels for roll-your-own products, while the SSI and Philip Morris, with little interest in the roll-your-own market, lobbied to reduce the tax gap between roll-your-own and factory made cigarettes. The NSO fought with BAT over the size of the retail margins on tobacco products sold in shops. The individual manufacturers have divergent interests and different views on lobbying strategy. Philip Morris stepped out of the SSI in 2005 because as market leader it could protect its interests better without needing to consult with the other tobacco producers.[1]

SCIENTISTS FOR HIRE

In 1964 the SSI set up the *Wetenschappelijke Adviesraad Roken en Gezondheid* (Scientific Advisory Council on Smoking and Health) (WARG) to counteract the health concerns that emerged after the first reports on smoking and health from the United States and the United Kingdom. WARG received large sums of money from the SSI to initiate scientific research into the effects of tobacco smoke on the lungs, much of it carried out at the CIVO in Zeist, part of *Nederlandse Organisatie voor Toegepast Natuurwetenschappelijk Onderzoek* (Netherlands Organisation for applied scientific research) (TNO). Some research money was also accepted by the Dutch Cancer Institute at the *Antoni van Leeuwenziekenhuis* (Emmelot, 1979; RJ Reynolds, 1978); in these years the tobacco industry was not yet widely regarded as morally "bad." After 15 years, WARG had published some 34 reports, 17 international scientific articles, and 1 PhD dissertation. Most of the research by WARG scientists was about reducing the carcinogenicity of tobacco smoke and determining acceptable threshold levels for exposure (Vossenaar, 1997). From 1973 onwards WARG operated a documentation centre that collected international scientific papers on smoking and health issues. Lists of selected publications with photocopies and summaries were widely distributed, finding their way to officials at the Ministry of Health (Emmelot, 1979). In 1979 alone, 46 such lists were distributed. WARG was disbanded in 1997, one year after the *British Medical Journal* and *The Lancet* declared that research funded by the tobacco industry would no longer be published. We do not know exactly how effective industry publications were in influencing the attitude of politicians and government officials towards the smoking problem, but it is likely that they contributed to some of the hesitance to act in these early years.

Recruitment of scientists continued after the disbandment of WARG. Philip Morris wanted to hold off smoking restrictions and started a concerted campaign "to prevent the imposition of smoking restrictions (...) based on the asserted health hazards of ETS to non-smokers. To realize this objective, three audiences had to be convinced that the health claims by anti-smoking forces concerning ETS were groundless. Those three audiences were the scientific community, regulatory authorities, and the general public" (Remes, 1988, p. 1). The strategy was to find scientists "who can attack the studies relied on by the anti-smoking forces to justify smoking restrictions on health grounds" (Remes, 1988, p. 1). At the core of the Philip Morris strategy was "mobilising in each market a corps of scientific consultants and engineers who can make the scientific case against smoking restrictions through articles in scientific journals and presentations at scientific conferences and symposia, through articles and interviews in the mass media, and through meetings with and appearances before regulatory authorities" (Remes, 1988, p. 2).

Philip Morris had some success in recruiting Dutch scientists. In 1993 a report from the US Environmental Protection Agency (EPA, 1992) attracted attention in the Netherlands. Toxicologist Freek de Wolff criticised the US Environmental Protection Agency (EPA) report (De Wolff, 1994b). De Wolff had served as an expert witness for Philip Morris, testifying against proposed rules on indoor air quality in the United States (De Wolff, 1994a), and had produced a report for Philip Morris with arguments against a European Union (EU) Directive that obliged the Dutch tobacco industry to declare the ingredients in their products (Wigand, 2005). Publications such as this made it easy for politicians to ignore the call for a workplace smoking ban, since they could label it a controversial issue with no apparent consensus on whether it was a problem important enough for the government to address.

Another attempt to normalise smoking was through Associates for Research into the Science of Enjoyment (ARISE), an industry-funded group of researchers. ARISE, active between 1988 and 1999, produced scientific papers and academic books promoting the idea that smoking is a harmless "everyday pleasure" comparable to drinking coffee or eating chocolate, improving the quality of life and reducing everyday stress (Elizabeth A. Smith, 2007). In 1995 ARISE held a conference in Amsterdam (ARISE, 1995b). The closing recommendation included the text, "people should live a life of moderate hedonism, so that they can live to the full the only life they are ever likely to have." The call to enjoy pleasures such as smoking without guilt received some positive press coverage in Dutch newspapers (ARISE, 1995a).

How the Industry Prevented Smoking Bans

By far the toughest battle between tobacco control advocates and the tobacco industry network was over smoking bans, a fight that started some 30 years ago. By the end of the 1980s most of the epidemiological evidence from international research supported the claim that passive smoking is harmful and causes lung cancer. Reports by the federal government of the United States, Australia, and WHO fuelled calls for better protection of non-smokers (National Research Council, 1986; O'NeillI, Brunnemann, Dodet, & Hoffmann, 1987; US Surgeon General, 1986). It was crucial for the industry's marketers to understand in which countries the threat of smoking bans was most imminent. In 1997 and 1998 Philip Morris collected public opinion data in all 57 countries where they were active. Representative samples of people in each were asked what they thought about the harm from passive smoking and whether they supported government regulations (GfK Great Britain, 1998). The researchers found that respondents were much more likely to support smoking restrictions when they were living in countries where there was more public concern about the health risks of ETS. The correlation coefficient was 0.72, quite high for this type of research. They also found an association between annoyance from second-hand smoke and the belief that smoking in public places is seen as a priority for governments. The level of felt annoyance in the Netherlands ranked remarkably low among the 37 countries where this item was measured: only 26% of Dutch non-smokers were "very annoyed" by people smoking around them. This suggested a high level of tolerance to smoking. Only Denmark was more tolerant (16%). The least tolerant were Greece (62%), Italy (57%), Ireland (45%), and the United Kingdom (45%). The industry used such data to tailor its normalisation efforts on a country-to-country basis. For the Netherlands, as tolerance was already high, it only needed to be boosted by tobacco normalising campaigns. In 1985 the SSI established a small professional communication bureau, the *Voorlichtingsbureau Sigaretten en Shag* (Cigarettes and Roll-your-own tobacco Education Bureau), renamed *Bureau Voorlichting Tabak* (Tobacco Education Bureau) (BVT) in 1994. This bureau was responsible for campaigns designed to influence public opinion about passive smoking (Table 8.1).

Through these campaigns, year after year, the public and politicians were bombarded with a simple message: smokers have the right to enjoy smoking and this should be tolerated and respected, not repressed. Such messages were well received by the Netherlands' pluralistic and permissive society.

In addition, Philip Morris ran programmes to accommodate smokers by either setting up smoking sections ("courtesy of choice" programmes) or promoting ventilation technology when separation was not possible. This started in 1995 in an effort to prevent smoking bans in public transport, the hospitality sector, and workplaces. In an internal memo,

Table 8.1 Tobacco industry tolerance campaigns in the Netherlands

Year	Campaign (translated from Dutch)
1978	Poster campaign "friendly smoking" targeted at city councils
1984	Campaign "There are smokers and non-smokers. Take each other into consideration"
1984	Letter campaign to parliamentarians and city councils "Smoking … a matter of give and take"
1984	Brochure to family physicians "Information about smoking and society"
1985–1987	Campaign "Smoking must be permitted"
1991	Campaign "Smoking? We work it out together"
1992	"Smoking as usual. Or not. We keep it sociable"
1995	Campaign "Enjoyment must be permitted"
1999	Campaign "Smoking? Ask for permission!"

industry representatives wrote that by 1999 such programmes had been rather successful:

> By any measure, the International Accommodation Program is very effective. This programme operates in 46 countries and more than 6600 establishments, is growing at 50% per year, has been used repeatedly to prevent or modify smoking restrictions, has generated no negative reaction, and effective coalitions have been built with the hospitality industry. (Goldberg, 1999b, p. 2074399558)

The memo further mentioned that the programmes in the Netherlands were "used by the Dutch hospitality industry to maintain a reasonable attitude. Courtesy of Choice is in operation in the Dutch Parliament in The Hague" (Goldberg, 1999b, p. 2074395548). Philip Morris had indeed organised smoking sections in the restaurant of the Dutch parliament building. This was a deliberate attempt to get to politicians, "another simple, yet very effective, strategy … to target places of influence" (Goldberg, 1999a, p. 2). What is remarkable is that the memo mentioned only the Dutch, Belgian, and EU parliament buildings in Brussels and Strasbourg, suggesting that the Dutch parliament was either an easy or an important target, or both.

While industry campaigns were well received in the 1980s and strengthened societal norms that smoking in public must be tolerated in the Netherlands, in the 1990s they were gradually losing the fight over smoking in public. Box 8.1 gives an example of how Philip Morris unsuccessfully attempted to sway public opinion on the risks of passive smoking during a time that passive smoking was already widely regarded as harmful.

Box 8.1 Philip Morris' failed "cookies campaign"
In June 1996 Philip Morris launched a Europe-wide attack on the growing concern about passive smoking. It ran large newspaper ads in nine European countries with the headline, "Second-hand tobacco smoke in perspective." Page-wide advertisements downplayed the risk from passive smoking by comparing it to presumed risks associated with drinking chlorinated tap water, consuming cookies, or eating hot pepper. The campaign was strongly condemned by Padraig

Flynn, the EU commissioner for health matters, and international health organisations challenged the campaign in court. The Union for International Cancer Control, a main European tobacco control lobbying organisation, faxed a document with a warning regarding the press release of the Philip Morris campaign and a detailed rebuttal of the claims that Philip Morris made in the advertisement to the *Stichting Volksgezondheid en Roken* (Dutch Smoking or Health Foundation) (STIVORO) (UICC, 1996). STIVORO was thus well prepared when Philip Morris presented the campaign at a press conference in The Hague, and on the day the campaign was launched issued a press statement in which STIVORO's director criticised the campaign to the press outside the conference room, claiming that the campaign was misleading (Nellen & De Blij, 1999). Health Minister Borst communicated the same message in reply to questions by parliament and through a press statement.[2] Dutch health organisations complained to the Advertising Control Board. Two weeks after the campaign started, Philip Morris had to withdraw the campaign prematurely.

Although it resulted in bad publicity for Philip Morris, and even brought them in conflict with other tobacco manufacturers, the "cookies campaign" still had some effect on Dutch public opinion regarding harm from passive smoking. According to survey data collected by STIVORO, before the campaign 60% of the Dutch believed that ETS could cause lung cancer, and this was 57% after the campaign (Nellen & De Blij, 1999). Research commissioned by Philip Morris showed that the proportion of Dutch who believed that environmental tobacco smoke was "a serious health risk" had gone down, from 21% to 18% (Wirthlin Group, 1996). However, the STIVORO survey showed that general public support for smoking bans had significantly increased, suggesting that the main goal of the campaign had failed. According to STIVORO, the campaign had "antagonised the Dutch government and the Health Commission of the European parliament ... it is likely that the campaign helped to reduce the tobacco industry's political and public support" (Nellen & De Blij, 1999, p. 222).

The Employers' Organisation VNO–NCW

A key supporter of the tobacco industry was the national employers interest organisation *Verbond van Nederlandse Ondernemingen en Nederlands Christelijk Werkgeversverbond* (Confederation of Netherlands Industry and Employers) (VNO–NCW). It was and is arguably the most powerful Dutch lobbying organisation. The three main Dutch tobacco lobby organisations (SSI, VNK, and NVS) have seats on its general board (Braam & Van Woerden, 2013) and its director is widely considered one of the most influential people in the country. According to Hans Hillen, former *Christen-Democratisch Appèl* (Christian Democratic Party) (CDA) senator, ex-minister for defence, and former advisor to British American Tobacco, "Everyone at a high position needs at least ten years to understand how Dutch governance works. Very few people have really mastered this and Niek Jan [van Kesteren] controls it to perfection. He is the spider in the web" (Van de Wetering, 2010). Some have called him the emperor of the *polder* (Korteweg & Huisman, 2016). In an interview, van Kesteren disclosed that all branch organisations in the tobacco sector regularly meet at VNO–NCW to discuss lobbying strategies (Braam & Van Woerden, 2013): "We are one of the few friends the tobacco industry has." VNO–NCW has a Brussels office and played a major role in opposing the revised Tobacco Products Directive (TPD-2). VNO–NCW preferably lobbies "through the inner line. The more silently, the better" (Andeweg & Irwin, 2009, p. 15). The Truth Tobacco Industry Documents database[3] contains many examples of letters from VNO–NCW on tobacco policy to Dutch government officials, including ministers. One example is a set of personal letters from VNO–NCW's Chairman Alexander Rinnooy Kan[4] to the minister for economic affairs and the minister for health in 1994 and 1995, pleading for self-regulation instead of a ban on tobacco advertising (Rinnooy-Kan, 1994, 1995a, 1995b).

Industry-Friendly Politicians

Lobbying through parliament is known as "the royal way," since it involves the instruments of democracy. CDA parliamentarian Wim van de Camp said in 1999, "The professionalism of the tobacco lobby in The Hague is remarkable. A strong, polished lobby, not obtrusive, very well organised. They monitor everything that is happening in the parliament quite well" (Bouma, 2012). If direct lobbying through contacts within the bureaucracy does not work, the industry puts pressure on the government through industry-friendly politicians who are willing to ask parliamentary questions. The one party that the industry can rely on to be generous in voicing concerns is the conservative–liberal *Volkspartij voor Vrijheid en Democratie* (People's Party for Freedom and Democracy) (VVD). VVD connections with the industry have been, and still are, close: for example, Ferry Houterman, political advisor to several VVD ministers, was supervisory director at Philip Morris for some years (Luyendijk, Verkade, & Heck, 2010). In the past VVD motions have often been supported by other liberal factions in parliament, especially the *Partij voor de Vrijheid* (Freedom Party) (PVV), and sometimes by *Democraten 66* (Democrats 66) (D66) and the CDA as well. These parties are in many ways different, but they share the values of preserving individual lifestyle choices and concerns that reducing the tobacco sector might result in negative consequences for (small) businesses.

The position of the CDA, a party occupying the middle of the political spectrum, is nuanced. Typical for the CDA approach is to advance tobacco control in small steps, taking the interests of small businesses into consideration. The CDA is ideologically conservative in that it usually opposes too much government interference, especially if it feels that an issue can be resolved by other means. The CDA played a key role in the tobacco industry lobby against legislation until the mid-1990s, and because it held strategic positions in ruling coalitions for many years it was an ideal vehicle for the industrial lobby. The CDA was always part of ruling coalitions, except in the Purple cabinets (1994–2002) and the Rutte II cabinet (2012–2017). Prominent CDA politician Joost van Iersel is often quoted for his remark in the 1980s: "We just run this country." One former civil servant remarked about the CDA in the 1980s and first half of the 1990s, "That was the old CDA of Lubbers and Brinkman who had close ties with VNO–NCW and Philip Morris, and who were against legislation."[5] Many key persons in the tobacco industry network were prominent members of the CDA. VNO–NCW Director Niek Jan van Kesteren and the various chairs of VNO–NCW were influential CDA members, and allowed the tobacco industry direct access to other powerful CDA people such as Fons van der Stee (Minister for Finance 1973–1982), Elco Brinkman (Minister for Health 1982–1989), Ab Klink (Minister for Health 2007–2010), and Prime Ministers Ruud Lubbers (1982–1994) and Jan Peter Balkenende (2002–2007). One ex-civil servant remembered how Health Minister

Ab Klink was played: "Niek-Jan van Kesteren phoned at the merest trifle. He had a hotline with Ab Klink, so to say. And what was the effect? That Ab inserted the idea of the parallel interests into the [tobacco] *nota*. That was all the doing of Niek-Jan van Kesteren."[6]

Former Health Minister Elco Brinkman was leader of the CDA faction in the second chamber of parliament from 1989 until 1994, and has been in the senate since 2011. Brinkman is a firm free-market proponent, very well connected in the business world. He explained in an interview why he believed that smoking should not be regulated: he was brought up "with a way of thinking that emphasises people's individual responsibility. I believe that smoking is a personal decision. Moreover, tobacco is a legal product."[7] These convictions reflect the core beliefs that are binding factors for the various parties in the tobacco network. Later in his political career he became commissioner for Philip Morris and vice president of VNO–NCW. In 2009 Brinkman helped the industry to change the official standpoint of the minister for finance about minimum cigarette prices in Europe.[8] There were also links between the industry and the CDA in Parliament. For example, Jan Schipper, a former director at Philip Morris, was a prominent CDA member and helped draft the list of members for CDA seats at the general elections in 1998 (Bouma, 2012).

Even when the CDA was in opposition between 1994 and 2002, the industry could still fall back on its connections to tone down the government's tobacco control policy intentions. In these years, advocates and left-wing politicians frequently accused the CDA of protecting tobacco industry interests. During the famous debate in the second chamber on 31 May 2001 about the amendments to the Tobacco Act, Labour Party politician Rob Oudkerk complained at one point, "When I hear the CDA, I hear the droning of the tobacco lobby. That is not a nice sound." At another moment in the debate, Agnes Kant (Socialist Party) remarked about the position of CDA and VVD, which tried to remove advertising and smoking bans from the Tobacco Act, "I must say that when I hear their position and their argumentation, I can still hear the tobacco lobby resounding in this house."

Smokers' Rights Groups

It was not only direct contacts with the government and politicians that helped the industry ward to off legislation. At times it is more effective to "speak as the smokers" (Smith & Malone, 2007). The main purpose of smokers' right groups was to keep smoking socially acceptable by framing the issue as one of individual rights, not health, and positioning smokers as defenders of freedom (Smith & Malone, 2007). In 1992 a Dutch national smokers' rights group *Stichting Rokers Belangen* (SRB) was founded by Philip Morris, with Ton Wurtz as chair and spokesperson. Philip Morris had high expectations of the group. The Dutch SRB formulated its aims in 1998 as follows: "We believe strict smoking bans and laws infringe on our individual rights, impede our society's principle of freedom of choice and reduce tolerance and respect within our society" (Forces USA, 1998). Philip Morris listed as one of the key issues for the Netherlands in 1994, to "continue to support and exploit to a maximum the Smokers' Rights Club. In doing so, develop regional chapters and make the Club a very active group and ally to the industry" (Philip Morris, 1994). According to Philip Morris corporate affairs experts, the SRB was an important media player in 1996, boasting huge numbers of members, and had some success in preventing smoking bans in workplaces and preventing higher tobacco taxes (Philip Morris, 1996a).

It is interesting to contrast this industry-led group with another group that was spontaneously founded on 7 January 1990 as a short-lived protest against the smoking ban that came into force on 1 January of that year. The group *Rokers Belangen Vereniging* (Smokers' Interest Society) was a colourful mix of Amsterdam-based artists, journalists, and intellectuals.[9] Its founders wanted to promote the image of the smoker as a "gentle, tolerant, freedom-loving, independent, undogmatic individualist" (Van Gelder, 1990). The group was disbanded soon after it was founded because of incompatible opinions about strategy and lack of interest from smokers.

The Dutch tobacco industry manages to keep the SRB alive to this day, which is remarkable since most smokers' right groups do not survive very long due to lack of support from smokers (Smith & Malone, 2007). While Philip Morris ceased to lobby against smoking bans in the Netherlands and lost interest in SRB, SSI and VNK continued to financially support SRB. Compared with similar organisations in Europe, the Dutch SRB has been a long-lasting force, more or less a one-man project of its director, Ton Wurtz. Wurtz's most successful initiative was when he, with help from the SSI, founded the small interest group *Stichting Red de kleine horecaondernemer* (Save the small hospitality entrepreneur) (Baltesen & Rosenberg, 2009). This foundation of bar owners played a crucial role in masterminding the revolt by pub owners against the smoking ban in 2008, which undermined legislation for several years. It was an example of astroturfing—the practice of deliberately staging activities that give the impression of spontaneous grass roots initiatives. The group received support from Wiel Maessen, chair of the Dutch libertarian group Forces, which fights against what it calls the "anti-tobacco industry"—a conspiracy theory in which "Big Pharma" is an omnipotent industry that pulls the strings in the tobacco control network.

THE MINISTRY OF ECONOMIC AFFAIRS

For many years representatives from the tobacco sector were natural and undisputed consultation partners for the Ministry of Economic Affairs on tobacco policy issues. The trade ministry was a long-time supporter of the tobacco sector because of the promise of employment and commerce: the industry promoted itself as major investor and job provider.[10] In 1969 Philip Morris established a company in Eindhoven and in 1981 opened the world's largest and most advanced cigarette production plant in Bergen op Zoom, conveniently close to Vlissingen and Rotterdam—Dutch harbours with facilities for the warehousing of tobacco from overseas. It is also close to Antwerp, the largest port for raw tobacco in mainland Europe. Bergen op Zoom was an economic development zone, which meant that the Ministry of Economic Affairs could offer attractive investment conditions. Through the Investment Account Act[11] the government subsidised the new production facility with 6.2 million guilders.[12] According to one civil servant, "The plant in Bergen op Zoom was constructed with enormous support from the government. The Ministry of Economic Affairs wanted that factory, because this would bring with it a lot of employment for people in the province of Brabant, where unemployment was high. So there was always a sort of understanding between Philip Morris and the trade minister."[13] Other tobacco producers (mainly located in the Northern provinces) also advanced the argument of being important to local employment and economy.

The Ministry of Economic Affairs was more powerful than the Ministry of Health. According to one former government official:

> If the minister for Economic Affairs wanted something to be done in these days, it just happened. And when the state secretary for Health wanted something, it did not happen. Economic Affairs tried to hold back all aspects of the tobacco dossier. So there was a continuous, big clash regarding

tobacco policy between the two ministries. There was minister Andriessen.[14] He was a real powerful trade minister. We wanted to get rid of the principle of self-regulation, but State Secretary for Health Hans Simons could not realise that as long as there was minister Andriessen. Andriessen was just more powerful. So we had to make do with what we had. Hans Simons had to go for the possible, for what was attainable.[15]

For the trade ministry, frequent contacts with the tobacco industry were business as usual. A civil servant from the trade ministry wrote a new year's wish to his contact with the VNK at the beginning of 1992: "There is no doubt that in the new year the branch organisations and Economic Affairs will again have to respond promptly to developments that may cause problems for the tobacco processing and cigar industries. Hopefully we will find each other again in a good cooperative spirit in 1992" (Ministerie van Economische Zaken, 1992).

Concrete threats that Philip Morris might withdraw its economic activities from the Netherlands were frequently voiced in the 1990s. For example, in 1995, when Health Minister Els Borst presented her public health policy intentions, the industry immediately argued that her plans would be devastating to the local and national economy (Vonk, 1995). In 1996 Philip Morris threatened not to expand its factory in Bergen op Zoom if the government's intention to increase tobacco taxation by 50 cents per pack was achieved.[16] Philip Morris organised an intimidating lobby, part of which was concerned letters to Prime Minister Wim Kok from a wide range of organisations, including labour unions in the tobacco processing sector (Philip Morris, 1996b), the municipality of Bergen op Zoom where the Philip Morris plant was located (Gemeente Bergen op Zoom, 1996), the local chamber of commerce (Hamers & Vermeulen, 1996), the governor of the province of Overijssel, and the Netherlands Trade Union Confederation (FNV) (Kok, 1996). The industry lobby could not stop the tax increase, but it did manage to have it spread over three years (1997, 1998, 1999), a much better outcome for the industry than the original plan.

Until 1996 it was normal practice that the ministers from Economic Affairs and the Ministry of Health, supported by top civil servants, met in person with the highest-ranking representatives from the industry (directors, CEOs). These were called executive meetings[17] and took place twice a year. In addition, administrative consultations,[18] where civil servants discussed and negotiated with the industry about the implementation of current policy and ideas for future policy, were held on a regular basis. Such meetings gave the industry a tremendous advantage to organise their lobbying apparatus in case the outcomes of negotiations were not to their liking. Box 8.2 describes how the tobacco industry was able to eliminate the most effective elements from the first Tobacco Act.

> **Box 8.2 How the industry crushed the first Tobacco Act**
> In 1979 the *Interdepartementale Commissie Beperking Tabaksgebruik* (Interdepartmental Committee for Reducing Tobacco Use) (ICBT) was set up by the government to draft a Tobacco Act. In December 1980 the ICBT committee organised confidential meetings with representatives from the tobacco sector to solicit their comments on two core elements of the proposed act: tobacco advertising and sales restrictions (Van Londen, 1980). Objections raised by the industry were acknowledged by the state secretary for economic affairs, and in particular objections against limiting tobacco sales to specialty shops.[19] The industry argued that the reduction of tobacco selling points must occur in a phased manner so that the market could slowly adjust, and argued that the number of specialty shops would be too small to accommodate the national demand for tobacco. After the ICBT report was presented, the government frequently organised meetings of the *Werkgroep Afspraken Tabaksbeleid* (Working Group on Agreements about Tobacco Policy) (WAT) to ensure that stakeholders from the tobacco industry sector could give further inputs and eventually endorse the Tobacco Act. The full tobacco sector was represented in WAT meetings: from retail organisations, the hospitality sector, tobacco wholesalers, and industry lobby organisations (NVS, SNK, SSI, NSO). The WAT meetings continued until at least 1995 and aimed at "making clear agreements on tobacco advertising, tobacco taxation, selling points, and smoking bans" (Ministerie van Economische Zaken, 1995). They were not open to representatives from health organisations.
> In March 1982 the Ministry of Economic Affairs sent a confidential first concept of the Tobacco Act to the Economic Institute for small- and medium-sized enterprises with the request to produce data that demonstrated the economic impact on businesses if the number of tobacco points of sale were drastically reduced (Ministerie van Economische Zaken, 1982b). In October 1982 the Ministry of Economic Affairs sent confidential letters about the government's

policy intentions regarding the Tobacco Act to WAT members, with an invitation to give feedback and comments (Ministerie van Economische Zaken, 1982a). They also met in person to hear their concerns. At that point the government still wanted to reduce sales to specialised tobacco retailers. In January 1983, in a meeting with the new State Secretary for Health Joop van der Reijden, SSI offered to remove cigarette vending machines from outdoor venues. In February 1983, WAT members met with the state secretaries for health and economic affairs to discuss the matter further,[20] and SSI and others were allowed to continue to make suggestions for change until the end of that month (SSI, 1983). This was all well in advance of the moment that the proposal for the Tobacco Act was presented to the cabinet for approval (July 1983) and to parliament (end of 1984). The drafting of the proposal was further delayed because the Ministry of Economic Affairs demanded that the text be scrutinised by the Commission Van der Grinten, a new commission that advised on how regulation could be streamlined in such a way as to "reduce legal regulations that hamper the recovery of the economy."[21,22] This gave the industry more time to organise its lobby. Business organisations involved with selling tobacco united and presented a study on the economic consequences of reducing the number of selling venues (Roos, 1985). The study suggested there would be damage to the food retail sector, especially small supermarkets, and argued that many would not survive without the sale of tobacco. This was reason for the Van der Grinten Commission to advise against the idea of restricting tobacco to specialty shops, and this was subsequently removed from the draft act (SSI & SNK, 1984). The other hot potato, a ban on tobacco advertising, was removed after several rounds of talks in which the industry and the state secretaries for health and economic affairs settled for a continuation of self-regulation by the industry (Evenhuis, 1988; Marres & Toet, 1987).

The obvious route of industry influence through the trade ministry was disrupted in 1996, when tobacco control became the prime responsibility of the Ministry of Health. This was possible because Minister of Economic Affairs Hans Wijers sided with Minister of Health Els Borst (both D66) after a collision with the industry—when the government's new tobacco control policy paper was extensively negotiated by Wijers and Borst in a confidential meeting with a broad representation of the industry sector (Borst-Eilers, 1996). Part of the negotiations was an agreement to set up a new "Platform Prevention of Youth Smoking," financed by the industry (Roelofs, 1996a). This would be a sort of clearing-house of scientific information about effective ways to tackle youth smoking. This platform turned out to be merely window dressing, a strategy to get more leverage over the government. The industry lobbied to prevent majority support in the parliament for Borst's policy intentions, and threatened that they would not finance the youth prevention platform if the major tax increase, announced by Borst soon after her tobacco control policy "*nota*" was issued, went ahead (Volkskrant, 1996). The industry regarded the tax increase as unjust and threatened to disband their "part of the deal" (Roelofs, 1996b; Van de Mortel & Roelofs, 1996), claiming that, in return for the industry's cooperation with the tobacco control intentions, the cabinet had promised not to increase tobacco taxes. This led to a quarrel between both ministers and industry lobbyists. On 2 September a large delegation from the industry discussed the disagreement with the two ministers, and the next day SSI issued a press statement with the title "Government breaches agreement" (Van Ronkel, 1996). SSI accused the government of having caused a breach of trust with the tobacco sector. Minister for Economic Affairs Hans Wijers was not amused, since in his eyes a deal with the industry to refrain from tax increases had not been made, and he threatened them: "There is always an alternative, which is regulation." In a snappy letter to the chairman of VNO–NCW he wrote, "Regarding the meeting with the industry I want to repeat what was said in parliament: there were no deals about tobacco taxes to which this cabinet could in any way be committed" (Wijers, 1996). From that moment, Wijers no longer opposed Borst's wishes for effective tobacco control (Van der Bles, 1996) and it became easier for the tobacco control officials at the health ministry to get tobacco control proposals approved in the cabinet, since they only had to try to get the health minister's signature for approval.

In the beginning of 1999, after the second Kok Cabinet was installed, Philip Morris contacted the new Minister of Economic Affairs Annemarie Jorritsma (VVD) to get her support in preventing Health Minister Borst from banning tobacco advertising altogether: "I thank you for your assurance that you will make sure that the interests of the concerned industries will be optimally protected when the European guideline concerning tobacco adverting will be implemented" (Schipper, 1999b). In June Jorritsma and Borst had an executive meeting with tobacco industry CEOs to discuss the industry's wish to resume "constructive dialogue" with the government (Schipper, 1999a). According to the industry, the ministers had promised to reinstall "regular executive level meetings," but two years later this had not yet occurred (SSI, 2001). In the meantime, employers organisation VNO–NCW complained to the minister of economic affairs that it was not doing enough to restrain Borst's plans for a revision of the Tobacco Act, which had just been sent for approval to parliament: "We find it difficult to understand that this kind of measures can be proposed with the support of the ministry of Economic Affairs, and cannot be stopped by Economic Affairs" (Blankert, 1999). Jorritsma wrote several "blue letters" (direct confidential letters between ministers) to Borst to try to restrain her, without success (Bouma, 2001, p. 94). When Borst asked the state attorney to study the possibility of suing the industry for the public health damage it had incurred, inspired by major court cases in the United States which had led to the 1998 Master Settlement Agreement,[23] the hostile attitude of the health minister and her staff was of great concern to the industry (discussed in more detail later in this chapter).

Despite tobacco control now being firmly in the hands of the Ministry of Health, and regular top-level meetings with the health minister had been terminated, the industry still tried to influence the ministry's tobacco control policy through the Ministry of Economic Affairs. Email exchanges between the Ministry of Economic Affairs and the Ministry of Health, found in the Truth Tobacco Industry Documents database,[24] reveal that the industry continued to maintain contact with officials from the trade ministry. An example of this, presented in Box 8.3, describes how the industry used the Ministry of Economic Affairs to extract information from the Ministry of Health about the Dutch position regarding the European Commission (EC) proposal for a council Recommendation on smoke-free environments in that year. The example illustrates how persistent and intensive the industry lobby at times was, even regarding what was initially thought to be a relatively unimportant matter such as a non-binding EU Recommendation. The industry was more up to date on the position of the various EU countries about upcoming legislation from Brussels than tobacco control advocates and politicians were (Algemene Rekenkamer, 2012).

Box 8.3 How the industry influenced the Dutch position on an EU Recommendation

The Recommendation on smoke-free environments (2009/C296/02) included the advice to support national smoking bans with specific additional measures. One of these was health warnings on cigarette packs. Much to the dismay of the industry, France proposed to turn this into a recommendation to consider plain packaging, and this led to a massive industry lobby both in the European arena and directed at national governments. The Netherlands was seen as crucial for a blocking minority, since the industry knew that Health Minister Klink (2007–2010) objected to graphic health warnings on cigarette packs, and would probably also not endorse the idea of plain packaging. In the Netherlands, civil servants at the Ministry of Economic Affairs, as well as at the Ministry of Health, and the health ministry's permanent representative in Brussels were approached by telephone and email, and letters were sent directly to Health Minister Klink, reminding him of his former statements about health warnings. Industry lobbyists asked Klink to object in the European Council of Health Ministers to the plain packaging advice. In reply to an email in which a lobbyist from Philip Morris pointed out industry concerns, a senior policy officer from the trade ministry replied, "Thank you for your mail. I appreciate very much that I am being informed about such signals from the business community. I will discuss this at short notice with my colleague at the Health Ministry. I'll give you an update afterwards" (Ministerie van Economische Zaken, 2009b). The official then did discuss the industry's concerns with his colleague at the Health Ministry, but from the emails it is clear that the official was uncertain if the issue was important enough for the trade ministry to act, since it was not immediately clear whether employment and cigarette production would be harmed (Ministerie van Economische Zaken, 2009a). The industry then contacted the state secretary for economic affairs directly, bypassing the civil servant: "I would appreciate it very much if you could have the matter looked into and if possibly take action against including plain packs in the proposed recommendation" (Ministerie van Economische Zaken, 2009c). In October the pressure was increased through a series of letters from industry stakeholders (SSI, VNK, VNO–NCW, PVT) directed at ministers and state secretaries for health, economic affairs, and finance, all urging the government to remove references to plain packs from the EU Recommendation. Philip Morris mobilised its contacts in parliament, resulting in an MP from the VVD asking parliamentary questions.[25]

Industry concerns increased when the plain packaging text was approved by the Working Party in the Public Health Commission (which prepares texts for the EU Health Council), despite objections by a minority of countries including the Netherlands. Next the proposal was to be discussed in the Committee of Permanent Representatives (COREPER), the highest preparatory body for meetings of the European Council of Ministers. The Dutch trade ministry considered taking extra steps to use its own network to influence EU countries which were neutral or still positive about plain packs: "Currently the Ministry of Economic Affairs examines (other) possibilities to change the minds of proponents of the Recommendation, for example through our economic diplomats network or by exploiting the argument of intellectual property" (Ministerie van Economische Zaken, 2009c).

At the COREPER meeting there was an intense debate between member states for or against an advice on plain packaging, with the Netherlands still against. Because this threatened the survival of the Recommendation, COREPER finally reached a compromise, which was to remove the advice to member states to implement plain packaging—a victory for the industry lobby. It is difficult to determine how influential the industry lobby was in achieving the end result, but it is reasonable to assume that, without its insistent pressure, countries such as the Netherlands might have given in to countries that were in favour.

Insistent industry pressure is very difficult for government officials to ignore. The example in Box 8.3 illustrates how the industry engages simultaneously at different levels: bureaucratic (targeting civil servants), political (targeting MPs), and governmental (targeting ministers); and that it does so in a coordinated fashion. It is unclear as to what extent this has changed, despite recent efforts from the government to improve the implementation of Article 5.3 FCTC, which aims to prevent industry interference with tobacco control policymaking (discussed in Chap. 6).

Around 2010, at the end of the ministership of Ab Klink, VNO–NCW made a stab at returning to the days when the Ministry of Economic Affairs had formal shared responsibility over tobacco control. It wrote to the ministry: "we would like to offer our help to increase the effectiveness of your department on several [tobacco] issues. ... VNO–NCW will take the initiative for a further meeting to prepare for strengthening of the role of your ministry" (VNK, NVS, SSI, & Philip Morris Benelux, 2010). In December 2010, soon after Health Minister Schippers entered office, VNO–NCW presented a memo by SSI in which it pleaded for a "strong and balanced role" for the trade ministry in the future formation of tobacco control policy, and asked that the trade minister once again co-sign new tobacco, alcohol, and food legislation and be consulted by other ministries on these topics (VNO–NCW, 2011b). VNO–NCW's director asked its high-level contact at the trade ministry to discuss this with "Maxim" [Minister for Economic Affairs Maxime Verhagen] and pointed out that the alcohol and tobacco industry had suffered from the "onesidedness of policy and the failure to understand their position. Would it not become time to restore the influence of the trade ministry to its old splendour?" (VNO–NCW, 2011a). Despite these attempts, Economic Affairs was content that the Ministry of Health handle the difficult tobacco policy dossier, as long as Economic Affairs was allowed to play a role from the side-line—that is, as long as it was consulted by the Ministry of Health about the impact of tobacco policy on the business sector through interdepartmental consultations.

Vanished Employability in the Tobacco Sector

While employment arguments might have been valid in previous decades, they have become hollow in recent years. Cigarette manufacturing is highly mechanised in the Netherlands, contributing little to the number of jobs. Throughout the twentieth century employment in the Dutch tobacco production sector became less and less important (Fig. 8.1). BAT produced cigarettes in Zevenaar until 2008, when the factory was closed and production moved to Eastern Europe. The Philip Morris facility was as good as closed in 2014, resulting in more than 1200 job losses. After the closing of this one factory, a civil servant at the Ministry of Economic Affairs confirmed that the importance of tobacco employment in the Netherlands had become "actually negligible" (Rijsterborgh, 2017).

With the disappearance of the huge production and export volumes of manufactured cigarettes of the past, the industry lost one of its leverages:

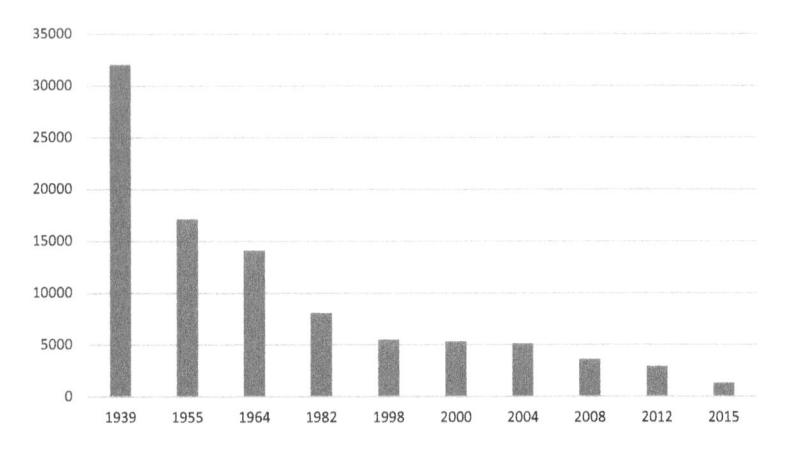

Fig. 8.1 Number of workers employed in tobacco production in the Netherlands since 1939. Sources: Van Proosdij (1957, p. 186) (data 1955), (Mantel & de Wolf, 1983) (data 1939, 1964, 1982), (De Steur) (data 1998), (Rijsterborgh, 2017) (data 2000, 2004, 2008, 2012, 2015, based on Statistics Netherlands StatLine)

its contribution to the national trade balance. In the mid-1980s the contribution of the Dutch tobacco industry to the national trade balance was still greater in the Netherlands than in other EU countries (Voorlichtingsbureau Sigaretten en Shag, 1986), but nowadays this is modest. Macro-economic considerations in relation to the tobacco manufacturing sector have therefore become unimportant to the Ministry of Economic Affairs. However, other arguments, such as threats to intellectual property as in the case of plain packaging, may still be used to get the ministry on its side.

Agreements with the Ministry of Finance

The tobacco sector has been cherished by the Ministry of Finance for many years because of the secure contribution of tobacco tax to the national state income. At the end of the 1970s, Philip Morris was pleased with the protection it enjoyed: "The strong influence of the Ministry of Finance and the complexity of the legislative process in Holland have aided in forestalling legislation to date" (Philip Morris, 1979). One former civil servant characterised the relationship that the government had with tobacco during the 1980s as "primarily a matter dealt with by the finance ministry. The Ministry of Health had to keep its mouth shut. If there is no tobacco control policy, all the better, because the incoming flow of money must not be disturbed."[26] He continued:

> The cheapest patient is a dead patient. That was what the industry told Finance and Economic Affairs, I am sure of that. … It is better for the state to do nothing. This will give you more revenues from tax. Smokers live shorter so we will have fewer costs. So for the state it is cheaper to do nothing against smoking. I have heard such points of view often when we had interdepartmental meetings. So it was always David against Goliath [the Ministry of Health against the other ministerial departments] in these early days.

When we look at the proportion of state income that comes from tobacco, we see a remarkably stable trend: tobacco tax revenues provide a steady state income, which has been between 0.5% and 1% of the total state income since 1995 (Fig. 8.2).

Despite the weak price elasticity, major price increases through substantial and frequent tobacco tax hikes are widely considered the most effective tobacco policy measure (Jha & Chaloupka, 2000; Nagelhout, Levy,

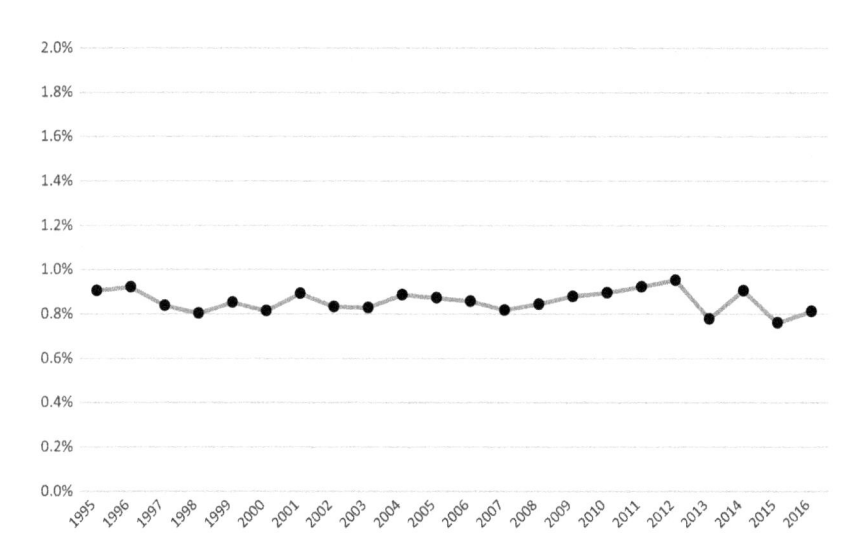

Fig. 8.2 State revenues from tobacco taxation (excl. VAT) as a proportion of the total state income per year. Source: CBS (Statistics Netherlands): http://statline.cbs.nl/Statweb/?LA=en

et al., 2012). However, the levying of excise duties originates from the *Wet of de Accijns* (Excise Duty Act) administered by the Ministry of Finance.[27] This means that the single most effective way to address the smoking problem is not under the direct control of the Ministry of Health—and the act does not mention health as a reason for tobacco tax increases. In 2014 representatives of the Tax and Customs Administration confirmed that the act's primary purpose is to raise revenue for the government (Loubeau, 2014). The positive effect of tobacco taxation on public health is regarded by most Dutch politicians as "a politically interesting side-effect" (Van Baal, Brouwer, Hoogenveen, & Feenstra, 2007). The Ministry of Health has to negotiate with the Ministry of Finance if it wants to use tobacco taxation as a way to protect health. This is what an ex-civil servant from the Health Ministry had to say: "Very often we tried to push for tax increases. But this was only possible when they [the Finance ministry] deemed that the time was right. I have always experienced this as very troublesome. A dialogue with the deaf."[28]

Tobacco manufacturers meet regularly with officials at the Ministry of Finance for "tobacco deliberations" (Ministerie van Financiën, 2011, p. 6). Because of the divergent interests of the various manufacturers regarding taxation, there are also separate contacts between individual businesses and the ministry.[29] According to one former Dutch industrial lobbyist, "The tobacco industry has much more knowledge about how taxation works. It is all very technical and quite a few people at the Ministry of Finance retired. So concerning technical knowledge, they had an information shortage. ... The industry is very capable of showing how specific types of taxation [e.g., gradual instead of abrupt] will be more effective for the treasury."[30]

For long, the Ministry of Finance has been receptive to suggestions by the industry on how tax increases might best be realised, as long as the end result is the same for the treasury (Philip Morris, 1989; SSI, 1991; VNK, 1991). Indeed, changes in taxation initiated by the government usually occur after consultation with the industry.[31] At irregular intervals, the government adjusts the taxation level if it temporarily needs to fill holes in the state budget. This requires changes to the taxation law, and parliamentary approval. This happened in 1991 (three gradual increases in 1992 and 1993), 1996 (three small increases from 1997 to 1999), 2001, 2004, 2006, 2008, 2010, 2011, 2013, and 2015. With the exception of 2004, 2008, and 2013,[32] the tax increases were small and intentionally imposed in a gradual manner, to minimise their effect on tobacco consumption.

The fact that tax increases are usually gradual rather than abrupt is a major success for the industry. For example, in 1991, at the height of national austerity measures, the government needed 500 million guilders extra income. The SSI made extensive preparations and presented a report with a proposal to realise the needed revenue for the state in an industry-friendly manner. The proposal was presented by industry representatives to the minister for finance (Klijn & Toet, 1991) and extensively discussed in parliament.[33] Although the tax was higher than the industry wanted, most of their other recommendations were adopted and tax levels were increased gradually (in three six-months intervals) to minimise behavioural effects that would undermine the net effect on the coffers or reduce industry profits.[34]

The industry had some other notable victories with the Ministry of Finance. Because the consumption of roll-your-own tobacco products increased dramatically between 1975 and 1985, while the consumption of the much more expensive manufactured cigarettes went down (Mindell & Whynes, 2000), cigarette manufacturers complained that the economic crisis affected them disproportionally, employment in their sector was threatened, and they needed a greater profit-earning capacity in order to survive. After lobbying from the cigarette manufacturers, a motion by VVD parliamentarian Jos van Rey supported by the Ministry for Economic Affairs (Ministerie van Economische Zaken, 1984) resulted in a decision by the Minister of Finance to *reduce* the tax on manufactured tobacco in 1984 (from 74% to 72%).[35] This enabled the industry to increase the price of a pack of cigarettes by 15 cents without the risk of losing customers. The industry was so pleased with this result that it organised an informal diner party at the high-class Hotel Des Indes in The Hague, inviting industry business organisations who benefited from the price increase and all involved officials from the Ministry of Economic Affairs and Ministry of Finance, including the state secretaries who helped to make it possible (SSI, 1984).

Tax increases are thus carefully fine-tuned after consultation with the tobacco sector. The industry frequently takes advantage of tax increases by increasing their wholesale price, while minimising the effect of tax increases on sale volumes. For example, the effect of the 2006 tax increase on smoking behaviour was neutralised by the industry, which simply reduced the number of cigarettes in a standard pack from 20 to 19. On other occasions the industry adjusted the volume of tobacco in roll-your-own pouches downward, to camouflage tax increases: in 2009 the weight of tobacco in roll-your-own packs was reduced from 50 grammes to 45 grammes. In 2011 it was 42.5 grammes and in the next year it was further reduced to 40 grammes of tobacco. Parliamentarians have repeatedly asked for a system where tax level is directly related either to the weight of tobacco, so that cigarettes and roll-your-own tobacco are equally taxed, or to the harmfulness of the product, so that products with higher tar and nicotine levels become more expensive.[36]

Dutch industry lobbyists not only put their stamp on national tax policy, but at times also use their contacts at the Ministry of Finance to influence European policy. For example in 1991, when the EU decided on a minimum tariff of 57% for tobacco products (Philip Morris, 1989), the Dutch Minister of Finance Wim Kok, who was chair of Ecofin (the Council of Ministers of Economic Affairs and Finance of all EU countries), was heavily lobbied on this issue by Philip Morris, which presented doomsday scenarios of job losses and negative effects on national trade balances (Philip Morris, 1989). The Minister of Economic Affairs asked Kok if he, in his capacity as chairman, could give ample speaking time and opportunity to the UK delegation to question the 57% tax ruling during the Ecofin meeting (Philip Morris, 1989). Afterwards the industry thanked the officials from the Ministry of Finance "for the efforts by the minister, the state secretary and yourself to bend the decision in, for the Dutch business community, a more acceptable direction" (Philip Morris, 1989). Another example of industry lobbying occurred between September 2008 and April 2009, when lobbyists visited the finance ministry nine times and also had a meeting with the State Secretary for Finance Jan Kees de Jager. The topic of the talks was the EC's wish to abandon minimum taxation levels for cigarettes (Algemene Rekenkamer, 2012). At first the government was in favour of the EC proposal, but after industry's lobbying efforts, it changed its position to neutral.

Targeting the Ministry of Health

Civil servants responsible for tobacco control policy in the Ministry of Health were main targets of tobacco industry lobbyists. In the 1980s and 1990s, there were only two civil servants dealing with tobacco control, and they had to divide their attention with other issues such as alcohol control and drugs. One government official described the government's relationship with the industry during these years: "There are frequent meetings between government and tobacco industry because of parallel interests … the government requests the industry to do certain activities (for example, self-regulation of advertising) and the same happens the other way around. The activities of the tobacco industry are important for the success of governmental policy regarding smoking" (Wever, 1988). It was normal practice that ideas for new tobacco legislation were discussed with sparring partners from the industrial sector. This suggests it was very much an insider game. Only when proposals had reached a certain level of incontrovertibility were broader consultation meetings organised. Symptomatic of the type of relationship was the fact that when two leading civil servants who were responsible for tobacco policy left the Ministry of Health in 1992, industry representatives were present at their farewell reception.[37]

The government continued to allow self-regulation of tobacco advertising by the industry well into the 1990s. As government officials needed to have contact with the industry to discuss details of the advertising code of conduct, this developed into a habit of seeing and meeting each other on a regular basis, which was a great advantage for the industry. At such meetings all aspects of tobacco control could be raised, and it became normal practice that proposals for new tobacco policy made by the Ministry of Health were sent directly, or through the Ministry of Economic Affairs, to the industry for scrutiny and comment, before they were sent to parliament (NVS, VNK, & SSI, 1990). Small steps in regulation and restrictions, especially regarding the many versions of the self-imposed code of conduct regarding tobacco advertising, were discussed endlessly with the industry, which treated these talks as if they were negotiations, while the government regarded them more as consultations. The industry presented their contributions as "concessions" and "giving in" to wishes of the government (Marres & Toet, 1987). In 1992 the code had to be renewed, and the Health Minister, Hans Simons, wanted it substantially improved, with fewer loopholes for the industry and termination of advertisements promoting positive images of smokers. This involved many meetings with the industry between 1992 and 1994 about the exact content of the new code. The industry's full support from the trade ministry, gave it a strong position during these talks, evidenced by the fact that they could get away with refusing to end tobacco advertisements. They continued advertising at the important international Formula 1 races in Zandvoort and at TT motorcycle events in Assen, a trade-off for the relatively unimportant termination of tobacco promotion through billboards at motorways.[38]

During the 1990s civil servants in the Ministry of Health became increasingly agitated by the arrogant attitude of the industry: "There is very little progress in the talks with the tobacco industry about reducing advertising through self-regulation. We do everything in our power to get concrete results, but the tobacco industry manages to sabotage everything, both regarding the content and regarding the process" (Wever, 1992). Another civil servant complained, "The tobacco advertising dossier has become rather extensive. The lobby by the (inter)national businesses (worldwide tobacco manufacturers, VNO–NCW, European employers, advertising agencies, publishers, media exploiters etc.) is immense" (Engelsman, 1992).

When Hans Simons was state secretary for health in the Lubbers III cabinet (1989–1994) the relationship with industry representatives began to stiffen, because Simons wished to intensify tobacco control. In 1994 he sent a summary of the outcomes of negotiations with the industry about the new advertising code to parliament, and received a prompt letter from SSI. The industry was outraged by what they saw as false representation of their intentions: "The industry is seriously disappointed and feels unjustly treated during the contacts with your department. This is all the more troublesome since this has happened already several times in the recent past" (Toet, 1994).

Industry Contacts During the Ministership of Els Borst

One year after Health Minister Borst (D66) began preparations to revise the Tobacco Act in 1994, she received an unambiguous signal from Alexander Rinnooy Kan, chairman of employee organisation VNO–NCW, that she was on a collision course with VNO–NCW (Rinnooy-Kan, 1995a, 1995b), and she was warned not to proceed with her intended plans. He wrote that VNO–NCW would not take it lightly if she dismissed self-regulation ("an agreement is an agreement") or if the advertising code was not continued for the full period of five years: "It must be clear to you that we do not accept a more paternalistic government."

The industry was intensely involved in the process of drafting the ministry's tobacco control policy document, which contained detailed proposals for a revised Tobacco Act, and industry spokesmen even made concrete suggestions for text changes (Van de Mortel, 1996)—the health sector was not consulted. Only after the text had been leaked to the press was STIVORO able to join in (Boudewijn De Blij, 1996a). In a letter to parliament, STIVORO's director Boudewijn de Blij noted, "It strikes me that the industry has been involved in every phase of the realisation. I expect STIVORO to be involved in such important decision making processes as well" (Boudewijn De Blij, 1996b). Parliamentarian Rob Oudkerk (PvdA) responded, "The tobacco industry relies on excellent lobbyists. They have accomplished a lot during 14 meetings with the cabinet, without any involvement from parliament. Cabinet and parliament have only debated about [the bill] twice" (Bruinsma, 1996).

As was discussed previously in Chap. 2 of this book, in 1996 routine meetings between the industry and the government to discuss tobacco policy were abandoned and the Ministry of Economic Affairs stepped back in favour of a more dominant role from the Ministry of Health, so the industry sought new ways to improve and strengthen communication with the tobacco policy officers at the Ministry of Health. They were not very successful. The relationship between industry representatives and the Ministry of Health at the time could best be characterised as distant and reserved, certainly not warm and welcoming.

In 1997 the ministry agreed to have "broad regular meetings" to which "other interested parties would also be invited, so that all aspects of comprehensive tobacco control policy could be discussed" (Van Hoogstraten, 1997a). This implied that not only would the tobacco industry be invited, as had been previous practice, but also representatives from the health sector. After the cabinet made its tobacco control policy intentions public, the Ministry of Health organised a broad consultation session in September 1997 (Van Hoogstraten, 1997b). The health sector including STIVORO, the Heart Foundation, Cancer Society, Medical Alliance Against Smoking, Clean Air Netherlands (CAN) and the *Gemeentelijke Gezondheidsdienst* (Association of Community Health Services) (GGD) was to be heard in the morning. Representations from civil society such as VNO–NCW, labour unions, NOC-NSF (the national sports federation), consumer organisations, the advertising sector, and the hospitality sector could present their arguments in the afternoon, followed by the tobacco industry sector, represented by lobbyists from LBT, SSI, VNK, NVS, and NSO. Soon afterwards Health Minister Borst received a letter from SSI, complaining that the Ministry of Health did not seem to take industry arguments seriously: "During these talks we brought a great number of concerns to the table. It is now clear that in no way whatsoever did you include any of our concerns in your policy" (Roelofs, 1998). VNO–NCW sent a critical letter to Borst demanding that "the wish list of this cabinet can be and must become considerably shorter" (Blankert, 1997). From these and other letters at the end of the 1990s it is clear that the industry had completely lost its inside grip on tobacco control policy and fell back on intimidation and external pressure.

For many years the tobacco team at the Ministry of Health was understaffed. Until 2000, only two public servants dealt with tobacco. They were not full-time dedicated staff, since they also had to deal with alcohol. In 1998, Minister Borst was asked in parliament why it took her so long to implement the tobacco control initiatives that she had presented two years earlier. She explained that the new tobacco control policy "contains in total more than 50 initiatives, intentions, projects and actions. ... All this work, in addition to the complete alcohol control policy, has to be done by just a few workers at my department."[39] Her predecessor, State Secretary Hans Simons, had also complained that he was so understaffed that negotiations with the industry about the advertising code of conduct were difficult and took too much time.[40] Sometime around 2000 the tobacco team was reinforced with three dedicated civil servants and a liaison officer from STIVORO to help adopt and implement the new Tobacco Act. Inspired and protected by Minister Borst, these officials were dedicated tobacco control advocates. The team worked closely with health organisations and kept contact with tobacco industry spokespersons to a minimum, but this did not mean that contact was rare. Officials and industry representatives continued to meet frequently to discuss technical aspects of regulation (such as specific allowances regarding advertising at points of sale), and industry representatives were given the opportunity to present their concerns and problems to the civil servants and sometimes to the director-general. A tobacco control officer said,

> You just wanted to allow all concerned parties to have their say. Did we write the correct text, are there any other ideas? Yes, you cannot write a product regulation proposal without ever having talked about it with the industry. ... It was common practice. ... I believe it is appropriate that we do it like that. This is sort of the consensus model that we have in the Netherlands: *polderen* and deliberating until we have a good outcome.[41]

VNO–NCW continued, unsuccessfully, to lobby for periodic regular meetings with the Ministry of Health (Schraven, 2001b).

Minister Borst Turns Her Back on the Tobacco Industry

In May 2000 the relationship between the industry and the Ministry of Health reached a dramatic low. Borst, in an interview with morning newspaper *De Telegraaf*, announced "rigorous measures" against tobacco and declared there was no future for tobacco in the Netherlands. The industry reacted furiously. Immediately the next day they sent an angry letter to her, with carbon copies to the ministers for social, economic, and financial affairs, and to parliament (Roelofs, 2000a), and a separate letter to prime minister Kok (Roelofs, 2000b). They blamed Borst for not talking with the industry: "This is not the first time that you have unilaterally launched proposals and ideas in public without first engaging in a constructive dialogue with us. ... Your approach to repeatedly confront the tobacco industry through the media with new measures and unfounded accusations is unacceptable to us." They demanded that the prime minister call Borst to account for "the way she chooses to deal with the tobacco and related sectors ... letters are not replied to, appointments are not kept and requests for executive meetings are ignored. ... We assume that you are willing to call upon your colleague from the Ministry of Health to normalise relationships with our sector."

A few weeks later, a meeting was indeed organised between VNO–NCW and Borst, accompanied by her top-level civil servants (Schraven, 2001a). They reached a compromise: there would be a dialogue between the Ministry of Health and the industry under independent chairmanship. Since this did not happen, VNO–NCW brought the matter up again a year later and proposed the possibility of an executive-level meeting once or twice per year between the industry and the ministers for health and for economic affairs (Schraven, 2001a). In addition they proposed regular tobacco policy expert meetings, open to both industry experts and experts from all involved societal organisations, ranging from STIVORO to smokers' right groups. However, Borst, who wanted to finalise her revision of the Tobacco Act before the end of her time in office, continued to hold off contact with the industry sector, despite many letters from the industry complaining that they were not heard. She allowed her civil servants to push the bill forward with limited opportunities for the industry to be consulted about the timing of its implementation (Horeca Nederland, 2002; Kalis, 2002).

Health Ministers Keep the Industry at a Distance

The SSI approached Borst's successor, Eduard Bomhoff, soon after he started work as the new minister for health. Bomhoff, a university professor in economics, had been a member of the Labour Party for many years, but was asked by the populist *Lijst Pim Fortuyn* (Pim Fortuyn List) (LPF) to take up the position of health minister in the first Balkenende Cabinet. SSI wrote him a long letter complaining about the "unacceptable way the Ministry of Health currently does not give meaning to a decent dialogue with the concerned industry sectors," demanding a resumption of "constructive dialogue" and requesting that the implementation of the Tobacco Act be put on hold (Monkhorst, 2002; SSI, 2002). Bomhoff replied in unmistakable terms that he wanted no personal contact with the industry, and was not willing to consider a respite in the implementation process (Bonhoff, 2002).

Bomhoff was minister for a very short period in 2002. Because of a fight between him and the Minister for Economic Affairs Herman Heinsbroek (LPF), the cabinet resigned. When his tasks were temporarily taken over by State Secretary Clémence Ross-van Dorp (CDA), VNO–NCW recognised an opportunity to bring the idea of regular executive meetings to her attention (Schraven, 2003a). Instead of granting the request, the ministry sent a short questionnaire to a large number of societal and business organisations with a stake in tobacco policy, asking them whether they were interested in being part of regular broad meetings about tobacco control policy (Kalis, 2003). When it became clear that these had also been sent to health organisations, the industry stepped down, not liking the prospect of having meetings with the ministry in the presence of tobacco control advocates. The ministry received replies from 26 of 67 organisations, insufficient for regular meetings (Hoogervorst, 2003b), and instead decided to continue the habit of granting meetings with individual stakeholders as circumstances required.

In the meantime, the industry and civil servants at the Ministry of Health had various meetings to discuss the ramifications of the transposition of the EU Tobacco Product Directive (TPD-1). The most difficult issue was the requirement that manufacturers submit lists of all additives used in the manufacture of their products, specifically at the level of each brand. The industry was not prepared to do this without a fight, claiming that the requirement infringed on company secrets. They tried to offer alternative formats that would entail a far smaller level of detail. State secretary Clémence Ross did not give in to their pressure, and after numerous letters and fruitless meetings between industry and government officials she published the regulation in the Bulletin of Acts and Decrees in April 2003.

Not only ministers Borst and Bomhoff but also their successor Hans Hoogervorst (health minister from 2003 to 2007) resented industry lobbyists. Hoogervorst made it clear that he had no intention of reinstalling the executive meetings (Hoogervorst, 2003b) and was not prepared to discuss the decision to make public the ingredients of cigarette brands (Hoogervorst, 2003a). A few weeks later the industry summoned the Dutch state to argue the ingredients matter in court.

Just after Hoogervorst took office, the Framework Convention on Tobacco Control (FCTC) treaty was signed by the Netherlands. This meant that the government was expected to refrain from interactions with the tobacco industry unless it was "strictly necessary to enable them to effectively regulate tobacco industry and tobacco products."[42] While Hoogervorst was minister, VNO–NCW was frustrated that regular meetings were not reinstated (Schraven, 2003b). Hoogervorst's policy regarding interaction with the industry was in line with the FCTC requirement: he only allowed contact about technical issues of implementation of tobacco regulation, of which he gave this example: "The government does not talk with the industry about whether there must be graphic health warnings on tobacco packages, but the government can initiate contact with the industry about practical matters such as the transition period that is necessary to adjust the packs."[43] Throughout his term in office Hoogervorst refused cooperation or meetings with the industry about general policy, explicitly referring to the FCTC (Dortland, 2005; Hoogervorst, 2006a, 2006b). However, the Ministry of Health allowed industry representatives to have bilateral contact with civil servants to discuss "concrete policy matters" (VWS, 2003). It is clear from the email correspondence published in the Truth Tobacco Industry Documents database[44] that the bureaucrats from the ministry did this reluctantly until around 2008, often using the formal "*u*" to address the recipient in emails, keeping the language aloof and business-like, while the industry used the informal "*je*" and was more direct and, at times, intrusive and pushy.

The Ministry of Health Resumes Contact with the Industry

In contrast to the three previous ministers, health ministers Ab Klink (2007–2010) and Edith Schippers (2010–2012) did not regard contact with the industry as inherently problematic. At first the ministry told the industry that the policy of the previous ministers, that there could be no collaboration between government and the tobacco sector regarding policy, would be continued (De Goeij, 2006), but this changed when Klink, after four months in office, granted a personal meeting with industry CEOs (Smid, 2007), followed by an "exceptionally constructive" (in SSI/VNK's words) meeting with SSI and VNK (SSI & VNK, 2007). Further meetings were planned to discuss industry ideas about such things as youth smoking prevention and new safer cigarettes (Klink, 2007). Minister Klink set the example and the norm for how government officials should communicate with the industry, and the number of contacts increased and emails between officials and industry representatives had a friendlier tone. Civil Servants fell back on the familiar habit of involving and consulting the sector. Symptomatic of the desire not to step on industrial toes was a reassuring response from one of Klink's tobacco control officers to a letter in which SSI expressed its concerns about the drafting of the guidelines to WHO Article 5.3, which could lead to full exclusion of the industry from the policymaking process: "First of all, I want to stress that it concerns non-binding guidelines. … Secondly, it is certainly not a matter of excluding the industry" (De Jager, 2008).

In March 2009, halfway through Klink's ministership, Director-General Hans de Goeij, who had a solid track record in tobacco control, was replaced by an economist who had less affinity with public health. The new Director-General for Health Paul Huijts, a former employee of the Ministry of Economic Affairs, set out to restore the dialogue with the industry that had gone astray under previous ministers. On 24 August 2009, after a meeting with the industry, Huijts looked back on "a useful and positive meeting, in which mutual interests and differences were well covered. … Future meetings … will have to contribute to mutual information exchange and the building up of mutual trust" (Huijts, 2009). Soon afterwards, the industry confirmed that it shared with the ministry the wish to come to a better understanding and was grateful that the ministry was again "open to any contacts, interventions, signals or questions" (NVK, NVS, SSI, & Philip Morris Benelux, 2010).

In 2009 Ministry of Health officials accepted an invitation from VNK to attend a "company day" (VNK & Ministry of Health, 2009). In the past, the industry had organised yearly small conferences around a specific theme, sometimes combined with a visit to a company or factory, for small groups of government officials. These meetings had been abandoned during the previous cabinets, but were reinstated under Huijts' leadership. The meeting took place in September 2009 and was attended by officials from three ministries (finance, economic affairs, and health) (VNK & Ministry of Health, 2009). In 2011 officials from the ministries of health, finance, and economic affairs visited a tobacco factory (VNK, 2011).

The responsive attitude towards the tobacco industry continued when Edith Schippers (VVD) became minister for health in October 2010. In reply to a congratulatory letter, Schippers confirmed to SSI and VNK, "I appreciate the intention to invest more in the coming time in an open and constructive exchange of thoughts about different international topics" (Schippers, 2010). The government's "generous" interpretation of the FCTC commitments, and in particular Article 5.3, lasted until 2016, when it felt obliged by a court case initiated by the Youth Smoking Prevention Foundation to rethink its policy regarding Article 5.3 and to settle for an implementation more in line with the spirit of the FCTC (discussed in Chap. 6).

Conclusion

In the first decades of tobacco control policymaking, the situation in the Netherlands was similar to that of the United Kingdom in the 1980s, where the tobacco industry survived, despite health concerns, under the protection of a "smoke ring" of tobacco-friendly individuals and organisations (Taylor, 1984). Such "iron triangles" were close-tied networks of lobbyists, advisory bodies, parliamentarians, and government officials who shared specific values and political ideology in line with industry arguments.[45] The industry felt protected through gentlemanly networks, able to lobby through direct contacts with ministers.

In the mid-1970s the iron triangle was challenged in the publication of the Health Council report *Measures to Reduce Smoking*. From then onwards, the industry had to defend its interests more proactively, to prevent the balance of power from shifting in an undesirable direction. This chapter has presented many examples of how the Dutch tobacco industry lobbied. Continued conflict with the industrial sector over regulation versus self-regulation was the main reason why it took until 2002 to revise the Tobacco Act. Until the mid-1990s the industry lobbied through direct contacts with ministers, while the health organisations had to rely on an outside lobby, most of the time relying on politicians who could not gather majorities in parliament. Well-known lobbyists who had worked for the industry for many years knew the ins and outs of tobacco policy better than most government officials, giving them an information advantage. Information asymmetry and dependence on information from the industry make it more difficult for the government to make independent, balanced policy decisions (Coglianese, Zeckhauser, & Parson, 2004).

What stands out is the perseverance of the industry lobby, which relentlessly voiced the same arguments and concerns over and over, exploiting diverse routes of influence. These included politicians, bureaucrats in various ministries, and third party contacts, especially the powerful employers' organisation VNO–NCW. They knew whom to contact at which point, and they approached policymakers at all levels, from low-ranking civil servants to ministers, and even the prime minister. The lobbying game was sometimes played simultaneously at national, European, and global levels.

Around 1996, when Health Minister Els Borst distanced herself from the tobacco industry, the industry lost some of its grip on the government, and moved to expand its influence through other parties. It forged coalitions with Royal Dutch Hospitality, smokers' rights groups, and the ventilation industry to fend off hospitality bans, and with supermarket and retail organisations to prevent sale restrictions. In later years VNO–NCW tried to normalise contacts with the Ministry of Health and to reinstate the practice of involving the industry in conceptualising and drafting tobacco control policy. They were somewhat successful between 2007 and 2012 under the ministerships of Klink and Schippers, but more recently, public outrage over the many violations of Article 5.3 FCTC tarnished the reputation of the Dutch tobacco industry and made direct contact between the government and the industry increasingly difficult. One former tobacco industry lobbyist lamented about more recent years, "the anti-tobacco lobby was much more effective than the tobacco lobby, much more effective, mainly because they have been very successful in holding off every contact between the government and the tobacco industry."[46]

Notes

1. Philip Morris, producer of best-selling brand Marlboro, became the market leader in the Netherlands around 1986.
2. Proceedings II, 1995–1996, Kamervragen, Aanhangsel 1428.
3. https://www.industrydocumentslibrary.ucsf.edu/tobacco/
4. Rinnooy Kan was proclaimed by the press as the most influential person in the Netherlands in the years 2007–2009.
5. Interview, 6 November 2015.
6. Interview, 6 October 2015.
7. Vrij Nederland, 23 November 2002.
8. Another example of the importance of the CDA to the industry was Rob Koreneef. He started in 1991 as political assistant to a CDA member of parliament. After that, he followed a similar career path as Wilhelmus: first working as public affairs consultant at Burson-Marsteller and then moving on to do similar work for tobacco manufactures (Imperial Tobacco and Philip Morris).
9. For example, Martin Bril, Drs. P., Max van Rooy, Martin van Amerongen, Jan Mulder (a non-smoker), and Theodor Holman.
10. This argument has become hollow over the years, as the Netherlands no longer had a noticeable cigarette manufacturing industry (see Chap. 5 for more details).
11. In Dutch: *Wet op de Investeringsrekening* (WIR). It was set up in 1978 by the Ministry for Economic Affairs to stimulate businesses to invest in company assets such as machines, and was in force until 1988.
12. Comparable to a sum of about €6 million in 2016.
13. Illustrative of the close links with the trade ministry is the fact that Jules Wilhelmus, information officer for that ministry between 1982 and 1987, left to work for some years with Burson-Marsteller, Philip Morris' main PR bureau, and continued his career as director of corporate affairs for Philip Morris from 1995 until 2005.
14. Minister of Economic Affairs from 1989 to 1994.
15. Interview, 26 April 2016.
16. Proceedings II, 1996–1997, 24743, nr. 3, p. 8.
17. Dutch: *bestuurlijk overleg*.
18. Dutch: *ambtelijk overleg*.
19. Parliamentary Papers II, 1982–1983, 17600, hoofdstuk XIII, nr. 36.
20. Proceedings II, 10 February 1983, 47^e meeting, p. 2241.
21. Proceedings I, 8 June 1983, 31^e meeting, p. 862.
22. See also Chap. 5 on the "better regulation" movement in the Netherlands.
23. Proceedings II, 31 May 2001, TK 82, 5216; Proceedings I, 26 March 2002, 24–1255.
24. https://www.industrydocumentslibrary.ucsf.edu/tobacco/

25. Parliamentary Papers II, 2009–2010, kv-2009Z17997.
26. Interview, 6 October 2015.
27. The Dutch Excise Duty Act dates from 1921 and has been modernised in 1961 and 1991.
28. Interview, 6 November 2015.
29. See for examples of such contacts in 2008 and 2010: https://www.industrydocumentslibrary.ucsf.edu/tobacco/docs/#id=xkxb0191
30. Interview, 22 February 2017.
31. See (SSI & Toet, 1972–1996) for a collection of correspondence between the industry and the government on tobacco taxation.
32. In 2004 there was a larger tax increase to support the workplace smoking ban. In 2008, with the introduction of the smoking ban in bars and restaurants, another higher-than-usual increase was realised. In 2013, tax increases resulted in consumer price increases of more than 10% for both cigarettes and roll-your-own tobacco.
33. Proceedings II, 1991–1992, 22351, nr. 4.
34. Parliamentary Papers II, 1991–1992, 22351, nrs. 5 and 7.
35. Proceedings II, 1983–1984, 18139, nr. 4.
36. Proceedings II, 24743, nr. 3, p. 4.
37. Interview with a former civil servant on 1 February 2017.
38. Proceedings II, 22 December 1993, 41–3246.
39. Proceedings II, 1997–1998, Annex 891.
40. Proceedings II, 1993–1994, 23400 XVI, 78, p. 6.
41. Interview on 18 November 2015.
42. Recommendation 2.1 of the implementation guidelines for Article 5.3 FCTC.
43. Parliamentary Papers II, 2005–2006, 22894, nr. 83.
44. https://www.industrydocumentslibrary.ucsf.edu/tobacco/
45. Such powerful networks that protect business interests are common in the Netherlands, not only in tobacco but in other areas such as education and agriculture as well (Trappenburg, 2005).
46. Interview on 22 February 2017.

References

Algemene Rekenkamer. (2012). *Bestrijding van accijnsfraude bij alcohol en tabak. EU-beleid: naleving en effecten.* Den Haag: Sdu Uitgevers.

Andeweg, R. B., & Irwin, G. A. (2009). *Governance and politics of the Netherlands* (3rd ed.). Hampshire: Palgrave Macmillan.

ARISE. (1995a). Living is more than surviving: The contribution of pleasure to everyday life—International media coverage 1995/96. *British American Tobacco Records*, Bates No. 500853324–500853394. Retrieved from https://www.industrydocumentslibrary.ucsf.edu/tobacco/docs/spmv0211

ARISE. (1995b). A summary of the workshop held in April 1995. Living is more than surviving. *RJ Reynolds Records*, Bates No. 511818234–511818241. Retrieved from https://www.industrydocumentslibrary.ucsf.edu/tobacco/docs/ppnm0089

Baltesen, F., & Rosenberg, E. (2009, June 22). Big tobacco pays Dutch opposition to smoking ban. *NRC Handelsblad*. Retrieved from http://vorige.nrc.nl/international/article2278646.ece/Big_tobacco_pays_Dutch_opposition_to_smoking_ban

Blankert, J. (1997). Wijzigingen tabakswet. *Dutch Tobacco Industry Collection*, Bates No. JB2074. Retrieved from https://www.industrydocumentslibrary.ucsf.edu/tobacco/docs/xjdp0219

Blankert, J. (1999). [Letter to Jorritsma]. *Dutch Tobacco Industry Collection*, Bates No. JB2377. Retrieved from https://www.industrydocumentslibrary.ucsf.edu/tobacco/docs/fsdp0219

Bonhoff, E. J. (2002). Brief van het ministerie van VWS aan de Stichting Sigarettenindustrie over het Tabaksontmoedigingsbeleid. *Dutch Tobacco Industry Collection*, Bates No. JB3527.

Borst-Eilers, E. (1996). Verslag overleg tabaksontmoedigingsbeleid. *Dutch Tobacco Industry Collection*, Bates No. JB2069. Retrieved from https://www.industrydocumentslibrary.ucsf.edu/tobacco/docs/txdp0219

Bouma, J. (2001). *Het rookgordijn: De macht van de Nederlandse tabaksindustrie*. Amsterdam: Veen.

Bouma, J. (2012, February 21). Tabakslobby op schoot bij minister Schippers. *Trouw*. Retrieved from http://www.trouw.nl/tr/nl/4516/Gezondheid/article/detail/3193743/2012/02/21/Tabakslobby-op-schoot-bij-minister-Schippers.dhtml

Braam, S., & Van Woerden, I. (2013, juni 27). De laatste vriend van de sigaret. *Vrij Nederland*.

Bruinsma, J. (1996, October 30). Alleen Jet Nijpels wijzigde standpunt na bezoek tabaksindustrie. Kamerleden ontkennen invloed lobby, *de Volkskrant*, p. 7. Retrieved from https://www.industrydocumentslibrary.ucsf.edu/tobacco/docs/thcp0219

Coglianese, C., Zeckhauser, R., & Parson, E. (2004). Seeking truth for power: Informational strategy and regulatory policy making. *Faculty Research Working Papers Series Harvard University, John F. Kennedy School of Government, RWP04-021*.

De Blij, B. (1996a). Letter to Wijers. *Dutch Tobacco Industry Collection*, Bates No. JB2517. Retrieved from https://www.industrydocumentslibrary.ucsf.edu/tobacco/docs/mxwp0219

De Blij, B. (1996b). Tabaksontmoedigingsbeleid. *Dutch Tobacco Industry Collection*, Bates No. JB2695. Retrieved from https://www.industrydocumentslibrary.ucsf.edu/tobacco/docs/gnfp0219

De Goeij, J. I. M. (2006). [Letter to VNK]. *Dutch Tobacco Industry Collection*, Bates No. JB3059. Retrieved from https://www.industrydocumentslibrary.ucsf.edu/tobacco/docs/jtwn0217

De Jager, J. H. (2008). Beleidsvoornemens tabaksontmoediging. *Dutch Tobacco Industry Collection*, Bates No. JB0562. Retrieved from https://www.industrydocumentslibrary.ucsf.edu/tobacco/docs/hkxb0191

De Wolff, F. A. (1994a). Comments on the OSHA proposed rule on indoor air quality, April 5. *Dutch Tobacco Industry Collection*, Bates No. JB1177. Retrieved from https://www.industrydocumentslibrary.ucsf.edu/tobacco/docs/hkxp0219

De Wolff, F. A. (1994b). Risico van longkanker door passief roken nog onbewezen. *Nederlands Tijdschrift voor Geneeskunde, 138*, 503–506.

Dortland, R. (2005). Brief van het ministerie van VWS aan de Stichting Sigarettenindustrie betreffende de Tabakswet. *Dutch Tobacco Industry Collection*, Bates No. JB3525. Retrieved from https://www.industrydocumentslibrary.ucsf.edu/tobacco/docs/fswn0217

Emmelot, P. (1979). Wetenschappelijke Adviesraad Roken en Gezondheid (WARG). *Dutch Tobacco Industry Collection*, Bates No. JB1400. Retrieved from https://www.industrydocumentslibrary.ucsf.edu/tobacco/docs/jqgp0219

Engelsman, E. (1992). Mondeling overleg tabaksontmoedigingsbeleid. *Dutch Tobacco Industry Collection*, Bates No. JB2031. Retrieved from https://www.industrydocumentslibrary.ucsf.edu/tobacco/docs/rmfp0219

EPA. (1992). *Respiratory health effects of passive smoking (also known as exposure to secondhand smoke or Environmental Tobacco Smoke—ETS)*. Washington, DC: U.S. Environmental Protection Agency (EPA).

Evenhuis, A. (1988). *Reclamecode sigaretten en shag Dutch Tobacco Industry Collection*, Bates No. JB2182. Retrieved from https://www.industrydocumentslibrary.ucsf.edu/tobacco/docs/fndp0219

Forces USA. (1998). The speakers of the 1997 Smokepeace International Conference. *Philip Morris Collection*, Bates No. 2073643759–2073643760. Retrieved from https://www.industrydocumentslibrary.ucsf.edu/tobacco/docs/nhbb0088

Gemeente Bergen op Zoom. (1996). Accijnsverhoging op tabaksproducten [letter to the prime minister]. *Dutch Tobacco Industry Collection*, Bates No. JB2646. Retrieved from https://www.industrydocumentslibrary.ucsf.edu/tobacco/docs/xywp0219

GfK Great Britain. (1998). ETS world report Philip Morris 1998. *Philip Morris Records*, Bates No. 2065221475–2065221544. Retrieved from http://legacy.library.ucsf.edu/tid/fnq90g00/pdf

Goldberg, H. (1999a). Accommodation programs. *Philip Morris Collection*, Bates No. 2072577224–2072577238. Retrieved from http://legacy.library.ucsf.edu/tid/otq59h00

Goldberg, H. (1999b). International accommodation programs. *Philip Morris Collection*, Bates No. 2074399542–2074399568. Retrieved from http://legacy.library.ucsf.edu/tid/thp11h00

Hamers, J., & Vermeulen, A. (1996). Tabakaccijns [letter to the prime minister]. *Dutch Tobacco Industry Collection*, Bates No. JB2670. Retrieved from https://www.industrydocumentslibrary.ucsf.edu/tobacco/docs/qpwp0219

Hoogervorst, H. (2003a). Regeling lijsten tabaksingrediënten [letter to SSI]. *Dutch Tobacco Industry Collection*, Bates No. JB3259. Retrieved from https://www.industrydocumentslibrary.ucsf.edu/tobacco/docs/nybn0217

Hoogervorst, H. (2003b). Regulier overleg tabaksontmoedigingsbeleid. *Dutch Tobacco Industry Collection*, Bates No. JB0278. Retrieved from https://www.industrydocumentslibrary.ucsf.edu/tobacco/docs/sjhb0191

Hoogervorst, H. (2006a). Antwoordbrief aan VNK en SSI. *Dutch Tobacco Industry Collection*, Bates No. JB0412.

Hoogervorst, H. (2006b). Brief van het ministerie van VWS aan de Vereniging Nederlandse Kerftabakindustrie. *Dutch Tobacco Industry Collection*, Bates No. JB3333. Retrieved from https://www.industrydocumentslibrary.ucsf.edu/tobacco/docs/ftwn0217

Horeca Nederland. (2002). Overleg Tabakswet [letter to Borst]. *Dutch Tobacco Industry Collection*, Bates No. JB3517. Retrieved from https://www.industrydocumentslibrary.ucsf.edu/tobacco/docs/flwn0217

Huijts, P. H. A. M. (2009). Gesprek 24 Augsutus jl. *Dutch Tobacco Industry Collection*, Bates No. JB0611. Retrieved from https://www.industrydocumentslibrary.ucsf.edu/tobacco/docs/hnxb0191

Jha, P., & Chaloupka, F. J. (2000). The economics of global tobacco control. *BMJ: British Medical Journal, 321*(7257), 358–361.

Kalis, A. W. (2002). Consultatie inzake inwerkingtreding van gewijzigde Tabakswet. *Dutch Tobacco Industry Collection*, Bates No. JB3519. Retrieved from https://www.industrydocumentslibrary.ucsf.edu/tobacco/docs/jkcn0217

Kalis, A. W. (2003). Regulier overleg tabaksontmoedigingsbeleid. *Dutch Tobacco Industry Collection*, Bates No. JB0272. Retrieved from https://www.industrydocumentslibrary.ucsf.edu/tobacco/docs/mjhb0191

Klijn, W., & Toet, R. L. J. (1991). [Letter to Ministry of Finance]. *Dutch Tobacco Industry Collection*, Bates No. JB2781. Retrieved from https://www.industrydocumentslibrary.ucsf.edu/tobacco/docs/mtwp0219

Klink, A. (2007). Tabaksontmoedigingsbeleid (letter to SSI). *Dutch Tobacco Industry Collection*, Bates No. JB0454. Retrieved from https://www.industrydocumentslibrary.ucsf.edu/tobacco/docs/qzhb0191

Kok, W. (1996, September 2). Verhoging tabakaccijns. Retrieved from https://www.industrydocumentslibrary.ucsf.edu/tobacco/docs/rywp0219

Korteweg, A., & Huisman, E. (2016). *Lobbyland: De geheime krachten in Den Haag*. Amsterdam: De Geus.

Loubeau, P. (2014). *An exploratory review of illicit tobacco trade in the Netherlands*. Den Haag: Alliantie Nederland Rookvrij.

Luyendijk, J., Verkade, T., & Heck, W. (2010). Het lobbywerk dat níét op de cv's van politici staat. Retrieved from https://www.nrc.nl/nieuws/2010/11/22/het-lobbywerk-dat-niet-op-de-cvs-van-politici-staat-11972720-a865044

Mantel, A., & de Wolf, P. (1983). Marktkoncentratie en internatialisatie in de Nederlandse tabaksindustrie. *Tijdschrift voor Politieke Ekonomie, 6*, 34–56.

Marres, E. A. H., & Toet, R. L. J. (1987). Voorstellen van de SSI en de VNK ter aanpassing van de reclamecode. *Dutch Tobacco Industry Collection*, Bates No. JB2179. Retrieved from https://www.industrydocumentslibrary.ucsf.edu/tobacco/docs/tmdp0219

Mindell, J. S., & Whynes, D. K. (2000). Cigarette consumption in The Netherlands 1970–1995: Does tax policy encourage the use of hand-rolling tobacco? *European Journal of Public Health, 10*(3), 214–219. https://doi.org/10.1093/eurpub/10.3.214

Ministerie van Economische Zaken. (1982a). Ontmoedigingsbeleid tabaksgebruik. *Dutch Tobacco Industry Collection*, Bates No. JB2449. Retrieved from https://www.industrydocumentslibrary.ucsf.edu/tobacco/docs/#id=fyfp0219

Ministerie van Economische Zaken. (1982b). Ontmoedigingsbeleid tabaksgebruik en alcoholbeleid. *Dutch Tobacco Industry Collection*, Bates No. JB2447. Retrieved from https://www.industrydocumentslibrary.ucsf.edu/tobacco/docs/mfwp0219

Ministerie van Economische Zaken. (1984). Wetsontwerp ter verlaging van accijns op sigaretten i.v.m. eenmalige accijnsvrije prijsverhoging. *Dutch Tobacco Industry Collection*, Bates No. JB2221. Retrieved from https://www.industrydocumentslibrary.ucsf.edu/tobacco/docs/snfp0219

Ministerie van Economische Zaken. (1992). [Brief van het ministerie van EZ aan de NVS betreft sigarenaccijns]. *Dutch Tobacco Industry Collection*, Bates No. JB2464. Retrieved from https://www.industrydocumentslibrary.ucsf.edu/tobacco/docs/hgwp0219

Ministerie van Economische Zaken. (1995). Tussenrapportage Werkgroep Afspraken Tabaksbeleid. *Dutch Tobacco Industry Collection*, Bates No. JB1037.

Ministerie van Economische Zaken. (2009a). E-mails over plain packaging. *Dutch Tobacco Industry Collection*, Bates No. JB3821. Retrieved from https://www.industrydocumentslibrary.ucsf.edu/tobacco/docs/rrbn0217

Ministerie van Economische Zaken. (2009b). RE: Generieke verpakkingen voor tabaksproducten. *Dutch Tobacco Industry Collection*, Bates No. JB0505. Retrieved from https://www.industrydocumentslibrary.ucsf.edu/tobacco/docs/mtxb0191

Ministerie van Economische Zaken. (2009c). Stand van zaken invoering "plain packaging" in de Aanbeveling van de Raad inzake rookvrije ruimten. *Dutch Tobacco Industry Collection*, Bates No. JB0512. Retrieved from https://www.industrydocumentslibrary.ucsf.edu/tobacco/docs/nzxb0191

Ministerie van Financiën. (2011). Various e-mails. *Dutch Tobacco Industry Collection*, Bates No. JB0402. Retrieved from https://www.industrydocumentslibrary.ucsf.edu/tobacco/docs/mrhb0191

Monkhorst, T. (2002). Brief aan het ministerie van VWS over tabaksbeleid. *Dutch Tobacco Industry Collection*, Bates No. JB3528. Retrieved from https://www.industrydocumentslibrary.ucsf.edu/tobacco/docs/xncn0217

Nagelhout, G. E., Levy, D. T., Blackman, K., Currie, L., Clancy, L., & Willemsen, M. C. (2012). The effect of tobacco control policies on smoking prevalence and smoking-attributable deaths. Findings from the Netherlands SimSmoke tobacco control policy simulation model. *Addiction, 107*(2), 407–416. https://doi.org/10.1111/j.1360-0443.2011.03642.x

National Research Council. (1986). *Environmental tobacco smoke: Measuring exposure and assessing health effects.* Washington, DC: National Academy Press.

Nellen, M. E. A. H., & De Blij, B. A. I. M. (1999). The "success" of Philip Morris' campaign on environmental tobacco smoke in the Netherlands. *Tobacco Control, 8*(2), 221–222. https://doi.org/10.1136/tc.8.2.221a

NVK, NVS, SSI & Philip Morris Benelux. (2010). [Letter to Huijts]. *Dutch Tobacco Industry Collection*, Bates No. JB0562. Retrieved from https://www.industrydocumentslibrary.ucsf.edu/tobacco/docs/#id=hkxb0191

NVS, VNK & SSI. (1990). [Brieven van de NVS, VNK en SSI aan het ministerie van VWS en het ministerie van EZ]. *Dutch Tobacco Industry Collection*, Bates No. JB2347. Retrieved from https://www.industrydocumentslibrary.ucsf.edu/tobacco/docs/nqdp0219

O'NeillI, K., Brunnemann, K. D., Dodet, B., & Hoffmann, D. (1987). Passive smoking: Environmental carcinogens. *IARC scientific publications* (Vol. 9). Lyon: International Agency for Research on Cancer (IARC).

Philip Morris. (1979). Smoking & health—Five year plan. *Philip Morris Records*, Bates No. 2501020542-2501020686. Retrieved from https://www.industrydocumentslibrary.ucsf.edu/tobacco/docs/yfhl0000

Philip Morris. (1989). Several lobby letters about tax increase. *Dutch Tobacco Industry Collection*, Bates No. JB2223. Retrieved from https://www.industrydocumentslibrary.ucsf.edu/tobacco/docs/gydp0219

Philip Morris. (1994). 1994 Action plans Benelux. *Philip Morris Records*, Bates No. 2501318291–2501318294. Retrieved from https://www.industrydocumentslibrary.ucsf.edu/tobacco/docs/pnbj0115

Philip Morris. (1996a). Corporate Affairs 1996/1997 The Netherlands. *Philip Morris Records*, Bates No. 2501076006–2501076023. Retrieved from https://www.industrydocumentslibrary.ucsf.edu/tobacco/docs/nzjl0112

Philip Morris. (1996b). Verhoging van de accijns op tabaksproducten. *Dutch Tobacco Industry Collection*, Bates No. JB2661. Retrieved from https://www.industrydocumentslibrary.ucsf.edu/tobacco/docs/hpwp0219

Remes, D. (1988). The PM EEC/EEMA ETS Project—Draft—20 Feb 1988. *Ness Motley Law Firm Documents*, Bates No. 2501474253–2501474259.

Retrieved from https://www.industrydocumentslibrary.ucsf.edu/tobacco/docs/psly0042
Rijsterborgh, I. J. (2017). *The importance of the tobacco industry for the Dutch economy*. Maastricht: Maastricht University.
Rinnooy-Kan, A. H. G. (1994). Letter to VWS. *Dutch Tobacco Industry Collection*, Bates No. JB2591. Retrieved from https://www.industrydocumentslibrary.ucsf.edu/tobacco/docs/jmwp0219
Rinnooy-Kan, A. H. G. (1995a). Letter to Minister Wijers. *Dutch Tobacco Industry Collection*, Bates No. JB2589. Retrieved from https://www.industrydocumentslibrary.ucsf.edu/tobacco/docs/hkfp0219
Rinnooy-Kan, A. H. G. (1995b). Letter to VWS. *Dutch Tobacco Industry Collection*, Bates No. JB2590. Retrieved from https://www.industrydocumentslibrary.ucsf.edu/tobacco/docs/xmwp0219
RJ Reynolds. (1978). Chapter 1 smoking and health. *RJ Reynolds Records*, Bates No. 500534913–500534931. Retrieved from https://www.industrydocumentslibrary.ucsf.edu/tobacco/docs/llmf0099
Roelofs, W. J. (1996a). Letter to VWS. *Dutch Tobacco Industry Collection*, Bates No. JB2175. Retrieved from https://www.industrydocumentslibrary.ucsf.edu/tobacco/docs/pmdp0219
Roelofs, W. J. (1996b). Tabaksontmoedigingsbeleid. *Dutch Tobacco Industry Collection*, Bates No. JB2687. Retrieved from https://www.industrydocumentslibrary.ucsf.edu/tobacco/docs/pqwp0219
Roelofs, W. J. (1998). Tabaksontmoedigingsbeleid. *Dutch Tobacco Industry Collection*, Bates No. JB2391. Retrieved from https://www.industrydocumentslibrary.ucsf.edu/tobacco/docs/psdp0219
Roelofs, W. J. (2000a). [Letter to Minister Borst]. *Dutch Tobacco Industry Collection*, Bates No. JB2402. Retrieved from https://www.industrydocumentslibrary.ucsf.edu/tobacco/docs/xtdp0219
Roelofs, W. J. (2000b). [Letter to Prime Minister Kok]. *Dutch Tobacco Industry Collection*, Bates No. JB0349. Retrieved from https://www.industrydocumentslibrary.ucsf.edu/tobacco/docs/hyhb0191
Roessingh, H. K. (1976). *Inlandse tabak: Expansie en contractie van een handelsgewas in de 17e en 18e eeuw in Nederland* (Doctoral dissertation), Landbouw Hogeschool, Wageningen.
Roos, M. J. (1985). Tabakswet. *Dutch Tobacco Industry Collection*, Bates No. JB2433. Retrieved from https://www.industrydocumentslibrary.ucsf.edu/tobacco/docs/pzdp0219
Schama, S. (1987). *The embarrassment of riches: An interpretation of Dutch culture in the Golden Age*. New York: Vintage Books.
Schipper, J. W. (1999a). [Brief van Philip Morris aan het ministerie van Economische Zaken betreft Overleg d.d. 14 juni 1999]. *Dutch Tobacco Industry Collection*, Bates No. JB2419. Retrieved from https://www.industrydocumentslibrary.ucsf.edu/tobacco/docs/ztdp0219

Schipper, J. W. (1999b). [Letter to Minister Jorritsma]. *Dutch Tobacco Industry Collection*, Bates No. JB2111. Retrieved from https://www.industrydocumentslibrary.ucsf.edu/tobacco/docs/gkdp0219

Schippers, E. J. (2010). Beleidsvoornemens tabaksontmoediging [letter to SSI and VNK]. *Dutch Tobacco Industry Collection*, Bates No. JB0562. Retrieved from https://www.industrydocumentslibrary.ucsf.edu/tobacco/docs/hkxb0191

Schraven, J. H. (2001a). [Letter VNO-NCW to Borst-Eilers]. *Dutch Tobacco Industry Collection*, Bates No. JB3560. Retrieved from https://www.industrydocumentslibrary.ucsf.edu/tobacco/docs/njwn0217

Schraven, J. H. (2001b). Regulier overleg tabaksontmoedigingsbeleid. *Dutch Tobacco Industry Collection*, Bates No. JB0271. Retrieved from https://www.industrydocumentslibrary.ucsf.edu/tobacco/docs/ljhb0191

Schraven, J. H. (2003a). [Letter VNO-NCW to Ross-van Dorp]. *Dutch Tobacco Industry Collection*, Bates No. JB3557. Retrieved from https://www.industrydocumentslibrary.ucsf.edu/tobacco/docs/sxdn0217

Schraven, J. H. (2003b). Regulier overleg tabaksontmoedigingsbeleid. *Dutch Tobacco Industry Collection*, Bates No. JB0269. Retrieved from https://www.industrydocumentslibrary.ucsf.edu/tobacco/docs/jjhb0191

Smid, E. (2007). [Letter to Ministry of VWS]. *Dutch Tobacco Industry Collection*, Bates No. JB3477. Retrieved from https://www.industrydocumentslibrary.ucsf.edu/tobacco/docs/gffn0217

Smith, E. A. (2007). 'It's interesting how few people die from smoking': Tobacco industry efforts to minimize risk and discredit health promotion. *The European Journal of Public Health*, 17(2), 162–170. https://doi.org/10.1093/eurpub/ckl097

Smith, E. A., & Malone, R. E. (2007). We will speak as the smoker: The tobacco industry's smokers' rights groups. *European Journal of Public Health*, 17(3), 306–313. https://doi.org/10.1093/eurpub/ckl244

SSI. (1983). Ontmoedigingsbeleid tabak. *Dutch Tobacco Industry Collection*, Bates No. JB2225. Retrieved from https://www.industrydocumentslibrary.ucsf.edu/tobacco/docs/#id=hydp0219

SSI. (1984). [Letter to Ministry of Economic Affairs]. *Dutch Tobacco Industry Collection*, Bates No. JB3980. Retrieved from https://www.industrydocumentslibrary.ucsf.edu/tobacco/docs/zzwp0219

SSI. (1991). [Correspondence with Ministries of Economic Affairs and Finance]. *Dutch Tobacco Industry Collection*, Bates No. JB2354. Retrieved from https://www.industrydocumentslibrary.ucsf.edu/tobacco/docs/tqdp0219

SSI. (2001). [Letter to ministries of VWS and Economic Affairs]. *Dutch Tobacco Industry Collection*, Bates No. JB3498. Retrieved from https://www.industrydocumentslibrary.ucsf.edu/tobacco/docs/pmcn0217

SSI. (2002). Tabaksontmoedigingsbeleid [Letter to Bomhoff] *Dutch Tobacco Industry Collection*, Bates No. JB3526. Retrieved from https://www.industrydocumentslibrary.ucsf.edu/tobacco/docs/hncn0217

SSI & SNK. (1984). Jaaroverzicht 1983. *Dutch Tobacco Industry Collection*, Bates No. JB2268. Retrieved from https://www.industrydocumentslibrary.ucsf. edu/tobacco/docs/#id=nfgp0219

SSI, & Toet, R. L. (1972–1996). Collection of industry lobby letters about tobacco price and taxation. *Dutch Tobacco Industry Collection*, Bates No. JB2000. Retrieved from https://www.industrydocumentslibrary.ucsf.edu/tobacco/docs/fxfp0219

SSI & VNK. (2007). Overleg met VNO-NCW en de tabaksindustrie (SSI, VNK en NVS). *Dutch Tobacco Industry Collection*, Bates No. JB0454. Retrieved from https://www.industrydocumentslibrary.ucsf.edu/tobacco/docs/qzhb0191

Taylor, P. (1984). *The smoke ring: Tobacco, money & multinational politics.* London: Sphere Books.

Toet, R. L. J. (1994). Reclamecode voor tabaksprodukten [letter]. *Dutch Tobacco Industry Collection*, Bates No. JB2533. Retrieved from https://www.industrydocumentslibrary.ucsf.edu/tobacco/docs/kjwp0219

Trappenburg, M. (2005). *Gezondheidszorg en democratie [inaugural lecture].* Rotterdam: Erasmus University.

UICC. (1996). Philip Morris campaign on passive smoking. *Dutch Tobacco Industry Collection*, Bates No. JB1186. Retrieved from https://www.industrydocumentslibrary.ucsf.edu/tobacco/docs/kkxp0219

US Surgeon General. (1986). *The health consequences of involuntary smoking.* Rockville: USDHHS.

Van Baal, P. H. M., Brouwer, W. B. F., Hoogenveen, R. T., & Feenstra, T. L. (2007). Increasing tobacco taxes: A cheap tool to increase public health. *Health Policy, 82*(2), 142–152. https://doi.org/10.1016/j.healthpol.2006.09.004

Van de Mortel, J. L. P. M. (1996). Reactie op de concept nota inzake tabaksontmoedigingsbeleid. *Dutch Tobacco Industry Collection*, Bates No. JB2518. Retrieved from https://www.industrydocumentslibrary.ucsf.edu/tobacco/docs/nxwp0219

Van de Mortel, P. M., & Roelofs, W. J. (1996). Concept-notitie interdepartementale werkgroep accijns. *Dutch Tobacco Industry Collection*, Bates No. JB2070. Retrieved from https://www.industrydocumentslibrary.ucsf.edu/tobacco/docs/zxdp0219

Van de Wetering, C. (2010). Niek Jan van Kesteren, directeur VNO-NCW. De onzichtbare onderhandelaar. Retrieved from http://www.pm.nl/artikel/640/niek-jan-van-kesteren-de-onzichtbare-onderhandelaar

Van der Bles, W. (1996). Boze Wijers treedt toe tot het gezelschap antirookmagiërs. Retrieved from http://www.trouw.nl/tr/nl/5009/Archief/article/detail/2632148/1996/09/06/Boze-Wijers-treedt-toe-tot-het-gezelschap-anti-rookmagiers.dhtml

Van Gelder, H. (1990). Rokers maken een vuist. Retrieved from http://www.nrc.nl/nieuws/1990/01/08/rokers-maken-een-vuist-6921081-a1190151

Van Hoogstraten, S. (1997a). Besluitenlijst overleg 'Aanscherping RvT'. *Dutch Tobacco Industry Collection*, Bates No. JB2196. Retrieved from https://www.industrydocumentslibrary.ucsf.edu/tobacco/docs/zxfp0219

Van Hoogstraten, S. (1997b). Gewijzigde definitieve verslag van de Hoordag op 2 September. *Dutch Tobacco Industry Collection*, Bates No. JB2079. Retrieved from https://www.industrydocumentslibrary.ucsf.edu/tobacco/docs/jpxp0219

Van Londen, J. (1980). Voorstellen ICBT inzake beperking tabakreclame en verkooppunten tabaksproducten. *Dutch Tobacco Industry Collection*, Bates No. JB1801. Retrieved from https://www.industrydocumentslibrary.ucsf.edu/tobacco/docs/ffdp0219

Van Oosten, R. (1996). Introductie landelijke belangenvereniging van tabaksdustributeurs Nederland. *Dutch Tobacco Industry Collection*, Bates No. JB2671. Retrieved from https://www.industrydocumentslibrary.ucsf.edu/tobacco/docs/pggp0219

Van Proosdij, C. (1957). *Smoking, its influence in the individual and its role in social medicine [Roken: Een individueel- en sociaalgeneeskundige studie]*. PhD thesis, University of Amsterdam, Amsterdam.

Van Ronkel, H. (1996). Overheid schendt gemaakte afspraken. *Dutch Tobacco Industry Collection*, Bates No. JB2174. Retrieved from https://www.industrydocumentslibrary.ucsf.edu/tobacco/docs/zqfp0219

VNK. (1991). [Brief van VNK aan het ministerie van EZ betreft Accijnsbrieven SSI/VNK]. *Dutch Tobacco Industry Collection*, Bates No. JB2780. Retrieved from https://www.industrydocumentslibrary.ucsf.edu/tobacco/docs/ltwp0219

VNK. (2011). [E-mails about visit to factory]. *Dutch Tobacco Industry Collection*, Bates No. JB3922. Retrieved from https://www.industrydocumentslibrary.ucsf.edu/tobacco/docs/mhcn0217

VNK & Ministry of Health. (2009). [various emails about VNK company day meeting]. *Dutch Tobacco Industry Collection*, Bates No. JB0066. Retrieved from https://www.industrydocumentslibrary.ucsf.edu/tobacco/docs/pmgb0191

VNK, NVS, SSI, & Philip Morris Benelux. (2010). Betreft: Gesprek 5 oktober jl. inzake ontwikkelingen tabaksbeleid. *Dutch Tobacco Industry Collection*, Bates No. JB0533. Retrieved from https://industrydocuments.library.ucsf.edu/tobacco/docs/lxxb0191

VNO-NCW. (2011a). alcohol en tabak [email from VNO-NCW to EZ]. *Dutch Tobacco Industry Collection*, Bates No. JB0539. Retrieved from https://www.industrydocumentslibrary.ucsf.edu/tobacco/docs/rxxb0191

VNO-NCW. (2011b). Economische impact tabaksector. *Dutch Tobacco Industry Collection*, Bates No. JB0537. Retrieved from https://www.industrydocumentslibrary.ucsf.edu/tobacco/docs/pxxb0191

Volkskrant. (1996, September 6). VVD en CDA tegen hogere tabaksaccijns. *Volkskrant*. Retrieved from http://www.volkskrant.nl/vk/nl/2844/Archief/archief/article/detail/425300/1996/09/06/VVD-en-CDA-tegen-hogere-tabaksaccijns.dhtml

Vonk, T. H. (1995). Verhoging Tabaksaccijns. *Dutch Tobacco Industry Collection*, Bates No. JB2657. Retrieved from https://www.industrydocumentslibrary.ucsf.edu/tobacco/docs/tywp0219

Voorlichtingsbureau Sigaretten en Shag. (1986). Jaaroverzicht. *Dutch Tobacco Industry Collection*, Bates No. JB2271. Retrieved from https://www.industrydocumentslibrary.ucsf.edu/tobacco/docs/qfgp0219

Vossenaar, T. (1997). Wetenschappelijke Adviesraad Roken en Gezondheid 1964–1997. *Dutch Tobacco Industry Collection*, Bates No. JB1390. Retrieved from https://www.industrydocumentslibrary.ucsf.edu/tobacco/docs/mhgp0219

VWS. (2003). Overleg 5/11/03 tabaksfabrikanten—VWS. *Dutch Tobacco Industry Collection*, Bates No. JB0266. Retrieved from https://www.industrydocumentslibrary.ucsf.edu/tobacco/docs/gjhb0191

Wever, L. J. S. (1988). Proces SVR/Tabaksindustrie. *Dutch Tobacco Industry Collection*, Bates No. JB0981. Retrieved from https://www.industrydocumentslibrary.ucsf.edu/tobacco/docs/yscp0219

Wever, L. J. S. (1992). Beperking tabaksreclame. *Dutch Tobacco Industry Collection*, Bates No. JB2156. Retrieved from https://www.industrydocumentslibrary.ucsf.edu/tobacco/docs/zldp0219

Wigand, J. S. (2005). Expert report on tobacco additives and validity of the Dutch decree on lists of tobacco ingredients. *Dutch Tobacco Industry Collection*, Bates No. JB0836. Retrieved from https://www.industrydocumentslibrary.ucsf.edu/tobacco/docs/glbp0219

Wijers, G. J. (1996). Tabaksontmoedigingsbeleid. *Dutch Tobacco Industry Collection*, Bates No. JB2701. Retrieved from https://www.industrydocumentslibrary.ucsf.edu/tobacco/docs/mrwp0219

Wirthlin Group. (1996). *ETS perceptions and attitudes: A review of available studies*, Bates No. 2065210430–2065210477. Retrieved from http://legacy.library.ucsf.edu/tid/txf83c00

Open Access This chapter is licensed under the terms of the Creative Commons Attribution 4.0 International License (http://creativecommons.org/licenses/by/4.0/), which permits use, sharing, adaptation, distribution and reproduction in any medium or format, as long as you give appropriate credit to the original author(s) and the source, provide a link to the Creative Commons license and indicate if changes were made.

The images or other third party material in this chapter are included in the chapter's Creative Commons license, unless indicated otherwise in a credit line to the material. If material is not included in the chapter's Creative Commons license and your intended use is not permitted by statutory regulation or exceeds the permitted use, you will need to obtain permission directly from the copyright holder.

CHAPTER 9

The Tobacco Control Coalition

Tobacco is the main contributor to three groups of disease: cancer, lung disease, and heart disease. Everywhere in the world, health charities fighting these illnesses became natural leaders in the field of tobacco control. The Netherlands is no exception. The Dutch Cancer Society, the Dutch Heart Foundation, and the Lung Foundation Netherlands have been fighting tobacco from the start of the Dutch tobacco control advocacy movement. The Dutch Cancer Society holds the oldest track record in tobacco control advocacy and has the largest financial resources.

This chapter describes the emergence, transformation, and accomplishments of the Dutch tobacco control coalition[1] and how it adapted to changes in the policy environment. It narrates how the three charities developed a tobacco control coalition with the *Stichting Volksgezondheid en Roken* (Dutch Smoking or Health Foundation) (STIVORO) as their main vehicle. STIVORO's accomplishments are described, with particular attention to its successes in the field of health education and smoking cessation and as the central tobacco control advocacy organisation in the Netherlands. It will also discuss the contribution to the tobacco control coalition of the medical community, the academic community, and governmental organisations. From the 1970s until the end of the 1990s the coalition fought a strong tobacco industry-dominated government, followed by a period in which tobacco control was supported by an activist tobacco control elite within the Ministry of Health. STIVORO and the

© The Author(s) 2018
M. C. Willemsen, *Tobacco Control Policy in the Netherlands*,
Palgrave Studies in Public Health Policy Research,
https://doi.org/10.1007/978-3-319-72368-6_9

charities collaborated with the ministry on its wish for stronger tobacco control. This changed around 2007 when new governments appointed health ministers who were more lenient towards the tobacco industry and several committed civil servants left the tobacco control team at the Ministry of Health, resulting in a temporary wakening of national tobacco control. The health charities later resumed their lead role, and recent years have seen a resurgence of a strong tobacco control coalition.

Early Days of Dutch Tobacco Control

The tobacco control movement in the Netherlands had a curious start in the 1960s, with two public figures who dominated the media: Robert Jasper Grootveld (Box 9.1) and Lenze Meinsma.

Box 9.1 Robert Jasper Grootveld, "anti-smoke magician"
One of the first activists was an initiator of the Provo youth counter movement in Amsterdam. Paradoxically, this well-known cult-figure, Robert Jasper Grootveld, started a crusade against the tobacco industry, but not against smoking, being a tobacco smoker and promoter of marihuana use. As a self-proclaimed *anti-rook magiër* (anti-smoke magician), he regarded the cigarette as the ultimate symbol of oppression by multinationals and their marketers, and provoked the tobacco industry and the Amsterdam police by writing the word "cancer" on tobacco billboard advertisements, for which he was repeatedly arrested—and once sentenced to jail (Duivenvoorden, 2009). Grootveld initiated famous weekly provocative "happenings" in Amsterdam, part of which was a purifying ritual involving the mass smoking of cigarettes and loud coughing. Other public protest performances were around a small bronze statue in the centre of Amsterdam dedicated to poor Amsterdam boys, called "Het Lieverdje"—a local tobacco manufacturer had donated the money for it. Grootveld used the statue as a symbol for the modern addicted consumer. These happenings, where participants were enticed to smoke collectively as a protest against smoking and the tobacco industry, were a commentary on the prevailing ethos, which was regarded as hypocritical. For decades, many who agitated against tobacco and the tobacco industry had been easily set aside as being *anti-rook magiërs*: fools not to be taken seriously.

The Dutch Cancer Society started tobacco education activities in the 1960s, years before the government took responsibility. Lenze Meinsma, director of the Cancer Society from 1953 until 1978, was a physician with a passion for the fight against tobacco. Meinsma became a public figure in 1963 through frequent appearances on television and other media, where he relentlessly warned against the dangers of smoking. He conducted campaigns aimed at teachers and pupils (known as *Actie Roken Jeugd*), which ran from 1964 to 1975. He also presented the first ideas about how tobacco should be tackled. He condemned the government for not doing enough, in the process turning into a well-known anti-tobacco activist.

In 1969 Meinsma published a small booklet, *Smoking and Risks* (Meinsma, 1969), which became known as Meinsma's "red book." In it, he presented a rough sketch of a comprehensive approach to the smoking problem. In addition to educating young people, he proposed that the government substantially increase tobacco taxation, put health warnings on cigarette packs, ban tobacco vending machines, restrict the sale of tobacco to specialty shops, initiate a ban on tobacco advertisements and promotion, ban smoking in government buildings and workplaces, ban smoking in restaurants and cinemas, ban smoking during sports events, and ban the sale of duty-free tobacco in airplanes and to military personnel. All in all, it was an ambitious package that proved to be far ahead of its time, despite the implicit endorsement of the state secretary from the Ministry of Health who in the preface to the book wrote that smoking was a "serious public health problem" responsible for about 30 daily deaths in the Netherlands.

Meinsma suffered the same fate as Robert Jasper Grootvelt. His activities received negative reactions from the public and experts, who felt his tone was too harsh and confrontational. He had become a lone wolf, howling in the dark. The charities learned from this that the fight against smoking could not be carried out by individuals, but required coordinated efforts from dedicated organisations and a cautious and diplomatic approach. In 1971 Meinsma negotiated with the Lung and Heart Foundations about collaboration with the Cancer Society—no easy task, as the three organisations were natural competitors in the charity market. Meinsma also approached medical specialist organisations. This resulted—in January 1971—in a letter from the scientific associations of four medical professional organisations appealing to the state secretary for health to take action and not leave tobacco solely to the charities. This led to a recommendation from the Health Council in 1975 to set up a national tobacco control organisation which became *Stichting Volksgezondheid en Roken* (Dutch Smoking or Health Foundation) (STIVORO), the national tobacco control organisation. The Health Council wrote, "Considering the number of yearly deaths caused by tobacco ... and the fact that smoking will continue to be a considerable problem for the coming 15 or 20 years, the creation of a dedicated institute to reduce smoking is justified" (Beernink & Plokker, 1975).

THE FOUNDATION OF STIVORO

In contrast to other countries, notably the United States and the United Kingdom, the health charities in the Netherlands wanted the government to take the lead in controlling tobacco.[2] However, the Dutch Health Council realised the danger of being too dependent on the government and advised that a national institute for the reduction of smoking should be set up in such a way that it could develop its own policy and be reasonably independent of its financers (Beernink & Plokker, 1975). It noted that the government had to weigh up multiple interests when it came to the smoking issue, including economic interests, so that it was undesirable that the government be solely responsible for the new institute, and advised that private organisations be the financial supporters and driving force. It also advised that the Dutch Cancer Society, Heart Foundation, and Lung Foundation take up this responsibility. These three organisations founded STIVORO on 24 December 1974, but were not willing to fully finance and remained dependent on governmental co-funding.

The foundation of STIVORO did not immediately result in a working organisation. During its first three years it was barely active, lacking the funds to appoint even a director, and the three founding charities could not agree on the best course of action to tackle the complex smoking problem.[3] In the first three years, STIVORO's activities were limited to distributing Meinsma's educational materials to schools, for which it received a governmental subsidy. As the government was accountable for STIVORO's activities to parliament, the state secretary assured critical libertarian politicians that each activity proposed by STIVORO would be analysed against the criterion of not overly restricting individual liberties.[4]

Three years after its foundation, STIVORO finally secured enough money to appoint a director and a small staff. It started to build up a network of academics who could advise on the scientific development of campaigns and overall strategy. A *Wetenschappelijke Adviesraad* (Scientific Advisory Council) was set up and in February 1978 Albert Pontfoort, the first director, presented STIVORO's policy programme to the press (STIVORO, 1978). The approach was to stimulate smokers to change their behaviour through campaigns that could be tailored to smokers' psychological determinants, applying methods and insights from psychology and the new fields of communication sciences and health education. Until then, STIVORO's activities had been restricted to informing the public about the health risks of smoking. The new approach was a direct translation of State Secretary Hendriks' *Tobacco Memorandum* (see Chap. 2). A comprehensive, long-term approach was proposed that included continued education of youth, protection of non-smokers against environmental tobacco smoke, and development of behavioural support for smokers who wanted to quit. Exposing tobacco industry strategies and lobbying for regulatory measures from the government were not explicitly mentioned.

At first the Ministry of Health did not want to structurally finance the new organisation, and limited subsidies to specific activities and ad hoc campaigns under more or less formal grant proposal conditions. In this way the government could control educational measures, which it regarded as its main responsibility in the fight against tobacco, without being responsible for a new semi-governmental organisation. This must be understood against the backdrop of a process in which the ministry explored ways to organise health education in the Netherlands. Health education was a new profession, and while the government wanted a national institute for the coordination of national and local health education activities, it had not yet decided if tobacco was going to be a part of this. Pending this decision, it was not prepared to structurally support STIVORO. It took three years before a compromise was reached, in which the three charities equally financed half of the bureau and the other 50% was financed by the government, but still in the form of project finance. The total budget for the organisation was one million guilders.[5] This understanding lasted until 1991, when the government began to finance STIVORO on a structural basis, not at 50%, but by the same amount that the three "mothers" each paid: 350,000 guilders. From 1991 onwards STIVORO was a semi-governmental organisation with one quarter of its core finance flowing from the Ministry of Health.

For many years the charities were not prepared to publicly operate as activist organisations. They were concerned that a too radical or confrontational approach would backfire, jeopardising the goodwill of donors (De Jong, 1989), remembering that Meinsma's rhetorical style had prompted negative reactions. Public opinion was antagonistic to a paternalistic approach, and the three organisations depended on private donations. By supporting STIVORO they could fight tobacco without standing directly in the spotlight.[6] The downside was that STIVORO had to walk a tightrope, balancing interests from three charities and the government.

Over the years STIVORO became more and more dependent on governmental subsidies. The Ministry of Health was on the management board, although it had no voting power. Internationally, the arrangement was unique, and typically Dutch: compromises between government and civil society were woven into the fabric of the organisation. Because of the collective financing arrangement, the three "mothers" and one "stepmother" (the state) held each other hostage, making it very difficult for any partner to withdraw its support. If one organisation wanted to pay less (or more), it had to convince the others to do the same, and if one wanted to withdraw altogether, the remaining three were unlikely to agree since they would then have to cover the costs of the dropout. However, this assured STIVORO of secure core funding for several decades, which can be considered as one reason for its success.

The Tobacco Control Coalition Expands

At the end of the 1970s the core of the Dutch tobacco control advocacy coalition consisted of the three charities, united in STIVORO, and their counterparts at the Ministry of Health. From the start it collaborated with Clean Air Netherlands (CAN; discussed in the next paragraph), which was founded in the same year as STIVORO. Over the years STIVORO expanded its network, mainly in the medical sector: in the mid-1990s through the Dutch Medical Alliance Against Smoking, and from the beginning of the 2000s through the Partnership Stop Smoking.

Clean Air Netherlands

The Club for Active Non-smokers, later dubbed Clean Air Netherlands (CAN), is a grass roots interest group founded in 1974 to protect the rights of non-smokers. From the beginning it received material and a small financial contribution from STIVORO, and in the first years the two organisations shared a post office box. It survived on donations and gifts from members and supporters. In 1979 analysts from the tobacco industry identified CAN and STIVORO as the two main Dutch anti-tobacco organisations (Unknown (Philip Morris), 1979). In their eyes CAN was immature, and "due to their inability and their rather passive attitude, they have played a non-effectual role." STIVORO was the "most active and serious anti-smoking group at this time, [but] as the personal freedom concept is widely accepted and supported in Holland, the anti-smoking cause is not exceptionally strong."

Despite its dismissal by the industry, CAN played a significant role in the fight for smoking bans. STIVORO collaborated with CAN if it needed an activist approach to put issues on the agenda, which it could not do under its own name. CAN exists to this day and has at times been an effective grass roots advocacy organisation, operating fairly independently of the broader STIVORO-led tobacco control coalition. It does not shy away from taking the government or companies to court. In 1995 CAN campaigned against national airlines (Transavia, Martinair, KLM) to ban smoking during flights. After 2004 it campaigned for a smoke-free hospitality sector. A major accomplishment was that they were the first organisation in the Netherlands to make use of a new right to citizens' initiative: anyone who can present 40,000 supporting signatures can put an issue on the official agenda of parliament. CAN handed in about 62,000 signatures to the president of parliament in May 2006, in an attempt to implement a smoking ban in bars and restaurants on the agenda. Parliament, however, did not discuss the topic because it had already debated several times on the smoke-free issue, and the citizens' initiative is not valid if the topic has been debated before. In 2007, in a collaborative action with STIVORO, CAN presented 60,000 letters from citizens who asked for a smoke-free hospitality sector, and presented these to the negotiators during the formation of the Balkenende IV cabinet, which contributed to the smoke-free hospitality sector becoming part of the coalition agreement of the cabinet. CAN's biggest success was the court case against the state over Minister Schippers' one-sided decision to exclude small bars from the smoking ban. The judge overruled the minister, who was defeated in the high court in 2013.

The Medical Sector

A remarkably weak link in the Dutch tobacco control health coalition was the passive stance of the medical community. After the initiative from medical specialist organisations in the beginning of the 1970s that resulted in the foundation of STIVORO, the medical establishment was happy to leave tobacco control advocacy to STIVORO. This may be because in the 1970s and 1980s smoking among physicians was very common. About half of all general practitioners smoked, and smoking rates were higher than in the general male population and much higher than what was normal in the higher social classes (Adriaanse, Van Reek, & Metsemakers, 1986; Vandenbroucke, Kok, Matroos, & Dekker, 1981). While in many countries smoking rates decreased earlier in the medical professions than in the general population, this was not the case in the Netherlands. In a review of data from 31 countries, only in France, Portugal, and the Netherlands did more physicians smoke than in the general population (Adriaanse, Van Reek, & Van Zutphen, 1986).

The passive stance of doctors may be further attributed to active lobbying by the tobacco industry. In 1979 the industry's Tobacco Education Bureau (BVT) began to distribute *Rookspectrum*, a periodical with "scientific information" on the smoking and health issue, to all Dutch family practitioners. *Rookspectrum* presented a selection of scientific news about smoking, downplaying the health risks of smoking and passive smoking. Its aim was "to defend issues concerning passive smoking" (RJ Reynolds, 1979). This free "service" to doctors continued for at least four years. In 1985 the industry boasted that, based on a survey they carried out among more than 1200 doctors, 70% said they were readers of the journal and 54% believed that *Rookspectrum* provided a meaningful contribution to the smoking and health discussion (SNK & SSI, 1985).

Surveys in the 1980s showed that Dutch general practitioners did not regard their exemplary role as particularly important (Adriaanse, Van Reek, & Metsemakers, 1986; E. Dekker, 1981). One in four family physicians smoked in the presence of patients (Dekker, 1981). Dutch physicians considered smoking a private lifestyle choice for which they were not responsible, were stoic about the need to fight the tobacco epidemic, and ignored the important role they could play (Knol, 1997).

The main medical organisation in the Netherlands is the *Koninklijke Nederlandsche Maatschappij tot bevordering der Geneeskunst* (Royal Dutch Medical Association) (KNMG), established in 1849. The KNMG represents all medical professions. In an editorial, the scientific journal of the KNMG called on the medical profession to become more actively involved in the political lobby (Van Es, 1987), but this did not result in a more activist role. In 2005 KNMG was asked to give its views on the government's tobacco control agenda. It briefly mentioned the need for a smoking ban in the hospitality sector, but emphasised the importance of smoking cessation, which they regarded as the main contribution the medical community could make (Rijksen, 2005); it did not mention tobacco control in its 2007 prevention policy document (KNMG, 2007). For decades the KNMG has not taken a particular interest in tobacco control advocacy and confined itself to being a member of the Partnership Stop Smoking. This situation lasted until 2016 when the KNMG felt certain enough to step forward with a distinctive and explicitly formulated tobacco control agenda, urging the government to do a better job of implementing WHO's Framework Convention on Tobacco Control (FCTC) measures (KNMG, 2016). The same lack of activism by the Dutch medical community was noticeable in the unremarkable role that the powerful *Landelijke Huisartsen Vereniging* (Dutch General Practitioners Association) (LHV)—established in 1946 to defend the interests of general practitioners—played in Dutch tobacco control.

In 1993, medical specialists founded the *Medische Alliantie tegen het Roken* (Medical Alliance Against Smoking), a Dutch branch of the European Medical Association Smoking or Health. The secretariat was provided by STIVORO. For many years the Medical Alliance was the only active medical tobacco control advocacy organisation, but it had no real political power, being a voluntary organisation with no resources, and dependent on the goodwill of a small number of engaged doctors and retired medical professors. Despite this, on various occasions the organisation was able to highlight failings in the self-regulation of tobacco advertising (Knol, 1995, 1996a, 1996b), sometimes together with the KNMG (Lanphen & Van Berkestijn, 1995). The most notable activity was a petition to the parliament, signed by 185 medical professors, asking for an advertising ban (Hilvering, Knol, & Wagener, 1995). This supported Health Minister Borst, who endeavoured to get a ban on tobacco advertising in the Tobacco Act. The Medical Alliance remained active until 2008 when it was dissolved, partly due to lack of interest from the medical community.

The Dutch doctors' passivity is in contrast with the important role that the medical community played in the United Kingdom. Early on, the UK

Royal College of Physicians published influential reports on the health risks of smoking and advocated for tobacco control measures, such as in their *Smoking and Health* report (Royal College of Physicians, 1962). It founded Action on Smoking and Health (ASH UK) in 1971 to lobby for better tobacco control by the government. Another strong medical force was the British Medical Association (BMA). In 1984, the BMA started an unprecedented attack against the tobacco industry in an attempt to eradicate tobacco advertising and promotion (BMA, 1986). Voluntary agreements to restrict advertising, comparable with those in place in the Netherlands, were not working, and the BMA realised that something had to be done to break the deadlock. The campaign carried the weight of the BMA's prestige and infrastructure (representing the majority of practising doctors in the United Kingdom), and one of the most highly organised professional bodies in the country, directly into a fight with the industry. It was a tremendous help for ASH UK, which, like STIVORO at the time, was a small organisation with only three full-time officials and five support staff. David Simpson, ASH's director, more than welcomed the help of the BMA, which had a reputation as one of the country's most powerful lobbying organisations: "It was like the Americans entering the Second World War" (BMA, 1986, p. 7). The campaign lasted several years, permeated the media with a general anti-tobacco climate, and put pressure on ministers to take the smoking problem more seriously. No such help from the medical community materialised in the Netherlands.

A Public–Private Partnership to Support Smoking Cessation

In 2000 STIVORO formed a coalition of organisations with expertise and interest in the treatment of smokers, under the name *Partnership Stop met Roken* (Partnership Stop Smoking). This was at the request of Health Minister Borst, who wanted to improve the quality of the treatment of tobacco addiction. The new coalition was launched in January 2002 as a public–private partnership and received financing from the Ministry of Health (€550.000 for the first two years).[7] The Partnership Stop Smoking included the KNMG, the Dutch Medical Alliance against Smoking, the Association of Doctors for Lung Disease and Tuberculosis, the Dutch Cardiology Association, the Dutch Institute for Psychologists, various addiction treatment organisations, health charities, scientific organisations, and several pharmaceutical companies. STIVORO initiated and coordinated the Partnership. Its main activity was to develop the first clinical guidelines for the treatment of tobacco dependence, following examples from the United States and the United Kingdom. It was hoped that such guidelines would encourage Dutch health-care professionals to motivate patients to quit smoking and also to engage more doctors in tobacco control activism. The Partnership identified its mission as placing the gravity of tobacco addiction and the urgent need to tackle this problem higher on the political agenda. Advocacy goals were a smoke-free workplace and hospitality sector, and reimbursement for smoking cessation, including for pharmaceutical treatment. The Partnership was the Dutch representative in the European Network for Smoking Prevention (ENSP). With support from the Partnership, the lobbying strength of the three charities and STIVORO improved considerably, because they were able to mobilise a much broader group of organisations.

In the first year of the Partnership, when STIVORO looked for overseas examples of how a network of tobacco control professionals could be organised, it identified Canada as a model. In November 2000 the Canadian activist Heidi Rathjen gave a workshop in the Netherlands to inspire the new Dutch coalition. Rathjen had founded the Quebec Coalition for Tobacco Control in 1996, a coalition of about 700 organisations that successfully pushed the government to make haste with drafting a Tobacco Act (Rathjen, 1999). In 2004 STIVORO, through the Partnership, called on the government to ratify the FCTC (Partnership Stop met Roken, 2004), which it did in 2005. In 2011 the Partnership campaigned for continuation of the national reimbursement for smoking cessation support, presenting a petition to politicians in the spring of 2011 and organising a press lunch with politicians at the end of that year. After this was accomplished, the Partnership Stop Smoking became an independent foundation which focused on further improving the quality of smoking cessation treatment in the Netherlands (see also Box 10.1 in the next chapter). The Partnership Stop Smoking was the first European organisation to develop clinical guidelines for the treatment of tobacco addiction, after the United Kingdom.

The Scientific Community

How much support did the Dutch tobacco control lobby get from the scientific community? Academics can have much influence on policymaking when they become media personalities, by appearing on radio and television, writing opinion pieces and popular books, and using the authority of scientific papers to tell their story (Chapman, 2017). Dutch academics did sporadically speak out for more effective tobacco control in the media, sometimes attracting attention from politicians. For example, the fact that the implementation of the Tobacco Act in 1990 was not followed by a noticeable impact on smoking rates (Dresscher, Elzinga & Koldenhof, 1991) led to critical remarks from prominent Dutch scientists about the national tobacco control policy (Barneveld, Dalesio, & van Leeuwen, 1992; Roscam Abbing, 1992). Johan Mackenbach, professor of public health at Erasmus University, regularly criticised the government for insufficient disease prevention and its weak tobacco control policy (Mackenbach, 2006, 2009, 2016; Mackenbach, Klazinga, & Van der wal, 2004). My own inaugural lecture was a catalyst for heighted attention to failed Dutch tobacco control policy (Willemsen, 2011, 2012; Willemsen, De Vries, & Van Schayck, 2009).

Over the years, STIVORO developed collaborations with various universities, predominantly concerned with building an evidence base for education, campaigns, and smoking cessation interventions—tobacco control advocacy was seldom the topic. The Netherlands has fewer research activists in the field of tobacco control than in some Anglo-Saxon countries. For example, the American tobacco control movement included notorious academic tobacco control advocates, committed to getting tobacco multinationals on their knees (Derthick, 2005). Tobacco control advocacy, at least when it is done through extensive and public media advocacy, is regarded by many in the Dutch academic community as difficult to reconcile with the scientific enterprise. When academics become too involved in activism, they may be perceived as pushy and stepping over the fine line of relationships in the Dutch corporatist system, where one needs to be part of the system to have influence.

Support from Governmental Agencies

The role of state agencies as an integral part of the tobacco control movement has been limited in the Netherlands. Dutch national governmental agencies such as the *Rijksinstituut voor Volksgezondheid en Milieu* (National Institute for Public Health and the Environment) (RIVM) and *Nederlandse Voedsel en Waren Autoriteit* (Netherlands Food and Consumer Product

Safety Authority) (NVWA) were (and are) not tasked to actively support and promote tobacco control activism at the state or local level. This contrasts with the United States, where federal governmental agencies such as the office of the Surgeon General, the National Cancer Institute, and the Center for Disease Control and Prevention played crucial roles. These organisations spent millions of dollars to fund advocacy efforts, disseminated scientific research findings in support of the health lobby, and provided training and technical assistance to advocates at local, state, and federal levels (Wolfson, 2001). For example, the National Cancer Institute, with support from the American Cancer Society, initiated and funded the multi-state project American Stop Smoking Intervention Study for Cancer Prevention (ASSIST), providing a massive injection of federal resources into state and local tobacco control advocacy (Wolfson, 2001).

THE GOLDEN YEARS OF DUTCH TOBACCO CONTROL

In 1987, parliament insisted that educational efforts to discourage smoking be intensified.[8] The goal of 20% smokers in 2000 could not be reached without more money for education, as tobacco promotion by the industry was still completely unregulated. The government agreed and brought together a group of experts to develop a multi-annual action plan. The proposal consisted of a comprehensive approach to youth education, smoking cessation, special attention to high-risk groups and protection of non-smokers, with yearly smoking cessation media campaigns as a core element, all to be coordinated and organised by STIVORO. This signified a change in STIVORO's focus, as it now became responsible for coordination and execution of national tobacco control action plans for the government. Its main activity was to organise yearly nation-wide smoking cessation campaigns in collaboration with national and local health organisations.

STIVORO's campaigns were highly successful and contributed to significant reductions in smoking in the Netherlands (see Box 9.2). Between 1986 and 2011, STIVORO organised 16 campaigns around smoking cessation. While the campaigns in the 1980s and the beginning of the 1990s still had an educational character (e.g., the 1986 campaign informed smokers about how misleading light cigarettes were), the campaigns after 1996 also went on to inform smokers about cessation support.

Box 9.2 STIVORO's great "smoke-outs"
Betweewn 1990 and 2008, STIVORO organised four large-scale media campaigns that involved entertainment-education strategies (such as TV shows) and stimulated between 20% and 30% of all smokers to make quit attempts (Willemsen, van Kann, & Jansen, 2012). The campaigns were accompanied by the introduction of cessation methods that were innovative for their time, such as a television cessation clinic (*Teleac*) in 1990–1991, a national telephone quit line and entertainment-education (TV entertainment shows) in 1999–2000, and a self-help cessation kit in 2003–2004.

The 1990–1991 campaign "Quit smoking together" featured a series of informative and entertaining television programmes showing celebrities trying to quit smoking, a TV cessation clinic, 73 cessation clinics conducted at the local level, a national quit line staffed by trained counsellors, and a comprehensive publicity campaign (Mudde & De Vries, 1999). The campaign contributed to a reduction in the proportion of smokers from 35% in 1990 to 34% in 1991. This seems modest at first glance, but is impressive when one considers the fact that between 1990 and 1991 the tobacco industry increased its expenditure on tobacco promotion and advertisements by 72% (from $66 to $113 million) (Mudde & De Vries, 1999).

The "I Can Do That Too" "millennium" campaign ran in 1999–2000 and was made possible through an extra subsidy by the Dutch Cancer Society, celebrating its 50th anniversary. During the period of the campaign more than 600,000 smokers attempted to quit: four times more than usual (Op de Weegh & Willemsen, 2003; Westerik & Van der Rijt, 2001). The campaign contributed to a reduction in national smoking prevalence from 34% to 33%.

The "Netherlands Start Quitting" campaign in 2003–2004 was financed by the Ministry of Health and aimed to accelerate the natural quitting that was expected to occur with the implementation of the workplace smoking ban. It was associated with a reduction in smoking prevalence from 27% to 25%, with more than a million quit attempts at or around New Year's Eve (Van den Putte, Yzer, Ten Berg, & Steeveld, 2005). In the same period, STIVORO ran campaigns to inform employees about the workplace ban and to motivate smoking parents to quit (*"Kinderen Kopiëren"*).

The last large campaign was the "In every smoker there is a quitter" campaign in 2008, financed by the three charities as part of the *Nationaal Programma Tabaksontmoediging* (National Programme of Tobacco Control) (NPT): the idea was that the implementation of the smoking ban in the hospitality sector in July 2008 would result in many smokers wanting to quit. The campaign ran between April 2008 and January 2009 and stimulated smokers to take the opportunity to quit. It is estimated to have contributed to between 1.1 and 1.4 million quit attempts, twice the number that would have quit normally during the same period (Nagelhout, Willemsen, van den Putte, Crone, & de Vries, 2009; STIVORO, 2009). Smoking prevalence dropped by 0.8% (STIVORO, 2009).

At the end of the 1980s, STIVORO began to coordinate smoking cessation initiatives at the local level through collaboration with municipal public health services and regional cancer centres. It set up a national council with representatives from municipal health services, home nursing organisations, and experts from several universities to coordinate and prepare annual cessation campaigns. In addition, it organised national meetings where scientists exchanged information on research findings. Over a period of three decades, STIVORO steadily extended and improved its repertoire of smoking cessation support. It became an internationally acknowledged example for other countries of how evidence-based cessation support can be integrated with yearly mass media cessation campaigns, and how to offer cessation support through the internet. An important feature of the Dutch system was that government funding allowed STIVORO to offer cessation support free of charge. Through close collaboration with the University of Maastricht, STIVORO became an international pioneer in evidence-based smoking cessation methods. These included self-help manuals; computer-tailored cessation materials; cessation protocols for use by general practitioners; specialised protocols for use with cardiac patients, lung patients, and pregnant women; and special programmes to motivate and support smoking employees to quit smoking at the workplace. Sometime around 2000 STIVORO set up a well-staffed smoking cessation telephone quit line. It was one of the leading partners of the European Network for Quitlines and, alongside

Sweden, the only quitline organisation that conducted scientific research to improve quitline counselling.

When the economy improved, the money that STIVORO could spend on campaigns was allowed to grow. It increased almost exponentially between 1993 and 2004, while the structural budget for the organisation remained fairly constant (see Fig. 9.1). The campaign budget reached a peak in 2003 with a total of €16 million. This large sum followed the resolution from Senator Werner that was key to getting approval for Minister Borst's Tobacco Act in the senate (discussed in Chap. 2). In 1996 STIVORO was already the best staffed and funded tobacco control organisation in Europe (Boucher, 2000), but the period from 1999 until around 2004 is considered by some to be the golden years of STIVORO, and Dutch tobacco control in general, as this period coincided with the adoption and implementation of the revised Tobacco Act.[9] STIVORO's size grew from around 9 employees in 1989, to 18 in 2000, and 46 in 2004.[10] The large number of employees from 2000 onwards reflected the many smoking cessation counsellors who worked in STIVORO's advice centre and smoking cessation quitline.

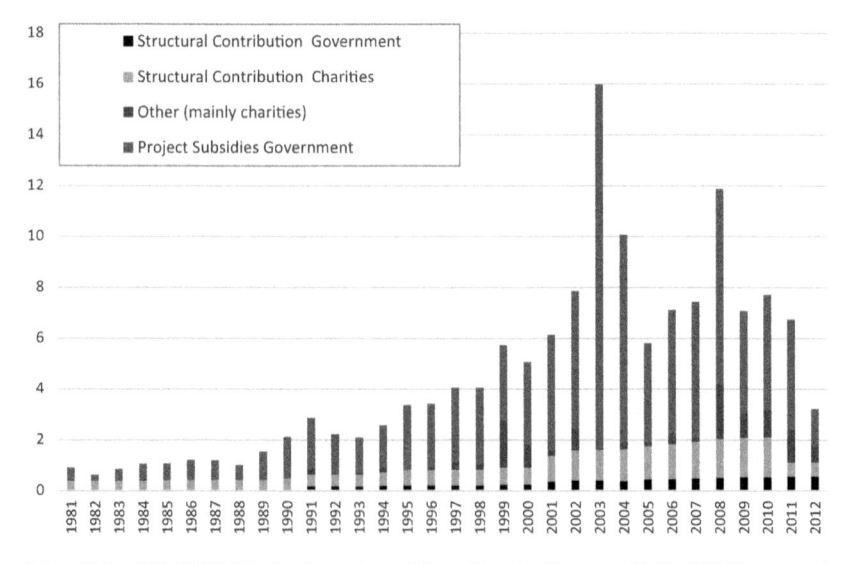

Fig. 9.1 STIVORO's budget (× million Euro). Source: STIVORO's annual reports 1981–2012

In the years between 2000 and 2008, the tobacco control team at the health ministry, which collaborated closely with STIVORO, was also rather large, and there was a strong team spirit, according to all interviewees. The team was supported by specialists from the ministry for such things as juridical and financial matters, and occasionally increased to a team of six to ten people.[11] In later years the team was downsized.[12]

Cracks in the National Tobacco Control Coalition

In the 40 years of its existence, STIVORO struggled with its mandate in tobacco control, trying to strike a balance between the sometimes competing interests and expectations of its three "mothers" and the government. The government and parliament regarded health education as STIVORO's sole task, but civil servants from the ministry and the charities expected STIVORO to lobby in parliament for better tobacco control policy, despite the fact that it had no professional lobbyists. A civil servant explained: "The lobby that the health organisations put up in the direction of the parliament was rather amateurish in our eyes. That was no reproach to anyone. We found that quite normal, since the business community was so much better in lobbying."[13] When judging the limited lobbying capacity of STIVORO, another civil servants observed: "STIVORO's people were of course constantly busy with education, with producing materials etc. They did not have the time, day in, day out, to gain skills in lobbying."[14] The more STIVORO became dependent on large subsidies from the government, the more difficult it was to criticise the government. Similar worries were felt in other countries. For example, ASH UK (STIVORO's counterpart in the United Kingdom) depended in the 1980s for 90% of its annual grants on the Department of Health. ASH "felt itself to some extent constrained in what it could say or do" (BMA, 1986).

Political parties opposing tobacco control criticised STIVORO's lobbying activities. For example, during a debate with parliament about the Ministry of Health's budget, the liberal–conservative representative of the *Volkspartij voor Vrijheid en Democratie* (People's Party for Freedom and Democracy) (VVD) criticised an advertisement that STIVORO had distributed protesting against tobacco advertising. The VVD argued that STIVORO must refrain from lobbying on the ground that taxpayers' money was being used for lobbying instead of health education. However, State Secretary for Health Hans Simons supported STIVORO as a matter of principle: "I think that subsidised organisations must have a large degree of liberty. ... I believe that such organisations must be able to critically express themselves about governmental policy. I firmly support that."[15] At the end of the 2000s, when such support from ministers was missing, criticism about the fact that STIVORO lobbied while it received government subsidies continued to be voiced by industry-friendly parliamentarians and eventually contributed to the government's withdrawal from the organisation.

The Three Health Charities Stepping Out of the Shadows

The adoption of the Tobacco Act in 1988, which led to more societal support for tobacco control, signified a first breach with the charities' taboo on tobacco control activism (De Jong, 1989). However, the largest change was with the implementation of the amended Tobacco Act in 2002. The successful smoking ban and advertising restrictions profoundly changed social norms about smoking in society. The charities began to feel more confident and stepped out of the shadows, hoping that their contribution to tobacco control would become more visible to the general public. Between 2001 and 2003, the Cancer Society started several high-profile smoking cessation campaigns targeted at pregnant women, and experimented with popular national "Quit & Win contests," where smokers who quit smoking would be eligible for a prize.

The year 2005 signified a major change within the health coalition. The three charities were no longer willing to give STIVORO carte blanche to play an advocacy role in tandem with civil servants from the Ministry of Health. The governing board of STIVORO (which consisted of representatives from the three charities, including their directors and representatives from the Ministry of Health) stepped down and was replaced by a board of trustees. The three charities could each nominate one candidate to the board. Former Health Minister Els Borst was one of the seven members; the ministry itself had no seats on the board. This allowed the charities to pursue their own agenda. In June of that year the directors of the three charities and Hoogervorst put their signatures to an intention document to collaborate closely in the National Programme Tobacco control (NPT 2006–2010). STIVORO's role was restricted to execution of the NPT, as "knowledge and expert centre, service and support provider and educator in the field of tobacco control" (Hoogervorst, Zoun, De Blij, & Hanselaar, 2005). In addition, the charities began to make STIVORO more accountable for the money they spent on tobacco control.

In Search of a New Strategy

During the four years that the NPT lasted, it became increasingly clear that the NPT coalition did not function well and that the goal of 20% smokers by 2010 would not be met (a more detailed discussed of the NPT programme can be found in Chap. 2). The three charities lacked a common vision on how tobacco should be tackled and the Ministry of Health lacked political support to pursue new tobacco control initiatives. In January 2007 the three charities desperately called on the government to make more money available for smoking cessation campaigns (STIVORO, 2007), but this was to no avail. Since Minister Klink was unwilling to deliver regulative measures, both STIVORO and the charities began to look out for other ways to advance tobacco control, trying to escape the deadlock. They explored new ways to denormalise the tobacco industry and tobacco use, to create a more coherent national policy, and to build societal support, inspired by best practices from California, Australia, Canada, and Finland (STIVORO, 2010a, 2010b). STIVORO presented its new vision in June 2010 at a symposium where it commemorated its 35-year anniversary. Reports presented to the press emphasised that Dutch smokers were still relatively unconcerned about smoking (ITC Project, 2010) and that more must be done, which led to headlines in the media such as "Are the Dutch too soft on smokers?."

In 2010 the NPT's goal of 20% smokers was not reached. With the failure of the NPT programme, the three charities decided to start a new alliance, and began preparatory talks. In December 2010 they announced that they wanted to withdraw their finances from STIVORO. On 6 January 2011 a small group of individuals from the three charities, STIVORO, CAN, Trimbos Institute, the Association of Municipal Health Services, and the *Stichting Rookpreventie Jeugd* (Youth Smoking Prevention Foundation) (SRJ) came together to discuss the next steps in Dutch tobacco control. There was an agreement that this time a proper coalition should be built, with the three charities taking the lead but supported by a wide range of organisations, and coordinated by a professional bureau. There should be ample room for grass roots initiatives, and the core activities would be empowerment, lobbying, and alliance building. The other existing alliance, the Partnership Stop Smoking, became an independent foundation in that same year and was destined to become part of the new alliance because of its important role in the quality assurance of smoking cessation treatments. STIVORO would be given the role of expert centre on tobacco control, but not lobbying, advocacy, and communication, which would be handled by the three charities.

In March 2011 STIVORO and the Dutch Cancer Society hosted the European Conference on Tobacco Control in Amsterdam. At the conference, the results of the Tobacco Control scale were presented. The Netherlands ranked 13 of 28, one place down from the previous measurement (Joossens & Raw, 2011). This supported the idea that the Dutch government could and should do more in terms of its FCTC requirements. In the aftermath of the European Conference, STIVORO organised a national "inspirational conference" to explore how the Dutch health network could be transformed into a more effective tobacco control alliance (Van Emst & Willemsen, 2011). Experts from Sweden and Ireland presented successful tobacco control alliances from their countries.

The End of STIVORO

On 25 May 2011, STIVORO received notification from the Ministry of Health that its structural subsidy would be cut by 25% in 2013 and by 50% in 2014. A month later another letter confirmed that all subsidies would end by 2013 and tobacco control would be integrated into the alcohol and drug prevention activities of the Trimbos Institute. This decision took STIVORO out of the equation, and paved the way for a new coalition. In the summer of 2011, after a study tour to the United Kingdom to find inspiration from how the British organised tobacco control advocacy, the charities understood that they had to broaden the fight for tobacco control by including societal organisations in a broad coalition. The alliance was to become a coalition of autonomous organisations that collaborated for a common goal with preservation of each one's identity and responsibilities. It was recognised that success was dependent on mutual trust and respect for each other's interests, a set of common goals that bound and unified, and formal and informal rules for mutual cooperation, including how to embed the alliance into the internal workings of the three charities. A professional management consultant was hired to lay the foundation.

At the end of 2013 STIVORO was officially disbanded. In January 2014 the *Alliantie Nederland Rookvrij* (Dutch Alliance for a Smokefree Society) (ANR) began to coordinate the tobacco control advocacy activities of the three charities, while STIVORO's budget and tasks regarding smoking cessation and educational were taken over by the Trimbos Institute.

The Youth Smoking Prevention Foundation

The failure of the NPT programme and the chaos in which the tobacco control coalition with STIVORO as centrepiece had found itself opened the way for other initiatives. In 2009 Wanda de Kanter and Pauline Dekker, two chest physicians, founded the SRJ, motivated by the fact that they were treating lung patients every day who were seriously sick or dying from smoking, while the cause (the tobacco industry) went unchallenged and the government failed to take appropriate measures to discourage new smokers. The two lung specialists built a coalition of organisations and individuals that became an inevitable new activist lobbying force in the Netherlands, operating fairly independently of the main tobacco control coalition. The group included journalists, lawyers, scientists, and influential people from the medical and political elite (Youth Smoking Prevention Foundation, 2014). De Kanter and Dekker became increasingly influential through media advocacy activities, including appearances in high-profile television shows and a strong presence in social media. In January 2011 they presented a manifesto, "Keep our youth smoke-free," co-signed by hundreds of physicians and sympathisers, to Health Minister Schippers, in which they called on her "to do all in her power to make tobacco addiction a thing of the past for future generations" (Youth Smoking Prevention Foundation, 2014). When Schippers rejected their proposals, they decided it was time for a more confrontational approach. In 2013 they began to explicitly name and shame tobacco industry representatives and people associated with the industry network through the website www.tabaknee.nl, and set out a programme for revealing tobacco industry tactics; for example, through investigative journalist pieces in Dutch magazines. Some of the revelations led to questions in parliament, putting more pressure on Schippers, who eventually in the second cabinet Rutte handed over the "hot" tobacco control dossier to State Secretary Martin van Rijn. See also Chap. 6, where the SRJ's successful attempt to take the State to court for violating Article 5.3 FCTC was described. In 2016 the Youth Smoking Prevention Foundation filed charges on behalf of lung cancer patient Anne Marie van Veen and Chronic Obstructive Pulmonary Disease (COPD) patient Lia Breed, against four tobacco manufacturers, accusing them of attempted murder and manslaughter, the first criminal case against the tobacco industry anywhere in the world (SRJ, 2017).

ACCOMPLISHMENTS OF THE TOBACCO CONTROL ADVOCACY COALITION

The preceding account might suggest that the tobacco control coalition led by STIVORO was not particularly effective in advocacy and lobbying since it was financially tied to the government and was preoccupied with educational and smoking cessation activities. Although its main contribution to reducing smoking rates was undoubtedly through mass media campaigns and the implementation and coordination of education and smoking cessation interventions, during its almost 40 year of existence its advocacy activities, which sometimes brought it in direct collision course with the tobacco industry, did have impact on the government's tobacco control policy as well.

Lobby and press contacts were the responsibility of STIVORO's directors, who had to combine these responsibilities with management tasks, so success with lobbying very much depended on the capacity and personal affinity of each director. STIVORO has had six directors since it was founded in 1974. The charities allowed them to decide lobbying strategy. Each director put a unique mark on the organisation and on the way the health network functioned. In the remainder of this section, I describe STIVORO's lobbying accomplishments, organised according to the leadership of the last four directors who left distinct marks on Dutch tobacco control.

Roch de Jong (1981–1995)

While the cabinet persisted in its unwillingness to regulate tobacco advertisements during the 1980s and 1990s, STIVORO just as persistently tried to keep the need for a tobacco advertising and promotion ban on the political agenda. STIVORO was a critical and persevering watchdog of the various centre–right-wing cabinets that did not invest in tobacco control. The driving force was Roch de Jong, director from 1981 until 1995.

De Jong had been a colonel in the TRIS, the former Dutch armed forces in Surinam. He was a strong personality, not afraid to confront the government or the industry. He transformed STIVORO from a passive to an active lobbying organisation. Jean Nelissen, a former marketer with the multinational Unilever, was hired for public relations. "With Nelissen, we took in a streetfighter," recalled Roch de Jong (Bouma, 2001). In 1983 Nelissen bought a pirated tape of the documentary *Death in the West*, an anti-Marlboro documentary that for many years was kept out of public view by lawyers from Philip Morris. Nelissen showed the film to State Secretary for Health Joop van der Reijden, who was impressed and said in an interview that the film should be broadcast in schools, and that he intended to take further measures against tobacco advertising (Bouma, 2000).

In the 1980s the government had no tobacco control policy to speak of. According to one former official,

> A real policy? I wouldn't even know. There might have been a letter to parliament on tobacco, but it rained incidents. The driving force was the dynamic coming from STIVORO's Jean Nelissen. Roch de Jong was also on my back all the time. He was often at the Department. But the Ministry of Health itself was non-existent on the tobacco dossier.[16]

Illustrative of STIVORO's approach in these years is a letter from De Jong in 1984 to parliament and cabinet, in which he criticised the government's long-awaited proposals for a Tobacco Act (De Jong, 1984; De Jong & Nelissen, 1984). He meticulously criticised the fact that the proposal did not include elements that would harm the industry. It was instead in line with the prevailing spirit of reducing the state deficit and putting sole priority on stimulating the economy. He demanded that the government abandon its passive stance, arguing that the current proposals would in no way contribute to effective tobacco control. Instead he listed the things that should be done: reducing the sale of tobacco to specialty shops, regulating tobacco advertising, substantially increasing the government's subsidy to STIVORO (he suggested reserving 0.1% of the tobacco tax revenues), increasing tobacco taxation, and involving STIVORO in all future preparation for a new tobacco policy.

Ben Baan, STIVORO's scientific officer, published a paper in the Dutch Medical Journal, criticising the weak draft to the Tobacco Act, in the same spirit as his director. Baan complained that STIVORO's educational efforts could not compete with tobacco advertising because the tobacco companies had enormous budgets while STIVORO was insufficiently funded by the government (Baan, 1986). He was transparent and open about STIVORO's new strategy: the former neutral focus on merely education was replaced by a more confrontational approach aimed at influencing the societal acceptance of smoking through media campaigns, targeted not only at smokers but also at the public and policymakers, so that they would take the issue of second-hand smoke more seriously. The new approach did not shy away from attacking the tobacco industry, or from political lobbying. In 1987, the year that parliament approved the Tobacco Act, STIVORO's lobby concentrated on influencing members of both houses of parliament and government officials through meetings and letters. STIVORO's 1987 annual report summarised the success of these lobbying efforts: "Much of our efforts can be found in parliament's proceedings." However, this did not lead to concrete improvements to the Tobacco Act. While the whole tobacco industry family had been intensively consulted and involved in the drafting of the act, STIVORO and other health organisations were left out.

In the 1980s STIVORO fought an uphill battle against the industry on the passive smoking issue. In 1981 it ran the campaign "Who smokes is not seen,"[17] on behalf of the Ministry of Health. The campaign morally supported non-smoking employees who longed for a smoke-free work environment. This reflected the cabinet's wish not to impose regulations but to leave it to employees and employers to work out solutions together. The industry's *Stichting Sigaretten Industrie* (Cigarette Manufacturers Association) (SSI) complained that STIVORO suggested in the advertisements that smokers endangered the health of non-smokers, and STIVORO was ordered by the Advertising Code Committee, which oversaw the appropriateness of advertisements, to refrain from similar advertising (Board of Appeal, 1982).

STIVORO was not intimidated and in 1984 ran another media campaign with large advertorials in the four main newspapers: "Ten million non-smokers ask for less."[18] The advertisement included an explicit statement that passive smoking is harmful to health. The SSI again filed a complaint, arguing that a causal association between passive smoking and disease had not been proven. The Advertising Code Committee requested STIVORO to refrain from similar statements in the future, but STIVORO refused. A similar complaint in 1985 by SSI and the *Vereniging Nederlandse Kerftabakindustrie* (Dutch Fine Cut Tobacco Industry Association) (VNK) was declared unfounded, and the industry appealed and won. STIVORO concluded publicly that the committee was not impartial, since members received tobacco industry advertising money.

In 1985 STIVORO published a blacklist summarising the tobacco industry's advertising and tobacco promotion tactics (STIVORO, 1985). Two years later it launched another campaign, "Who will relieve the non-smoker from smoking?"[19] The campaign consisted of newspaper advertisements and letters to employers aimed at swinging public opinion towards support for smoking bans, explicitly stating that passive smoking is harmful to health. STIVORO and civil servants from the Ministry of Health regarded this as a crucial campaign, because once it was recognised and broadly accepted that passive smoking is not merely a nuisance but damaging to health, it would open the way to smoking bans in the public domain. The tobacco industry reacted furiously and launched a counter-campaign, "Who will relieve the workplace from a discussion?" casting doubt on the causal link between passive smoking and disease. SSI and VNK filed a successful complaint about STIVORO with the Advertising Code Committee. STIVORO neglected the committee's demand to cease and continued its campaign into 1987 and 1988. The industry, in a collaborative action of 14 tobacco manufacturers, took STIVORO to court, leading to a three-year legal battle that put a strain on STIVORO's resources and challenged the determination of its board. In 1991 STIVORO won the case convincingly, since it could prove that exposure to second-hand smoke does cause disease. However, deterred by the prospect of continued legal battle in a higher court (legal costs had already reached 400,000 guilders, paid by the government), STIVORO's board accepted an offer by the industry to settle the case. Much to their dismay, the industry immediately sent out a misleading press statement claiming victory and proclaiming that "The Court of Justice at The Hague concluded that scientific investigations have not established which facts concerning passive smoking are correct and which are incorrect. The matter is a controversial one and opinions about it differ" (Cigarette shag information bureau, 1991).

In 1991 at a press conference, STIVORO called on the government to support the European Commission's (EC) proposal for a tobacco advertising directive. The director of the Dutch Heart Foundation, who was chair of the European Heart Network at the time, wrote a letter to ministers and parliament, asking them to adopt the advertising ban and arguing that health and wellbeing must prevail above economic interests (Vermaat, 1995). In September 1993 STIVORO's director De Jong visited the leaders of the main factions in parliament to further lobby for the ad ban, and in December STIVORO published a large newspaper advertisement with the title, "Where is our politicians' common sense? Eight million Dutch say 'no' to tobacco advertising." The ad featured a cartoon of a Marlboro-type cowboy riding an ostrich with its head in the sand. The three health charities and the newly founded Medical Alliance Against Smoking wrote letters to the parliament. At the 9th World Conference on Tobacco or Health in 1994 in Paris, the governments of the Netherlands, the United Kingdom, and Germany were called upon by conference organisers to give up their blocking minority position in the European Union (EU): "Their governments' action in blocking the implementation of the Directive on Tobacco Advertising in the European Union is an international scandal" (Tubiana, 1994).

Boudewijn de Blij (1994–1999)

STIVORO's director Boudewijn de Blij had experience with Dutch politics in a former position as secretary of the supporting organisation of the Labour Party's faction in the Dutch parliament. He eschewed the confrontational and activist style of De Jong, convinced that it was better to entertain good contacts with representatives from the ministry:

> We trusted each other. We collaborated. If they needed a critical letter from us, we immediately produced that. But at the time no one was allowed to know this arrangement. I think that we were calling each other two or three times per week. I wanted to know what was happening at the ministry, or he [his counterpart at the ministry] needed something from me, sometimes just information.[20]

De Blij was successful in securing money from the ministry because he knew exactly when and how to ask for more through his contacts. "I found this much more effective than publicly picking fights with your friends. That is how I did it."[21] A civil servant, when contemplating STIVORO's different directors, commented, "I think Boudewijn manoeuvred most cleverly of all. He operated as much as possible in a low profile manner."[22]

De Blij regularly wrote letters to the government to ask for improvements in tobacco control: for example, in 1996 he made a plea to the cabinet to limit tobacco sales to specialty shops and to ban vending machines (Boudewijn De Blij, 1996). He personally wrote amendments to the new Tobacco Act that were put forward by Labour politicians in parliament because "that was my old profession, so I was quite familiar with how to do it."[23]

On one occasion De Blij agitated the industry by commissioning a report examining how much money the industry spent on tobacco advertising and checking on whether it was correctly paying taxes. This resulted in a remarkable finding: the industry was allowed substantial permanent interest-free sums of money (more than a million euros free to re-invest) because there was a larger time delay then necessary between the delivery of cigarettes to the market and having to pay tax and VAT to the Ministry of Finance (Okkerse, 1997). The report led to media attention, parliamentary questions, proposals from parliament to amend the tobacco taxation law,[24] and even protests from the tobacco retail sector NSO about unfair treatment of the manufacturers at the cost of the retailers. Although the Ministry of Finance reconsidered its agreement with the industry, not much changed. Nevertheless, a few years later the matter still bothered the industry, which again had to deny that it received "state finance" (Roelofs, 2001).

When Minister Els Borst came into office in 1994, the first tobacco control proposals were not very innovative, especially concerning tobacco advertising. STIVORO intensified its lobby, calling on the new minister to come up with the strongest possible tobacco control programme. When Borst presented her prevention *nota* to parliament, De Blij wrote her a letter, copied to the minister of economic affairs, remarking that the European Advertising directive was not mentioned in the *nota* and that Borst must support an EU advertising ban (De Blij, 1995). In addition, the chair of the KNMG wrote a letter to cabinet and parliament urging them to support the ad ban proposal (Lanphen & van Berkestijn, 1995), and the Dutch Medical Alliance Against Smoking called on the cabinet to regulate tobacco advertising in a petition signed by 185 professors. When the Dutch industry distributed a report highlighting the negative economic consequences of advertising and marketing restrictions (it claimed that 651 jobs would be lost in the marketing and advertising sector), STIVORO quickly replied by commissioning the research firm Science & Strategy to list the many marketing activities that the industry uses to reach young people (Science & Strategy, 1996). Other organisations were also rounded up by De Blij to put more pressure on the government. For example, in 1996 the youth organisations of the *Christen-Democratisch Appèl* (Christian Democratic Party) (CDA), the Green–Left Party, the Labour Party, D66, and the small Christian parties, wrote a long letter to the leaders of their factions in the parliament arguing for an advertising ban (De Poorter, 1996). They gave many examples of how the industry continued to target students (through university magazines and sponsoring activities on campus, for instance), and called on their parties to ban tobacco advertising in addition to increasing taxation levels and reducing the number of tobacco selling points.

The following year, Borst said she had changed her position regarding tobacco advertising. The new Labour government in the United Kingdom had stopped resisting the ban, releasing the government from a commitment dating back to 1993 to oppose the EU advertising ban as long as the British voted against it (see also Box 6.1). This paved the way for national legislation in the Netherlands. The intensified lobbying for an advertising ban by the national tobacco control coalition led by STIVORO was important, but what ultimately made the difference was the change in the United Kingdom's position, which opened up a window of opportunity for Borst to give the advertising ban its final push.

De Blij did not shy away from direct confrontations with the industry. Inspired by news from the United States that the industry had known for years that tobacco was addictive and had lied about it, De Blij explored the costs and viability of taking the tobacco industry to court in a product liability court case, claiming incurred damage to society because of tobacco use (Geus & Van der Lee, 1997). However, considering the enormous cost, necessary perseverance, and other constraints on the organisation, STIVORO's board decided against legal action.

Trudy Prins (1999–2006)

Trudy Prins had a background in public relations at the Ministry of Agriculture. Her biggest distinguishing element was that she used the media as a lobbying tool. Most often she did this in tandem with civil servants at the ministry. Critique through the media on the slow working of the bureaucracy helped her counterparts at the ministry speed things up or come up with stricter regulative proposals than might have been possible without such public attention.

One of Prins's first actions was to have STIVORO organise a lobby campaign to support the governments' intention to increase tobacco taxation in 2004 by at least 10%. Directors of six national institutes for public health co-signed the letter to the minister of Finance (Prins, 2003). The Ministry of Health simultaneously pleaded with the finance minister to increase taxation for public health reasons. It is unclear how instrumental the lobbying was to this, but in 2004 tobacco taxation increased by 14%.

During Prins' time as director, STIVORO had its biggest success. Prins with help from STIVORO's network succeeded in securing majority support in parliament for an amendment by the Green–Left party to include the workplace smoking ban in the new Tobacco Act in 2002. Part of the reason for Prins' success was that STIVORO, together with CAN and the Lung Foundation, had supported post office employee Nanny Nooijen about her right to work in a smoke-free environment. The fact that Nanny Nooijen won her case convincingly was important in encouraging politicians to support the ban.

With Health Minister Els Borst the government was committed to stronger tobacco control STIVORO was given an important role in executing the governments' tobacco control agenda, and the organisation grew considerably to handle its new tasks. STIVORO transformed into a national expert centre on tobacco education and cessation support, with a staff fully dedicated to developing evidence-based education, cessation interventions, and campaigns. These were STIVORO's 'golden years'.

Lies van Gennip (2006–2012)

At the time that Lies van Gennip, a biologist with a PhD and management experience in health research organisations, began working as director of STIVORO, the three charities were reconsidering their relationship with STIVORO and were already experimenting with their own tobacco control activities. The governing board of STIVORO was replaced by a board of trustees and the health ministry no longer had a seat on the board. STIVORO was given the task of executing the NPT programme and the charities began to make STIVORO more accountable for the money they spent on tobacco control. Van Gennip was charged with the task of reorganising the organisation and making STIVORO more efficient and accountable.

At the request of the charities, STIVORO hired Van Oort & Van Oort Public Affairs, a professional lobbying firm, to support advocacy activities. At that time the third Balkenende cabinet had just fallen, and new elections were called. Van Oort organised a broad lobby to get three goals into party programmes and into the coalition agreement: a smoke-free hospitality sector, a tax increase, and reimbursement of smoking cessation support. In a few months STIVORO was able to secure support from 40 societal and medical organisations around one united call for political commitment to a smoke-free hospitality sector. In addition, it supported CAN to initiate the first civil society initiative to get smoke-free bars and restaurants on the political agenda, by helping CAN collect 62,000 signatures.

In 2007, when the smoking ban in the hospitality sector was to be discussed in the cabinet, van Gennip sent a letter to Prime Minister

Balkenende with arguments as to why a smoking ban was good for public health (Van Gennip, 2007). The letter was accompanied by a DVD featuring interviews with experts from several European countries, all of whom testified to the successes and positive experiences with similar bans in their home countries. The lobbying effort was successful, and the introductory dossier for the new minister of health listed all three goals (Bekker, 2007), and a smoke-free hospitality sector was included in the coalition agreement of the fourth Balkenende cabinet to fast track the smoking ban in bars and restaurants. Van Gennip and the directors of the three charities met with the new Health Minister Ab Klink, but this did not result in further commitments from the government to initiate new tobacco control measures (Rutgers, Hanselaar, Stam, & Van Gennip, 2007). The clumsy and ambiguous implementation of the smoking ban in cafés by Minister Klink unleashed an unprecedentedly aggressive response by groups and individuals who regarded the ban as an infringement on individual liberties. They took their anger out on STIVORO, which was confronted by angry smokers, sometimes fuelled by organisations such as pro-smokers group Forces and the smokers' rights group *Stichting Rokers Belangen* (SRB), but also from anonymous sources on the internet.

Gradually the unwillingness of the government to take further action on tobacco control, coupled with the determination of Lies van Gennip to obtain results, led to polarisation and a hostile atmosphere. The charities were not comfortable with this because it jeopardised the relationship they enjoyed with the government. As a lobbyist from one of the charities said, "We were very much bothered by the unpleasant and harsh tone of voice that STIVORO was using. As a result, the government was closing its doors to us."[25]

STIVORO's successes and the tight connections between STIVORO and the tobacco control officers at the health ministry did not go unnoticed. According to an ex-civil-servant:

> The industry was horrified by all this ... Eventually with other ministers, with another political winds of change, it began to affect STIVORO. I belief that STIVORO was ultimately judged on this; the questions that were raised in parliament by MP Schippers... At a certain moment it also began to vibrate within the ministry, especially under 'minister] Klink: STIVORO was no longer allowed to run campaigns ... STIVORO began to be seen as patronising and as the 'anti's'.[26]

In May 2009 Van Gennip received a phone call from the industry's VNK with the threat that if STIVORO continued its assertive lobbying, VNK would use its influence at the ministry through VNO–NCW to make sure that STIVORO was harmed. Soon afterwards a civil servant from the Ministry of Health told STIVORO's director that it must cease advocacy activities because STIVORO was losing its support from the ministry. A month after the threat from VNK, in June 2009, STIVORO received a letter from the ministry that its yearly subsidy would be cut.

One example of the intensive lobbying activities that STIVORO was capable of during this time were letters delivered personally to the officials responsible for forming a new ruling coalition in July 2010 (Bensing, Brand, & Borst, 2010). The letter was co-signed by 34 national and international experts, and informed the officials that the previous government had invested too little in tobacco control, causing a stagnation of the decline in smoking prevalence rates, and that they advised the new government to adopt a tobacco control policy based on three pillars: a substantial tobacco tax increase, allocation of the revenues to more education, and making the denormalisation of tobacco use a central issue.

When Health Minister Schippers entered the arena in 2010 and tobacco control was reversed, STIVORO fired up its advocacy activities while fighting for its own survival—a move that distanced it even more from the three charities. STIVORO tried to win an increasingly lost cause by continuing the strategy of presenting facts and science against ideology, using the public health frame to emphasise tobacco's deathly effects. For example, it launched a website where statements by Schippers about tobacco and tobacco policy were rebutted. The website was introduced with these lines:

> Every year tens of thousands of people die because of smoking. Smoking is the number one cause of death in the Netherlands. One in two dies from its addiction. It is harsh to put it this way, but it is a policy choice. Choosing for no policy or a minimal policy is choosing for these numbers. That is what this website is about.

STIVORO was determined to fight the reversal of the smoking ban and to push for a California-inspired activist model: "clearly, the challenge for the public health community is to stand firm and continue to press for the successful model already working so well in many other countries. Where the protection of non-smokers is at stake, "going Dutch" is simply not an option" (Van Bladeren, 2011). But by now STIVORO's cause was lost, for it had lost its support from the charities, which wanted to re-organise tobacco control advocacy and take the lead themselves.

Conclusion

The Dutch tobacco control coalition was organised in a unique way. The core of the advocacy network consisted of the three charities that financed STIVORO to fight smoking on their behalf, while the Ministry of Health was also on the board of the organisation. The organisations were united in a joint fight against the tobacco industry. The arrangement was typically Dutch: compromises between government and civil society were locked into the fabric of the organisation of STIVORO. For many years this worked well: especially under Minister Els Borst, the relationship between STIVORO and the tobacco control unit at the Ministry of Health was very good and mutually reinforcing, and STIVORO was allowed to prosper and grow into an internationally acclaimed tobacco control expert centre, while ever-increasing subsidies from the government and occasional large donations from the charities made it possible to organise large-scale smoking cessation media events that motivated many smokers to quit smoking. The flip side was that, since the government was accountable for STIVORO's activities to parliament, the tobacco control coalition was unable to set up a professional lobbying apparatus. Professional lobbying was not integrated into the overall action plans of the organisation until around 2006, when a professional lobbying firm was hired to coordinate advocacy activities.

Over time the tobacco control coalition expanded, in the mid-1990s through the Dutch Medical Alliance Against Smoking and at the beginning of the 2000s through the Partnership Stop Smoking. Despite the fact that this strengthened the coalition's advocacy capacity, help from the broader medical community did not materialise in the Netherlands as it did in the United Kingdom, where medical organisations were key to cultivating a social climate more conducive to tobacco control while putting pressure on ministers to take the smoking problem more seriously.

During periods when the government opposed or delayed tobacco control, the lobby led by STIVORO was more assertive towards the government. This happened in the 1980s and beginning of the 1990s (Van Agt and Lubbers cabinets), and between 2007 and 2012 when Klink and

Schippers were ministers of Health. During periods when the government showed more willingness to control tobacco, the collaboration with STIVORO relaxed. The tobacco control coalition had several important lobbying successes. Most important probably was its support of the small understaffed tobacco control unit at the ministry of health leading up to the revised Tobacco Act. Notable was the inclusion of the important workplace smoking ban in the revised Tobacco Act, which was a direct result of coordinated lobbying of parliamentarians by STIVORO. In 2007, STIVORO was successful in pushing the government to extend the workplace smoking ban to bars and restaurants, but it failed to prevent the tobacco lobby from sabotaging the implementation, leading to a temporary reversal of the ban.

Around 2005 a major shift took place in the Dutch tobacco control coalition when the three charities were no longer willing to play second fiddle and wanted a more proactive tobacco control advocacy role. However, it took another 8 years before STIVORO, which had been the central tobacco control organisation since 1975, was disbanded, during which time the three charities gradually increased and professionalised tobacco control advocacy.

Notes

1. "Coalition" is used here in terms of the Advocacy Coalition Framework.
2. The three big charities in the United States built the "Coalition on Smoking OR Health," in which lobbyists from the charities worked together under a single coordinator, independent from the government (Derthick, 2005).
3. Parliamentary Papers II, 1977–1978, 14,800, XVIII, nr. 34.
4. Proceeding, II 1976–1977, 14,360, nr. 2.
5. About €910,000 at current monetary value.
6. This was not a typical Dutch concern at the time. For example, in the United States, the health charities faced similar constraints. They felt that they needed to protect their image as a mainstream, legitimate organisation, which limited the way they could lobby openly for controversial goals (Wolfson, 2001).
7. Proceedings I, 26 March 2002, EK 24–1263.
8. Proceedings II, 24 June 1987, 91–4639.
9. Interview on 16 June 2016.
10. Source: STIVORO's annual reports.
11. Interview on 20 October 2015.

12. Interview on 29 October 2015. The current size of the core team is three officials: one team leader (who may also be responsible for other issues), and two officers—one responsible for international-level tobacco policy and one for national-level tobacco policy. It is supported by trainees or officials from "flex pools."
13. Interview on 16 April 2016.
14. Interview on 26 April 2016.
15. Proceedings II, 9 December 1993, 36–2773.
16. Interview with a former civil servant on 6 October 2015.
17. In Dutch: "Wie rookt is niet gezien."
18. In Dutch: "10 miljoen niet-rokers vragen of het wat minder kan."
19. In Dutch: "Wie helpt de roker van het roken af?"
20. Interview 17 June 2016.
21. Interview 17 June 2016.
22. Interview 26 April 2016.
23. Interview 17 June 2016.
24. Tweede Kamer, 2000–2001, 26,472, nr. 23.
25. Interview on 15 March 2017.
26. Interview, 6 November 2015.

References

Adriaanse, H., Van Reek, J., & Metsemakers, J. (1986). Smoking behaviour of Dutch general practitioners in the period 1977–1983. *Scandinavian Journal of Primary Health Care, 4,* 151–156.

Adriaanse, H., Van Reek, J., & Van Zutphen, W. (1986). Rookgewoonten van artsen wereldwijd: Een overzicht van 100 onderzoekingen naar tabaksgebruik onder artsen in 31 landen in de periode 1951–1985. *Nederlands Tijdschrift voor Geneeskunde, 130,* 2224–2229.

Baan, B. (1986). Strategieen ter bevordering van het niet-roken. *Nederlands Tijdschrift voor Geneeskunde, 130,* 1232–1139.

Barneveld, J. T. A., Dalesio, O. B., & Van Leeuwen, F. E. (1992). Een ontmoedigend tabaksontmoedigingsbeleid: Pleidooi voor een integrale aanpak. *Medisch Contact, 47,* 943–944.

Beernink, J. F., & Plokker, J. H. (1975). Maatregelen tot beperking van het roken. Advies van de Gezondheidsraad. *Verslagen, Adviezen, Rapporten* (Vol. 23). Leidschendam: Ministerie van Volksgezondheid en Milieuhygiëne.

Bekker, R. (2007). *Introductiedossier nieuwe bewindspersonen Ministeries van VWS.* Den Haag: VWS.

Bensing, J., Brand, P., & Borst, E. (2010). Brief aan de informateurs [letter to the inquirers]. Retrieved from http://www.ggdghor.nl/media/filebank/557bea2 639e542e8843db5db9797445c/stivorobrief.pdf

BMA. (1986). *Smoking out the barons: The campaign against the tobacco industry. A report of the British Medical Association Public Affairs Division*. Chichester: Wiley & Sons.

Board of Appeal. (1982). Decision in the case of Dijkstra/Public Health and Smoking Foundation. *Dutch Tobacco Industry Collection*, Bates No. JB1457. Retrieved from https://www.industrydocumentslibrary.ucsf.edu/tobacco/docs/#id=zkgp0219

Boucher, P. (2000). Rendez-vous with Trudy Prins. Retrieved from http://archive.tobacco.org/News/rendezvous/prins.html

Bouma, J. (2000). Echo's uit de prairie. *Dossiers Onderzoeksjournalistiek*. Retrieved 29 July, 2017, from https://www.villamedia.nl/journalist/n/dossiers/onderzoekphilipmorris.shtm

Bouma, J. (2001). *Het rookgordijn: De macht van de Nederlandse tabaksindustrie*. Amsterdam: Veen.

Chapman, S. (2017). Why researchers have a duty to try and influence policy. Retrieved from The Conversation website: https://theconversation.com/why-researchers-have-a-duty-to-try-and-influence-policy-71081

Cigarette shag information bureau. (1991). STIVORO trial ended: Tobacco Industry satisfied with court verdict. *Dutch Tobacco Industry Collection*, Bates No. JB1025. Retrieved from https://www.industrydocumentslibrary.ucsf.edu/tobacco/docs/xqfp0219

De Blij, B. (1995). [Brieven van Stivoro aan de ministeries van EZ en VWS]. *Dutch Tobacco Industry Collection*, Bates No. JB2574. Retrieved from https://www.industrydocumentslibrary.ucsf.edu/tobacco/docs/nlwp0219

De Blij, B. (1996). Amendement Tabaksaccijns. *Dutch Tobacco Industry Collection*, Bates No. JB2691. Retrieved from https://www.industrydocumentslibrary.ucsf.edu/tobacco/docs/tqwp0219

De Jong, R. (1984). Commentaar op de ontwerp tabakswet [letter]. *Dutch Tobacco Industry Collection*, Bates No. JB2104. Retrieved from https://www.industrydocumentslibrary.ucsf.edu/tobacco/docs/hpfp0219

De Jong, R. (1989). Notitie met het oog op de uitvoering van het meerjaren voorlichtingsprogramma niet-roken. *Dutch Tobacco Industry Collection*, Bates No. JB1425. Retrieved from https://www.industrydocumentslibrary.ucsf.edu/tobacco/docs/kzhp0219

De Jong, R., & Nelissen, J. G. M. (1984). [Brief van Stivoro aan de voorzitter en Leden der Staten-Generaal]. *Dutch Tobacco Industry Collection*, Bates No. JB2305. Retrieved from https://www.industrydocumentslibrary.ucsf.edu/tobacco/docs/mpdp0219

De Poorter, J.-P. (1996). [Brief van de Nationale Jongerenraad voor Milieu en Ontwikkeling aad de Tweede kamer fractie van CDA]. *Dutch Tobacco Industry Collection*, Bates No. JB1948. Retrieved from https://www.industrydocumentslibrary.ucsf.edu/tobacco/docs/jjbp0219

Dekker, E. (1981). De huisarts en het rookpatroon. In STIVORO (Ed.), *Trekt de rook langzaam op? Voordrachten van het symposium*. Den Haag: STIVORO.
Derthick, M. A. (2005). *Up in smoke: From legislation to litigation in tobacco politics* (2nd ed.). Washington, DC: CQ Press.
Dresscher, I., Elzinga, A., & Koldenhof, E. (1991). *Evaluatie tabakswet en zelfregulering tabaksreclame*. Zoetermeer: Research voor Beleid.
Duivenvoorden, E. (2009). *Magiër van een nieuwe tijd: Het leven van Robert Jasper Grootveld*. Amsterdam: De Arbeiderspers.
Geus, M., & Van der Lee, J. (1997). STIVORO/Produktaansprakelijkheid. *Dutch Tobacco Industry Collection*, Bates No. JB1011. Retrieved from https://www.industrydocumentslibrary.ucsf.edu/tobacco/docs/ftcp0219
Hilvering, C., Knol, K., & Wagener, D. J. (1995). Petitie tot strenge beperking tabaksreclame. *Dutch Tobacco Industry Collection*, Bates No. JB2550. Retrieved from https://www.industrydocumentslibrary.ucsf.edu/tobacco/docs/gggp0219
Hoogervorst, H., Zoun, J. P. M., De Blij, B. A. J. M., & Hanselaar, A. G. J. M. (2005). Intentieverklaring tabaksontmoediging. *Dutch Tobacco Industry Collection*, Bates No. JB3189. Retrieved from https://www.industrydocumentslibrary.ucsf.edu/tobacco/docs/kgdn0217
ITC Project. (2010). *The International Tobacco Control Policy Evaluation Project: ITC Netherlands National Report*. Ontario, The Hague: ITC Project, University of Waterloo, Canada.
Joossens, L., & Raw, M. (2011). *The tobacco control scale 2010 in Europe*. Brussels: Association of European Cancer Leagues.
KNMG. (2007). *Volksgezondheid en Preventie De visie van de KNMG*. Utrecht: KNMG.
KNMG. (2016). *Tobacco discouragement: Towards a smoke-free society*. Utrecht: Royal Dutch Medical Association.
Knol, K. (1995, January 11). Kinderen doelwit van tabaksreclame. *Trouw*. Retrieved August 19, 2017, from http://www.trouw.nl/tr/nl/5009/Archief/article/detail/2663243/1995/01/11/Kinderen-doelwit-van-tabaksreclame.dhtml
Knol, K. (1996a). [Brief van Knol aan Borst]. *Dutch Tobacco Industry Collection*, Bates No. JB1947. Retrieved from https://www.industrydocumentslibrary.ucsf.edu/tobacco/docs/ytvp0219
Knol, K. (1996b). Medische Alliantie tegen het roken. *Dutch Tobacco Industry Collection*, Bates No. JB2673. Retrieved from https://www.industrydocumentslibrary.ucsf.edu/tobacco/docs/spwp0219
Knol, K. (1997). De toekomst van de strijd tegen het roken. *Medisch Contact, 52*(25), 803–804.
Lanphen, J.M.G., & Van Berkestijn, Th.M.G. (1995). [Brief van de Koninklijke Nederlandse Maatschappij tot Bevordering de Geneeskunst aan de leden van het Kabint en de leden vande Tweede Kamer der Staten Generaal]. *Dutch Tobacco Industry*, Bates No. 2057. Retrieved from https://www.industrydocumentslibrary.ucsf.edu/tobacco/docs/lxdp0219

Mackenbach, J. P. (2006). Antirookbeleid moet anders. *Medisch Contact, 13*, 512–514.
Mackenbach, J. P. (2009). Echte minister van Gezondheid gezocht. *Volkskrant.*
Mackenbach, J. P. (2016). Nederland rookvrij: dokters spreken zich uit: Nu de politiek nog. *Nederlands Tijdschrift voor Geneeskunde, 160*, D310.
Mackenbach, J. P., Klazinga, N. S., & Van der wal, G. (2004). Preventie vraagt ambitieuzere aanpak. Reactie op de kabinetsnota 'Langer gezond leven 2004-2007; ook een kwestie van gezond gedrag. *Nederlands Tijdschrift voor Geneeskunde, 148*(15), 704–707.
Meinsma, L. (1969). *Roken en risico's.* Lochem: De Tijdstroom.
Mudde, A. N., & De Vries, H. (1999). The reach and effectiveness of a national mass media-led smoking cessation campaign in the Netherlands. *American Journal of Public Health, 89*(3), 346–350. https://doi.org/10.2105/AJPH.89.3.346
Nagelhout, G. E., Willemsen, M. C., van den Putte, B., Crone, M., & de Vries, H. (2009). *Evaluatie 'in iedere roker zit een stopper' campagne: tweede nameting.* Den Haag: STIVORO.
Okkerse, W. D. (1997). *De sigarettenindustrie in Nederland: Uit (de) Balans?* Rijswijk: ITLC Associate.
Op de Weegh, J. M. J., & Willemsen, M. C. (2003). *Dat Kan Ik Ook!: De stoppen met roken millenniumcampagne.* Den Haag: STIVORO.
Partnership Stop met Roken. (2004). *Beleidsaanbevelingen voor de behandeling van tabaksverslaving.* Den Haag: Partnership Stop met Roken.
Prins, G. J. J. (2003). Verhoging tabaksaccijns. *Dutch Tobacco Industry Collection*, Bates No. JB0600. Retrieved from https://www.industrydocumentslibrary.ucsf.edu/tobacco/docs/mmxb0191
Rathjen, H. (1999). *The coalition. How to build a coalition in connection with a public health campaign to obtain tobacco control measures.* Quebec: Coalition Québécoise pur le contrôle du tabac.
Rijksen, W. (2005). Evaluatie van het tabaksontmoedigingsbeleid [letter KNMG]. *Dutch Tobacco Industry Collection*, Bates No. JB2971. Retrieved from https://www.industrydocumentslibrary.ucsf.edu/tobacco/docs/qsdn0217
RJ Reynolds. (1979). Summary of the PR Program of the Dutch Cigarette Manufactures Association. *RJ Reynolds Records*, Bates No. 500877429–500877431. Retrieved from https://www.industrydocumentslibrary.ucsf.edu/tobacco/docs/jrpj0096
Roelofs, W. J. (2001). Accijnskrediet. *Dutch Tobacco Industry Collection*, Bates No. JB1755. Retrieved from https://www.industrydocumentslibrary.ucsf.edu/tobacco/docs/xkcp0219
Roscam Abbing, E. W. (1992). Tabaksbeleid: rookgordijn voor massamoord. *Medisch Contact, 47*, 931.
Royal College of Physicians. (1962). *Smoking and health.* London: Royal College of Physicians of London.

Rutgers, M., Hanselaar, T., Stam, H., & Van Gennip, L. (2007). Letters to Klink. *Dutch Tobacco Industry Collection*, Bates No. JB0455. Retrieved from https://www.industrydocumentslibrary.ucsf.edu/tobacco/docs/rzhb0191

Science & Strategy. (1996). Inventaristatie van de martketingactiviteiten van de tabaksindustrie. *Dutch Tobacco Industry Collection*, Bates No. JB1537. Retrieved from https://www.industrydocumentslibrary.ucsf.edu/tobacco/docs/jmbp0219

SNK & SSI. (1985). Jaaroverzicht 1984. *Dutch Tobacco Industry Collection*, Bates No. JB2269. Retrieved from https://www.industrydocumentslibrary.ucsf.edu/tobacco/docs/yfgp0219

SRJ. (2017). Smokers bring case against the tobacco industry. Retrieved from http://www.stichtingrookpreventiejeugd.nl/over-rookpreventie-jeugd/english/item/86-smokers-bring-case-against-the-tobacco-industry

STIVORO. (1978). *Een gulden per jaar: Beleidslijnen van de Stichting Volksgezondheid en Roken*. Den Haag: STIVORO.

STIVORO. (1985). *Reclame als pacemaker van de tabaksindustrie*. Den Haag: STIVORO.

STIVORO. (2007). 7,4 miljoen te weinig om gewenste daling rokers te halen [press release 9 januari 2007]. In STIVORO (Ed.). Den Haag: STIVORO.

STIVORO. (2009). *Terugblik 2008 [Year report]*. Den Haag: STIVORO.

STIVORO. (2010a). Tabaksontmoediging moet anders [newsletter] *STIVORO.nl* (Vol. 14). Den Haag: STIVORO.

STIVORO. (2010b). *Van onderop en van bovenaf: De toekomst van tabaksontmoediging in Nederland 2011–2020*. Den Haag: STIVORO.

Tubiana, M. (1994). [Letter from Tubiana to Borst-Eilers and Prime Minister Kok]. *Dutch Tobacco Industry Collection*, Bates No. JB2584. Retrieved from https://www.industrydocumentslibrary.ucsf.edu/tobacco/docs/hphp0219

Unknown (Philip Morris). (1979). *Smoking & health—Five year plan*, Bates No 2501020542–2501020686. Truth Tobacco Industry Documents.

Van Bladeren, F. (2011). Netherlands: Going backwards [news analysis]. *Tobacco Control, 20*, 4–7.

Van den Putte, S. J. H. M., Yzer, M. C., Ten Berg, B. M., & Steeveld, R. M. A. (2005). *Nederland start met stoppen/Nederland gaat door met stoppen. Evaluatie van de STIVORO campagnes rondom de jaarwisseling 2003–2004*. Amsterdam: Universiteit van Amsterdam, ASCOR.

Van Emst, A. J., & Willemsen, M. C. (2011). *Naar een nieuwe structuur voor tabaksontmoediging in Nederland: Verslag van een inspirational conference*. Den Haag: STIVORO.

Van Es, J. (1987). Roken. *Medisch Contact, 42*, 259.

Van Gennip, E. M. S. J. (2007). Brief STIVORO aan Ministerie van Algemene Zaken over beleidsvoornemen om de horeca-rookvrij te maken. *Dutch Tobacco Industry Collection*, Bates No. JB0344. Retrieved from https://www.industrydocumentslibrary.ucsf.edu/tobacco/docs/snhb0191

Vandenbroucke, J. P., Kok, J. F. J., Matroos, A., & Dekker, E. (1981). Rookgewoonten van Nederlandse huisartsen vergeleken met die van de bevolking. *Nederlands Tijdschrift voor Geneeskunde, 125*(1), 406.
Vermaat, H. (1995). *Een piece de résistance: De tabaksreclame en de lobby van de Nederlandse hartstichting voor een verbod* (Doctoral thesis), Vrije Universiteit Amsterdam.
Westerik, H., & Van der Rijt, G. A. J. (2001). *De millenniumcampagne 'Stoppen met roken 2000': Evaluatie van een campagne onder Nederlandse rokers*. Nijmegen: Katholieke Universiteit Nijmegen.
Willemsen, M. C. (2011). *Roken in Nederland: De keerzijde van tolerantie [inaugural lecture]*. Maastricht: Maastricht University.
Willemsen, M. C. (2012). Pak de tabakslobby keihard aan. *de Volkskrant*, 31.
Willemsen, M. C., De Vries, H., & Van Schayck, O. (2009). Wat ging er mis met rookverbod in de horeca? [Why only the Dutch resist the smoking ban?]. *NRC Handelsblad*.
Willemsen, M. C., van Kann, D., & Jansen, E. (2012). Stoppen met roken: ontwikkeling, implementatie en evaluatie van een massamediale campagne. In J. Brug, P. v. Assema, & L. Lechner (Eds.), *Gezondheidsvoorlichting en gedragsverandering*. Assen: Van Gorcum.
Wolfson, M. (2001). *The fight against big tobacco: The movement, the state, and the public's health*. New York: Aldine de Gruyter.
Youth Smoking Prevention Foundation. (2014). *Five years of action for a smoke-free country*. Amsterdam: Youth Smoking Prevention Foundation.

Open Access This chapter is licensed under the terms of the Creative Commons Attribution 4.0 International License (http://creativecommons.org/licenses/by/4.0/), which permits use, sharing, adaptation, distribution and reproduction in any medium or format, as long as you give appropriate credit to the original author(s) and the source, provide a link to the Creative Commons license and indicate if changes were made.

The images or other third party material in this chapter are included in the chapter's Creative Commons license, unless indicated otherwise in a credit line to the material. If material is not included in the chapter's Creative Commons license and your intended use is not permitted by statutory regulation or exceeds the permitted use, you will need to obtain permission directly from the copyright holder.

CHAPTER 10

Problem Identification and Agenda Setting

Tobacco is a highly contested topic. Lobbyists present their policy solutions to politicians and government officials who weigh the evidence against what they believe is feasible or desirable, much like solving a complex puzzle (Kingdon, 2003). Such puzzles take considerable time. In the meantime, the many other concerns that a government is confronted with compete with tobacco control for a place on the policy agenda. The public policy literature distinguishes different stages of agenda setting: issues move from the public agenda to the political agenda, move again to the formal (sometimes called institutional or governmental) agenda, and finally reach the decision agenda. The public agenda consists of issues that have achieved a high level of public interest and visibility, while the formal agenda lists the topics that decision makers are actually working on (Cobb, Ross, & Ross, 1976). For an issue to reach the formal agenda, decision makers must be aware of the underlying problem, and consensus must be reached that acting upon the problem is possible and necessary and that the solution falls within the government's responsibility.

This chapter starts with an examination of the process of problem identification, which is the first step in agenda setting. Problem definition is central to understanding agenda setting, and refers to what Rochefort and Cobb (cited in Cairney (2012)) describe as "what we choose to identify as public issues and how we think and talk about these concerns." Attention from the government is often drawn to an issue when new statistics surface

© The Author(s) 2018
M. C. Willemsen, *Tobacco Control Policy in the Netherlands*,
Palgrave Studies in Public Health Policy Research,
https://doi.org/10.1007/978-3-319-72368-6_10

which show that the issue is problematic. This will be explored for Dutch tobacco control by looking at the presentation of four-yearly data from the *Rijksinstituut voor Volksgezondheid en Milieu* (National Institute for Public Health and the Environment) (RIVM) on the public health status of the population and how successive governments translated this into quantitative national targets for tobacco control. I then consider why tobacco control seems to be a "low issue" topic most of the time and explore the reasons for this. Is it not seen as urgent? Is smoking not regarded as a legitimate target for state interference? This brings me to consider if the low urgency for tobacco control might be explained by the political orientation of Dutch governments (left/progressive vs. right/conservative), and whether it might be further explained by a related factor, which is how governments deal with times of economic recession. I present evidence that the Dutch governments least active in tobacco control were at the time preoccupied with economic crises.

Government attention is not automatically directed at what the facts tell us, but depends on how successful various interests groups are in drawing attention to an issue. This chapter therefore closes by discussing how framing of the smoking issue influenced agenda setting. Framing is "a strategy that interest groups employ to further their interests by generating powerful beliefs and ideas which function as a framework for the public's way of thinking" (Grüning, Strünk, & Gilmore, 2008). How was smoking framed by tobacco control organisations and by the tobacco industry, and which was most successful? Some attention will also be paid to the role of media advocacy as an important tool in communicating specific frames and in setting agendas.

Problem Identification

For something to become a policy issue, it must first come to the attention of policymakers. This may be triggered by the publication of new statistics (Kingdon, 2003). Main statistical indicators in our case are the proportion of smokers in the adult and youth population and smoking-related morbidity and mortality statistics. The Netherlands was one of the first countries to build its public health policy in a systematic manner on epidemiologic data. Following the Public Health Act, every four years the *Rijksinstituut voor Volksgezondheid en Milieu* (National Institute for Public Health and the Environment) (RIVM) publishes *Volksgezondheid Toekomst Verkenning* (Public Health Status and Foresight) reports (VTV). Since 1992 these comprehensive and detailed reports have outlined the public health priorities of the next four years for the Ministry of Health.[1] The first was Health Minister Els Borst's *Healthy and well* policy document (VWS, 1995), which identified specific conditions that must be met before a topic may be identified as a policy priority: the health problem must concern a serious problem that concerns a large group of people, it must be preventable and modifiable, efficacious prevention methods must be available, prevention must result in improvement in public health, and the policy methods must be legally, ethically, and societally acceptable.

To date, six VTV reports have been issued. Table 10.1 summarises the main statements about the tobacco problem.

In the first three RIVM reports smoking was singled out as a public health problem to be addressed urgently. These reports included alarming messages, since adult and youth smoking was not going down and compared unfavourably with other countries. RIVM experts warned that the Netherlands had lost its top position regarding general life expectancy in Europe and was facing the possibility that life expectancy might decline for the first time in history (RIVM, 2002). Later VTV reports noted a decline in tobacco use following the implementation of the revised Tobacco Act in 2002, and characterised trends in adults and youth in a less alarming manner, although smoking rates were still regarded as high compared with those of other countries and smoking remained the most important preventable cause of death and disease. A consequence was that the feeling of urgency for tighter tobacco control became less poignant.

NATIONAL TARGETS FOR TOBACCO CONTROL

The Ministry of Health's policy documents with intentions in the field of public health and disease prevention, listed in Table 10.2, carry political weight and are discussed in parliament. The first was the *Nota 2000* of 1986 (WVC, 1986). The report recognised that the Dutch tobacco policy lagged behind other countries, especially Scandinavian countries. Despite smoking being recognised as the number one cause of death, and the setting of an aspirational target of reducing the smoking population to 20% in 2000, tobacco control was not yet mentioned as a national policy priority. The government was hesitant, wanting to wait until the Tobacco Act was implemented in 1990 in the hope that this would increase public support for new measures. In 2003 the prevention documents included a list of unhealthy lifestyle behaviours that were the priority targets for the next four years: smoking was listed next to obesity and diabetes (VWS, 2003). In 2006 the list was extended to include alcohol and depression (VWS,

Table 10.1 Tobacco problem indicators in the Public Health Status Forecasts reports by the National Institute of Health and the Environment (RIVM)

Year	Title of report (translated in Dutch)	Problem indicators (as they are formulated in the report)	
		Smoking prevalence	Smoking and health
1993	Public Health Forecast: The health of the Dutch population in the period 1950–2010 (RIVM, 1993)	– While tobacco use continues to decline in various European countries, it stagnates in the Netherlands at around 40% in men and more than 30% in women. – Among youth, it seems to start to rise.	– Smoking constitutes the largest demonstrable contribution to total mortality in the Netherlands (about one-quarter of all deaths). – Smoking is responsible for about 29,000 deaths in 1990.
1997	The sum of the parts (RIVM, 1997)	– An unfavourable development in the adult population is that the number of smokers has not gone down for a number of years. – There are clearly unfavourable developments in youth smoking, where the number of smokers has started to increase (already 28% of 10–19-year-olds are smoking).	– A major cause of mortality can be attributed to smoking (circa 23,000 per year).
2002	Health on track? (RIVM, 2002)	– The long-term reduction in smoking rates in the adult population (1980–2000) has halted. The trend is unfavourable. – Smoking rates in women in low socioeconomic groups are increasing. – Smoking rates among young people are a cause for concern. – The Netherlands occupies the sixth position in the EU concerning the proportion of smokers who are 15–16 years old (36% are smokers).	– Lung cancer deaths in men remain one of the highest in Europe. In women it increases faster than the European average. Women die more often from chronic lung disease. Both diseases are primarily attributable to smoking. – The difference in life expectancy between low and highly educated men is five years.

Table 10.1 (continued)

Year	Title of report (translated in Dutch)	Problem indicators (as they are formulated in the report)	
		Smoking prevalence	Smoking and health
2006	*Care for health* (RIVM, 2006)	– The trend is favourable: smoking is going down among both men and women (1990–2004). – However, smoking, especially among women, still compares unfavourably to the average in the EU. – Notable is the widening of differences in smoking rates between those of high and low education between 1990 and 2007. – Trends are much less positive for the young. Many young people smoke.	– Smoking is the single most important cause of death and disease, responsible for 20.9% of lost life years, 7.1% of total sick years, and 13% of the disease burden.
2010	*From health to better* (RIVM, 2010)	– The general trend in smoking seems favourable. – Over the past four years a minor improvement can be reported with respect to smoking, but that does not change the fact that the Dutch still smoke more than those living in countries nearby. – The ambition in the previous prevention *nota* to reduce smokers to 20% in 2010 has not been accomplished. – Despite policy efforts, health differences between the high and low educated have not diminished in recent years, and with respect to smoking the differences have widened.	– Smoking causes the greatest disease burden. If no one smoked, the healthy life expectancy of the population would increase by two years.

(*continued*)

Table 10.1 (continued)

Year	Title of report (translated in Dutch)	Problem indicators (as they are formulated in the report)	
		Smoking prevalence	Smoking and health
2014	*A healthier Netherlands* (RIVM, 2014)	– For many years now the percentage of smokers has declined. The percentage of Dutch male smokers is now slightly lower than in other EU countries, and the percentage of female smokers is about average. – People with low education have a 1.5 times higher rate of smoking than those with high education, a disparity that has widened slightly from 1990 to 2012. – Youth smoking is going down. The proportion of 10–19-year-olds who smoke has reduced from 27% in 2000 to 18% in 2012.	– Smoking remains by far the major cause of death and illness, causing 13% of the disease burden.

Table 10.2 Quantitative goals for tobacco control in national prevention policy documents

Year	Minister/state secretary	Prevention policy document	Proportion of smokers in the year preceding the policy document (%)	Policy goal	Result	Ambition[a]
1986	Joop van der Reijden	Nota 2000 (WVC, 1986)	40	20% smokers in 2000 (WHO target)	Failed	−1.4
1991	Hans Simons	Health with tact (WVC, 1991)	31 (women) and 39 (men)	25% female smokers and 32% male smokers in 1993	Failed	−2 (women) and −2.3 (men)
1995	Els Borst	Healthy and well (VWS, 1995)	34	No new target	–	–
2001	Els Borst	Policy agenda 2001 (VWS, 2002)	33	28% smokers in 2004	Succeeded	−1.3
2003	Hans Hoogervorst	Live a longer healthy life (VWS, 2003)	31	25% smokers in 2007	Failed	−1.2
2006	Hans Hoogervorst	Choosing healthy living (VWS, 2006b)	28	20% smokers in 2010	Failed	−1.6
2007	Ab Klink	Being healthy, staying healthy (VWS, 2007a)	28	No targets	–	–
2011	Edith Schippers	Health close to people (VWS, 2011)[b]	26	18% in 2025	–	−0.6

(*continued*)

Table 10.2 (continued)

Year	Minister/state secretary	Prevention policy document	Proportion of smokers in the year preceding the policy document (%)	Policy goal	Result	Ambition[a]
2013	Martin van Rijn, Edith Schippers	National Prevention Programme "Everything is health"[c] (VWS, 2013)	23	No targets	–	–

[a] "Ambition" is the intended reduction in percentage of smokers per year

[b] The 2013 prevention document does not mention a concrete target, but in response to questions from parliament, a long-term goal of 30% reduction in smoking prevalence in adults in 2025 was mentioned, referring to a voluntary agreement with WHO at the 66th World Health Assembly (WHO, 2013). This amounts to 18% smokers in 2025

[c] Proceedings II, 2013–2014, 32,793, nr. 114

2006b). These five topics were repeated in the two following prevention documents (VWS, 2007a, 2011). The most recent document added physical activity and emphasised the importance of exercise, diluting the relative importance of tobacco control as a public health policy goal despite the fact that smoking continued to have the greatest impact on the disease burden in the Netherlands (RIVM, 2014). While smoking continues to be listed in the prevention policy documents as one of the priorities, this has not yet resulted in new action plans for tobacco control since the failed *Nationaal Programma Tabaksontmoediging* (National Program of Tobacco Control) (NPT) of 2006 (VWS, 2006a). Time will tell if this well happen with the upcoming 2018 prevention policy document.

Of the nine public health policy documents since 1986, six stated quantitative targets for tobacco control but only one has ever been reached. Table 10.2 includes the tobacco control policy goals as stated by the government. Levels of ambition should be compared with the long-term trend of a declining smoking rate, which was on average −0.7% per year between 1958 and 2006 and less than −0.5% between 1990 and 2010 (Willemsen, 2010). Health Minister Borst was able to accelerate this to a staggering −1.3% per year, from 33% in 2000 to 28% in 2004. She was the only minister who ever succeeded in reaching a tobacco control target.

The NPT programme during the office of Minister Hoogervorst aimed at an unrealistic reduction of 1.6% per year, more an aspirational target than a realistic one, but one of the reasons why the NPT programme was destined to fail. Such unrealistic short term ambitions inevitably lead to disappointment. More recent cabinets did not want to set targets or resorted to extremely unambitious goals, with a projected trend which did not even challenge the naturally occurring downward trend (VWS, 2011).

The most recent *Everything is health* prevention policy programme projected that the proportion of smokers would be 19% in 2030 (from 23% in 2012) if no new initiatives were undertaken (VWS, 2013). It aimed to improve this "significantly" but did not mention a concrete goal, despite an explicit and urgent call in August 2010 from the *Raad voor de Volksgezondheid en Zorg* (Council for Public Health and Health Care) (RVZ)[2] that "the cabinet [should] commit to a quantifiable target ... and a balanced mix of instruments with which it can obtain visible results in 2020" (RVZ, 2010, p. 39). The RVZ report referred to data from the Organisation for Economic Co-operation and Development (OECD) that showed that the prevalence of smoking in the Netherlands was higher than the OECD countries average, which signalled a need for the government to initiate a tobacco control policy with concrete targets. Another report from the RVZ emphasised that setting quantifiable targets for smoking is certainly feasible, given the high quality level of monitoring data available in the Netherlands (RVZ, 2011). The tobacco control coalition had started to collect reliable yearly population data about smokers in 1978, through the *Stichting Volksgezondheid en Roken* (Dutch Smoking or Health Foundation) (STIVORO). The fact that smoking rates were collected from the 1970s onwards, and that they were conducted with sufficient statistical power to be able to detect increments of 1% in the yearly adult smoking rate, was unique.

The absence of targets in tobacco control in the Netherlands seems symptomatic of the lack of political will in recent years. Through ambitious but realistic targets, governments can show leadership and provide a sense of strategic direction and focus to the policy domain, while they can be held politically accountable (Van Herten & Gunning-Schepers). A prerequisite "is political will and daring. Without political commitment and the will to execute a health target approach, a policy will be doomed to fail" (Van Herten & Gunning-Schepers). Political will and daring are indeed crucial, since setting quantifying targets in public health is sometimes seen as "political suicide" (RIVM, 2006). Political will is linked to ideology: whether one believes in the idea of a malleable society and whether one believes that achievement of a goal is sufficiently under the control of the state (Maarse, 2011).

Tobacco a "Low Politics" Issue

As shown in Chap. 3, tobacco control follows policy cycles that may last for a decade or more, so the policy process is slow, complex, and contested. There is continuous tension between the recognition that smoking remains a public health problem for each new government, evidenced by VTV reports that the government cannot ignore, and the realisation that there is no easy, quick fix.

The issue of smoking slumbered in the background of day-to-day concerns of politicians and policymakers ever since it became a societal issue in 1964. It is rare that Dutch politicians identify tobacco as an urgent problem: the notable exception was the administration under the leadership of Health Minister Els Borst, who was confronted with stagnating smoking rates and increased smoking among young people. Smoking does not involve fundamental or key questions relating to the state's national interests or security. Issues such as the national economy and urgent foreign political matters are sometimes referred to as "high politics" (Walt, 1994), while smoking is a typically "low politics" concern.

Although the smoking rate is regarded as a chronic condition, it is relatively insensitive to policy measures and remains a low-profile issue on governmental agendas (Studlar, 2007b). In the eyes of policymakers, the chance that a "condition" will turn into a problem is greatest when there is a crisis (Kingdon, 2003, pp. 94–100). There is the perception of a crisis when policymakers feel that failure to act will lead to an even greater disaster. With tobacco control, policymakers rarely feel that this is the case. Smoking rates tend to go down most of the time, giving policymakers the impression that doing a little bit is good enough. There was a downward trend between 1960 and the end of the 1980s, and again between 2000 and 2014. However, the flywheel model of tobacco control (see Chap. 4) predicts that the decline in smoking rates will slow and stop in the absence of new impactful tobacco control measures. This is indeed what happened in the long period in the 1990s when no measures were taken and what we also seem to witness in most recent years.

The time lag between cause and effect is decades, so the benefits of policy measures only become noticeable long after a cabinet has resigned.

This has been mentioned as one explanation for the Dutch administrations' lack of enthusiasm in dealing with smoking (Meijerink & Vos, 2011). The treatment of smoking-related, life-threatening illness such as heart disease has steadily improved, and this may have further reduced any feeling of urgency in controlling tobacco (Meijerink & Vos, 2011).

A related reason why politicians and policymakers tend to underestimate the seriousness of the smoking problem is that smoking kills quietly: deaths of smokers go relatively unnoticed. People who have a chronic smoking-related disease such as emphysema hardly get out of the house, and out of sight is out of mind. This is why many people, including politicians, find it hard to imagine that smoking causes suffering on the grand scale as the statistics indicate.

Legitimacy

One of the main reasons why governments are unwilling to address certain topics may be a lack of perceived legitimacy (Hall, Land, Parker, & Webb, 1975). This means that the government feels an issue is not something that the state should be involved in. The line between what the Dutch government sees as its responsibility and what is not is subtly drawn, but most of the time in the background is the wish not to interfere with freedom of choice. For example, when the government defended her proposal to ban smoking in private workplaces (31 May 2001), Health Minister Borst said about cultural venues and theatres:

> It doesn't necessarily need to be totally smoke-free. Ideally yes, but through self-regulation theatres can make arrangements so that there will be no complaints. Dressing rooms are not open to the public. Men who sing as Louis Armstrong can continue to sing with a nice hoarse voice. That is not something that we want to interfere with.

On another occasion, when she defended her bill in the senate, she tried to reassure liberal–conservative politicians:

> One of our guiding principles is that grown-ups, people who are well educated and who know the risks but want to smoke anyway, should be left in peace as long as they don't bother other people. The [proposed] measures are aimed at protecting youth against the temptation to smoke. They are

further aimed at protecting the non-smoker. A third goal is to help those who wish to quit smoking.[3]

In 2007 an influential advisory report in the Netherlands analysed whether and how prevention policy can be made more efficient (Werkgroep IBO preventie, 2007). The report, written by an interdepartmental workgroup, the *Interdepartementaal Beleidsonderzoek* (Interdepartmental Policy Research) coordinated by the Ministry of Finance,[4] identified two rationales that legitimise governmental interference in unhealthy lifestyles. The first is if an information shortage leads to a situation in which people cannot make informed decisions. The second is if a person's unhealthy behaviour affects other people. In the case of smoking, the workgroup noted that the information shortage is less relevant, as the message that smoking is harmful is widely known. It concluded that the only time the government may intervene is to protect non-smokers from passive smoking (protection from an external threat), to protect young people or to target low-educated smokers if the government considers the existence of health inequalities a problem. Indeed, in liberal societies such as the Netherlands and the United Kingdom, "an important dimension of public health policy is ... to balance the liberal emphasis on choice and autonomy with the imperative to support those who do not have the opportunities to choose, because of, for instance, poverty or dependency" (Nuffield Council on Bioethics, 2007). The government took the report by the workgroup as its starting point for prevention policy from 2007 onwards (VWS, 2007b). It relied heavily on citizens' self-reliance and ability to make good choices, and stressed that "a free lifestyle choice must not be impaired, the balancing of positive (pleasure) with negative (cost and health) aspects is surely a personal one to make" (VWS, 2008, p. 14). However, the government was criticised by the *Wetenschappelijke Raad voor het Regeerbeleid* (Scientific Council for Government Policy) (WRR), an independent think tank of the government, for having unrealistic expectations about citizens' coping capabilities and self-control (WRR, 2017). The WRR argued that the government is especially legitimate in helping young people's determination not to smoke by limiting the instances when they are confronted with temptation to smoke or buy cigarettes.

Left–Right Orientation of the Government

If ideology is important, one might expect that left-wing governments are more likely to adopt strong tobacco control programmes since they are most open to imposing legislative measures to protect public health.[5] Several international studies have looked at the relationship between a government's political orientation and its tobacco policy. There is anecdotal evidence from Canada and Australia that provinces or territories controlled by the left are more likely to adopt tobacco control measures, although the relationship is not very strong (Studlar, 2007a). In the United Kingdom, conservative governments opposed tobacco control regulation between 1979 and 1997, while subsequent Labour governments introduced a range of measures which resulted in the United Kingdom becoming Europe's tobacco control leader (Asare, Cairney, & Studlar, 2009). In the United States, associations are found between Republican dominance at state level and lower cigarette taxes (Morley & Pratte, 2013), and between a legislator's being Republican and his or her intention to vote against tobacco taxes (Flynn et al., 1998). In Europe, in the period between 1996 and 2003, left-wing governments were more likely to adopt tobacco control measures than were right-wing governments (Bosdriesz, Willemsen, Stronks, & Kunst, 2014).

To the extent that a left-wing political orientation in government is beneficial for tobacco control, the Netherlands has not been in a very good position to advance tobacco control. Between 1972 and 2017 the Netherlands had 15 governments and in all of them either the conservative–liberal *Volkspartij voor Vrijheid en Democratie* (People's Party for Freedom and Democracy) (VVD) or the *Christen-Democratisch Appèl* (Christian Democratic Party) (CDA),[6] or both, was part of the ruling coalition. The Labour Party was only involved in seven instances, while the CDA took part in 12 cabinets and the VVD in 10. What is more important, perhaps, is that the Netherlands has had only one truly "progressive" cabinet, which was the Den Uyl cabinet (Labour Party), which lasted from 1973 until 1977. It had ten ministers from left-wing parties, six from Christian parties, and no liberal–conservative ministers. In Chap. 2, I narrated how this cabinet presented the most comprehensive set of tobacco control ambitions ever in Dutch history, but was not in power long enough to realise any of it.

Tobacco Control in Times of Economic Recession

An interesting question is whether tobacco control policy is lower on the political agenda during periods when the government struggles with economic hardship. In such times, Dutch governments tend to resort to a policy of budget cuts, privatisation of government tasks, and economic stimulation by introducing business-friendly policies. Although the obsession with wealth and economy is increasingly criticised by politicians from the left (Klaver, 2015; Thieme & Engelen, 2016), economic considerations and citizens' purchasing power continue to dominate the political discourse in the Netherlands. The following is an account of the economic situation of the various cabinets since the early 1970s (Van den Braak & Van den Berg, 2017) in relation to their accomplishments in tobacco control.

The Den Uyl (Labour party) government (1973–1977) was confronted with a blow to the national economy when Arab countries boycotted the Netherlands in 1973 by increasing the price of petrol and reducing the supply (the "oil crisis"), which was followed by an economic crisis, staggering inflation, and alarming prognoses of unemployment. However, the Den Uyl cabinet ignored the crisis and increased spending. It developed a far-reaching tobacco control agenda, in line with the ideology of the *maakbare samenleving* (a just and modifiable society).

The conservative Van Agt (CDA) cabinets (1977–1982) had to deal with a second oil crisis (1979) and exploding unemployment; and in 1982, at the end of the second Van Agt cabinet, the Netherlands was in its deepest recession since the 1950s. Extra budget cuts were deemed necessary at around 13 billion guilders (a value of around €11 billion in 2016). Under these conditions it was not politically feasible to increase spending on tobacco control. The feeling was that any execution of a tobacco control agenda would hurt the economy and employment.

The first Lubbers (CDA) cabinet (1982–1986) regarded it as its mission to get the economy back on track. This was done through a neoliberal "no nonsense" austerity programme with a pledge to cut seven billion guilders (around €6 billion), far-reaching privatisation of the public sector, and a business-friendly policy of deregulation. Despite economic growth, the second Lubbers cabinet (1986–1989) was unsuccessful in addressing the high unemployment rate. This led to a further decision to cut state spending in the beginning of the 1990s, which was also in response to demands from the European Union (EU) to reduce the state budget deficit. In 1991 the third Lubbers cabinet (1986–1989) announced new drastic cuts in government spending and increased burdens on citizens, such as higher taxes and fewer subsidies, which lasted until 1994. Tobacco control was put on the back burner during these cabinets. A Tobacco Act was adopted and implemented in 1990, but was insufficient to control smoking since it relied strongly on industrial self-regulation. Smoking rates went up between 1988 and 1996.

The first Purple cabinet Kok (Labour) (1994–1998) was an economic success, enjoying a miraculous growth in employment and a budget surplus. This was partly ascribed to the successful outcome of negotiations between employers and employees (the *polder* model). During this cabinet, Health Minister Els Borst and Minister of Economic Affairs Hans Wijers presented unprecedented tobacco control policy intentions. The economy was still booming during the first years of the second Kok cabinet (1998–2002). This opened up another window of opportunity to advance the tobacco control agenda. The fact that state finances allowed for a more generous budgetary allocation to tobacco control, in the way of extra campaigns and education, was crucial in getting support from the CDA for the most far-reaching legislative part of the new Tobacco Act: the workplace smoking ban.

During the first Balkenende (CDA) cabinet (2002–2003), economic growth came to a virtual standstill, resulting in considerable budget cuts, limits on state spending, and reforms of social security and the health-care sector. The last Balkenende cabinet (2007–2010) was faced with the international financial crisis of 2008. Spending on tobacco control was less than in the previous cabinet, and no new legislation was realised. The first Rutte (VVD) cabinet (2010–2012) regarded its main task to be fighting the crisis through cuts in government spending and reducing the size of the government. During this cabinet, all health promotion non-governmental organisations (NGOs) were confronted with cuts in governmental subsidies, while support for the *Stichting Volksgezondheid en Roken* (Dutch Smoking or Health Foundation) (STIVORO) was completely withdrawn and financial reimbursement to smokers for smoking cessation counselling was discontinued. The second Rutte cabinet (2013–2017) continued to emphasise getting government finances in order, partly through reforms to the health sector. There was little room for new tobacco control initiatives on the part of the government.

From the preceding description it might be concluded that during economically prosperous times the government is more generous and interested in a tobacco control agenda, although this is somewhat confounded by the political orientation, discussed in the preceding paragraph, which offered an alternative explanation. In any case, when "the economy" is at the top of cabinets' agendas, it seems more difficult to advance tobacco control.

Framing the Smoking Problem

In the previous chapter I explored the importance of research and statistics, and concluded that there is a gap between knowledge about effective tobacco control and if and when it appears on the government's executive agenda. It is not so much that the evidence does not find its way to the policy deciders; rather, it is determined by the ways in which arguments and evidence are constructed and framed by policy networks, and whether and how they resonate with policymakers (K. E. Smith, 2013). Coalitions differ in their capacity to discover and use such issue frames (Shiffman et al., 2015). Indeed, "if the tobacco control community is disbelieved, it may not be the result of being wrong, but rather from a failure to frame ourselves in such a way that our goals and our approaches resonate with the public" (Fox, 2005). Policy frames have been described as "weapons of advocacy" (Weiss, 1989). Unfortunately, the framing of tobacco control by Dutch pro- and anti-tobacco coalitions has not yet been subjected to systematic scientific research. The following is an attempt, based on a reading of official documents and reports of debates with health ministers in the parliament, to reconstruct the major changes to how the smoking problem was portrayed by the tobacco industry on the one hand and the Dutch tobacco control community on the other. The results are summarised in Table 10.3.

The government's take on smoking was first aligned with the industry framing that smoking was good for the economy. Until the 1980s, the tobacco industry and the government formed a policy monopoly in which tobacco was portrayed as a positive contributor to the economy. The government continued to use industry frames way into the 1990s. This monopoly was challenged by medical specialists who used a medical frame: that smoking is harmful to individuals. In the 1980s and especially in the 1990s the debate increasingly turned to the issue of the danger of passive smoking. Health organisations framed smoking as a problem for non-smokers, while the industry used a "tolerance frame": common courtesy between smokers and non-smokers should solve most problems. This

Table 10.3 How smoking has been framed in the Netherlands by the tobacco control coalition, the government, and the tobacco industry

Years	Ministers	Tobacco control coalition	Government	Tobacco industry
1950s–1970s		Medical frame: Smoking is harmful to individuals.	Economic frame: Smoking is good for business and the economy.	Economic frame: Smoking is good for business and the economy.
1980s	Joop van der Reijden, Dick Dees	Public health frame: Smoking is harmful to the population and to non-smokers.	Mixed public health and economy frame: Smoking is harmful to public health but good for business and the economy. Personal freedom frame: Smoking is one's own responsibility.	Economic frame: Smoking is good for business and the economy. Personal freedom frame: Smoking is one's own responsibility. Tolerance frame: Common courtesy between smokers and non-smokers solves most problems with tobacco.
1989–1998	Hans Simons, Els Borst	Public health frame: Smoking is harmful to the population and to non-smokers. Non-smokers are cool.	Combination of a public health frame and a personal freedom frame: Smoking is harmful to the population and non-smokers, while tobacco use remains an adults' own responsibility.	Personal freedom frame: Smoking is one's own responsibility. Tolerance frame: Common courtesy between smokers and non-smokers solves most problems with smoking.

(*continued*)

Table 10.3 (continued)

Years	Ministers	Tobacco control coalition	Government	Tobacco industry
1998–2003	Els Borst, Eduard Bomhoff	Public health frame: Smoking is harmful to the population and to non-smokers.	Public health frame: Smoking is harmful to the population and to non-smokers. Youth frame: Measures are necessary to protect youth.	Legal and libertarian frames: Tobacco is a legal product and smoking is a free choice for adults.
2003–2006	Hans Hoogervorst	Public health frame: Smoking is harmful to the population and to non-smokers. Addiction frame: Tobacco is addictive, not a free choice.	Public health frame: Smoking is harmful to the population and to non-smokers. Economic frame: Smoking is bad for the economy and for employers.	Legal and libertarian frames: Tobacco is a legal product and smoking is a free choice for adults.
2007–2010	Ab Klink	Public health frame: Smoking is harmful to the population and to non-smokers.	Fairness frame: Tobacco control measures must be implemented fairly.	Legal and libertarian frames: Tobacco is a legal product and smoking is a free choice for adults.
2010–2013	Edith Schippers	Public health frame: Smoking is harmful to the population and to non-smokers. Tobacco industry demonising frame: The tobacco industry is deceptive and capitalises on the addiction of children.	Libertarian frame: Smoking is a free choice for adults.	Legal and libertarian frames: Tobacco is a legal product and smoking is a free choice for adults.

(continued)

PROBLEM IDENTIFICATION AND AGENDA SETTING   289

Table 10.3 (continued)

Years	Ministers	Tobacco control coalition	Government	Tobacco industry
2013–2017	Martin van Rijn	Youth frame: Children deserve to grow up in a smoke-free environment.	Youth frame: Children deserve to grow up in a smoke-free environment.	Legal and libertarian frames: Tobacco is a legal product and smoking is a free choice for adults. Health frame: Smoking is harmful: The best solution is to reduce its harm by product innovations by the industry. Effectiveness frame: Tobacco control might be supported as long as it is evidence-based.

industry frame resonated well in the Dutch society. In these years the government approached the issue with a mixed economic and health frame: tobacco control is good for public health but must not harm business and the economy. This ended at the end of the 1990s when the World Bank published its influential report *Curbing the Epidemic*, which concluded that tobacco control is good not only for public health but also for national economies. In 1991 State Secretary Hans Simons emphasised that smoking substantially contributes to societal costs.[7] This was calculated for 1987 at around one billion guilders per year, two-thirds in the health-care sector and one-third through productivity loss (Meijer & Tjioe, 1990). For Simons this was an important reason to intensify tobacco control.[8] Around 1996 the industry could no longer use the tolerance frame, since Philip Morris lost all credibility in a failed campaign where it compared the risks of passive smoking to that of eating cookies (see Box 8.1 in Chap. 8). The government adopted the passive smoking frame of the health coalition, which carved the way for smoking bans.

One particularly powerful industry frame is the notion that smoking is an adult's personal lifestyle choice, which must be respected at all times as long as the smoker does not harm others. For many years the industry succeeded in presenting smoking as an adult "guilty" pleasure, no worse than coffee, good food, or a moderate alcohol intake. At the basis of this notion lies the idea that smoking is a habit, a learned behaviour that can be unlearned. Internationally, this conception was gradually replaced in the 1980s by the notion that smoking is a true addiction. This became more widely accepted in Europe at the end of the 1990s, and this made it easier for conservative politicians and the medical sector to support tobacco control initiatives. The Dutch tobacco control coalition was relatively late in promoting the addiction frame (see Box 10.1).

> **Box 10.1 Smoking is an addiction**
> International recognition that smoking is addictive did not occur overnight. It was preceded by a period in which researchers tried to find and answer to the question of why it was so difficult for people to quit (Krasnegor, 1979), and in which the industry denied that nicotine is addictive. This was an important issue for the industry: "We can't defend continued smoking as 'free choice' if the person is 'addicted'" (Knopick, 1980). The breakthrough came when the US Surgeon General's report on the addictive properties of tobacco concluded in 1988 that nicotine addiction was an addictive disorder to which the same standards applied as to heroin, cocaine, and other drugs (U.S. Department of Health and Human Services, 1988). The tobacco industry continued to deny the addictiveness of tobacco, culminating in 1994 when the heads of the major US tobacco companies gave sworn testimony before the US Congress that they did not believe nicotine was addictive. The revelation that they lied under oath was a devastating blow to the industry's reputation. US experts understood that the evidence—that smoking is addictive and that most smokers start smoking during childhood—morally legitimises a youth-centred tobacco control strategy (Lynch & Bonnie, 1994). In 1996 US President Bill Clinton declared nicotine an addictive drug, and addiction was regarded by scientists as "a brain disease" (Leshner, 1997). This challenged the mantra of free choice and went against the public's view that people who cannot

quit smoking are weak or bad, unable to break the habit. In Europe the breakthrough came with the publication of clinical guidelines for the treatment of tobacco addiction in England (Raw, McNeill, & West, 1998). Soon after, the Royal College of Physicians published a report, *Nicotine Addiction in Britain* (Britton et al., 2000), and WHO presented recommendations on how to treat tobacco dependence (WHO, 2001). A Dutch guideline, similar to the UK one, was published some years later by the Partnership Stop Smoking (CBO, 2004, 2006). It was endorsed by 19 professional organisations covering all medical disciplines. The Dutch guideline "deliberately [chose] a different perspective: not that of the smoker who is responsible for his own behaviour, but that of an addiction for which help is necessary."(CBO, 2006, p. 11)

The dominant "public health frame" adopted by the government was effective until around 2006. Health Minister Els Borst (D66) (1994–2002), a medical doctor, was most outspoken about the public health dangers of smoking. On many occasions she talked about smoking as the number one cause of death, more deadly than alcohol, drugs, traffic accidents, and HIV combined.[9] In a debate in parliament she used the image of crashing jumbo jets, each week causing 441 deaths,[10] and pointed out that smoking is the biggest epidemic that humankind has called upon itself, that death and disease by smoking are avoidable, and that government has a duty to act, especially to protect young people. She urged tobacco control using a combination of arguments: the high number of deaths, the health risks for non-smokers, the fact that smoking rates were not going down and were higher than in many other European countries, the notable increase in youth smoking, the high economic costs to society, and the heavy burden on the health-care system. She supported this with statistics made available by STIVORO. She made the problem tangible:

> These seem emotionless statistics, but this changes if one looks at them differently: 23,000 deaths means 23,000 times a premature death, so 23,000 times a man or a women, often of middle age, who leaves behind a partner or a family. A dear family member, a valuable partner, friend or lover who passes away before his or her time has come. It is a great drama, first of all for the smoker who often dies in miserable conditions, and second for those who are left behind.[11]

Irritated by the obstinate stance of the liberal–conservative VVD party, she added at one point in the debate, "Confronted with 23,000 deaths, the government cannot remain aloof and say: the people have to sort it out themselves. A minister of health who does not try to do something against such a great number of deaths is not worth a penny." As a liberal-democratic politician, Borst choose her wording carefully and avoided being associated with nannyism. The solution was to present her proposals as policies to protect youth, since "for adults … we think these matters are not very sensible, but for them one's own choice is paramount and, in addition, adults can do some things moderately, making it less harmful to them."[12] The next minister, Eduard Bomhoff (LPF) (2002), adopted Borst's position that tobacco had created the biggest epidemic that humankind had ever called down upon itself. His temporary replacement, State Secretary Clémence Ross-van Dorp (CDA) (2002–2003), also used the general public health frame of 23,000 deaths caused by smoking.

At the beginning of the 2000s, in an attempt to retrieve its battered reputation, the tobacco industry initiated corporate social responsibility programmes, using their own version of health frames (Tobacco Free Initiative, 2003). The industry publicly acknowledged that smoking is harmful, and tried to promote an image of responsibility by declaring an interest in reducing youth smoking (McDaniel, Cadman, & Malone, 2016). Industry representatives approached the government with offers to cooperate with preventing young people from smoking (See Chap. 8, where the industry's "Platform Prevention of Youth Smoking" was discussed).

Health minister Hans Hoogervorst (VVD) (2003–2007), whose previous appointment was as minister of finance, frequently framed the need for tobacco control in economic terms. He occasionally mentioned the serious public health consequences of tobacco use and the need to protect non-smokers, and sometimes applied an addiction frame, but was most convincing when pointing to the fact that smoking substantially contributes to total health-care costs and is bad for employers (at the time estimated at €105 extra costs per smoking employee) (Hoogervorst, 2005). Tobacco control is good for the economy since "health generates wealth" (VWS, 2005), a frame he hoped would appeal to his VVD rank and file.

Health Minister Ab Klink (CDA) (2007–2010) seldom used a public health or addiction frame. He distanced himself from anti-tobacco statements and was reluctant to initiate new policy that did not fit his wish to deliver "positive stimulants" to smokers (Klink, 2008). Instead he was most comfortable with a fairness frame. One of his biggest challenges was the implementation of the smoking ban in the hospitality sector. He took non-smoking employees' right to work in a smoke-free environment and "level playing field" considerations between small and large bars as starting point, but seldom talked about health risks.[13]

Minister Edith Schippers (VVD) (2010–2012), who was trained as a political scientist, consistently used a libertarian frame, emphasising that state interference with tobacco use is nannyism, and consenting adults must decide for themselves if they want to smoke or not. She said, "If adults decide on Friday evening to smoke together with their glass of beer in a small pub, who am I to forbid this?" (VARA, 2011).

During most of the time, the tobacco control coalition continued to use a general public health frame of deaths caused by smoking. When its appeal was worn-out, the tobacco industry demonising frame was used as well. In some countries, tobacco control advocates have been successful in challenging the tobacco industry frames through counter-frames such as protection of the vulnerable against a merciless industry (Cohen et al., 2000; Fox, 2005; Jacobson & Banerjee, 2005; Katz, 2005). The tobacco industry has been effectively portrayed as a deceptive industry that capitalises on addiction, and such portrayal invokes anger and activism (Malone, 2014). Such a frame was used by the tobacco control organisations in the Netherlands around 2011, when Schippers was portrayed in a TV documentary as "minister of tobacco" (VARA, 2011) and the *Stichting Rookpreventie Jeugd* (Youth Smoking Prevention Foundation) (SRJ) began to name and shame everyone with affiliations to the tobacco industry. SRJ used the addiction frame to make the case that children are hooked on nicotine by the tobacco industry. This gave renewed impetus to viewing tobacco and the tobacco industry as morally bad, which made it more difficult for the industry lobbyists to find the ear of policymakers and politicians.

Most recently, with the advance of the *Alliantie Nederland Rookvrij* (Dutch Alliance for a Smokefree Society) (ANR), tobacco control in the Netherlands has been framed in terms of protecting young people, which appeals to the general public and a wide range of societal organisations, and also to local and national government. The Ministry of Health adopted the idea of a "smoke-free generation" and State Secretary Martin Van Rijn (Labour party) (2013–2017) used the phrase "smoke-free generation" in communications with parliament.[14] In the meantime, the tobacco industry tried to show goodwill by promoting less harmful product innovations such as electronic cigarettes and heat-not-burn products. They also employed an effectiveness frame: tobacco control measures are acceptable, but only when their effectiveness is proven beyond any doubt.

One may conclude that Dutch tobacco control advocates have not been very successful in setting the agenda by issue framing, struggling to find a frame that resonated with policymakers, politicians, and the public during times when the government was less open to tobacco control, too long holding on to a general public health frame.

A Health Inequality Frame?

It is remarkable that the portrayal of smoking as a fundamental cause of health inequalities has rarely been used in the Netherlands. The social gradient in smoking emerged as an important policy problem in most European countries in the 1990s, and again at the beginning of the twenty-first century (Brown, Platt, & Amos, 2014). The Netherlands is no exception. Health inequalities are substantial: life expectancy among low-educated people is six years shorter than among the highly educated (RIVM, 2014). A reduction in health disparities was considered an important task for the Dutch government around 2005 (VWS, 2006b, 2008). Dutch politicians on the left who valued social equality argued that tackling inequalities in smoking helped to reduce health inequalities, and urged the government to act.[15] This did not result in concrete tobacco control policy proposals from the government; although it acknowledged that the differences are substantial: while only 17% of the highest educated smoke, the rate is 31% among low-educated groups (VWS, 2013). Recent data (covering the years until 2011) show that inequalities in smoking have further increased (Bosdriesz, Willemsen, Stronks, & Kunst, 2015).

The dominant right-wing governments in the Netherlands have not been receptive to the argument that smoking must be targeted as a means to reduce health inequalities. This is in contrast to the United Kingdom (Department of Health, 2011) where this argument has broadened support for tobacco control in society (K. Smith, 2013) and has resulted in a national budget to set up smoking cessation support programmes in disadvantaged areas. In response to calls for a prevention policy that reduces health inequalities, the Dutch government did set up broad community-based projects in municipalities (*Kracht wijken*),[16] similar to the "New deals for communities" programme in the United Kingdom, but without specific aims for tobacco. The government has further integrated the issue of health inequalities into its decentralised health strategy *Everything is health* (VWS, 2013), which aims to stimulate integrated local health promotion initiatives. A recent initiative is a national incentive programme, *Healthy in the City*, which supports local approaches to tackling health inequalities. A total of €44 million was made available between 2014 and 2017, most of which went directly to the municipalities, which were given ample freedom to choose programmes and measures that they believed were best tailored to the problems they encountered in their respective communities (Van Berkum, 2016). There were no distinct incentives to tackle smoking. The programme is illustrative of the current approach to health promotion and disease prevention in the Netherlands: to give optimal responsibility and freedom at the local level without setting national targets or providing blueprints for local targets (see also Chap. 5 on decentralisation). Time will tell if this approach is effective.

Media Advocacy

According to the agenda-setting theory, if a topic is covered frequently and prominently by the media, the general public will regard it as important. In the words of one of the founders of the agenda-setting theory, "elements prominent on the media agenda become prominent over time on the public agenda. The media not only can be successful in telling us *what to think about*, they also can be successful in telling us *how to think about it*" (McCombs, 2005, p. 546). Activists and lobbyists try to persuade the mass media to adopt their take on a problem and to promote their policy solutions. The media can also magnify movements that have already started (Walt, 1994), and can be especially important in encouraging government to act on low-level political issues such as smoking (Buse, Mays, & Walt, 2012). A study of how newspaper coverage affects support for tobacco control in the Netherlands (Nagelhout, Van den Putte, et al., 2012) found that most newspapers wrote in a negative manner about the smoking ban for pubs and restaurants implemented in July 2008, mostly approaching the topic from an economic perspective and highlighting potential negative economic effects. Readers of these newspapers adjusted their support for the ban downwards. The tobacco control network missed an opportunity to influence public opinion about the ban because it lacked a good media advocacy counter-strategy. Pro-smoking interest groups were able to dominate the media by focusing attention on staged "problems" with the ban and presumed resistance from small bar owners (discussed in Chap. 8). This was relatively easy, since problems are more newsworthy than successes.

Politicians and policymakers are sensitive to how an issue is covered in the press, and can hardly ignore media attention. Newspaper coverage is often a trigger for parliamentarians to ask questions to the responsible minister or state secretary. The influence of the media on the parliamentary agenda in the Netherlands has grown considerably over time (Van Noije, Kleinnijenhuis, & Oegema, 2008). Dutch parliamentary questions are, indeed, almost always inspired or influenced by media attention (Van Aelst & Vliegenthart, 2013). Figure 10.1 shows the number of written questions asked by Dutch members of parliament about tobacco control.[17] I counted the number of parent questions (they typically consist of three to seven sub-questions) submitted at one point in time by a member of parliament.

The number of questions is remarkably modest, considering the major health consequences associated with smoking. It is also modest in comparison to the total number of parliamentary questions, which is between 1400 and 2600 per year, with recent years seeing more activity. Until 2008 there were few questions on tobacco, with the exception of the year 2000 when liberal–conservative parliamentarians questioned Health Minister Els Borst regarding her attacks on the tobacco industry. The first peaks occurred in 2008 and 2009, caused by media attention to the troublesome implementation of the smoking ban in bars. About half the questions were by the opposing right-wing populist *Partij voor de Vrijheid* (Freedom Party) (PVV). Soon after the Rutte cabinet (2010–2012) was installed at the end of 2010, and Edith Schippers became health minister, Socialist and Labour party members asked parliamentary questions about Schippers' presumed ties to the tobacco industry in 2011. The year 2012 continued with more questions on tobacco industry lobbying, prompted by a series of critical articles in the media. The peak in 2013 was partly caused by concerns about the electronic cigarette.

When the Labour party (28), Socialist Party (25), Green–Left party (2), Christian Union (3), and D66 (6) are taken together, there were 74 questions from the left/progressive flank. On the right/conservative flank, I counted 38 questions (13 by PVV, 12 by CDA and 13 by VVD). This suggests that tobacco control coalition organisations have been more successful in putting pressure on the government by raising the attention of parliamentarians, especially through the Labour and Socialist Parties.

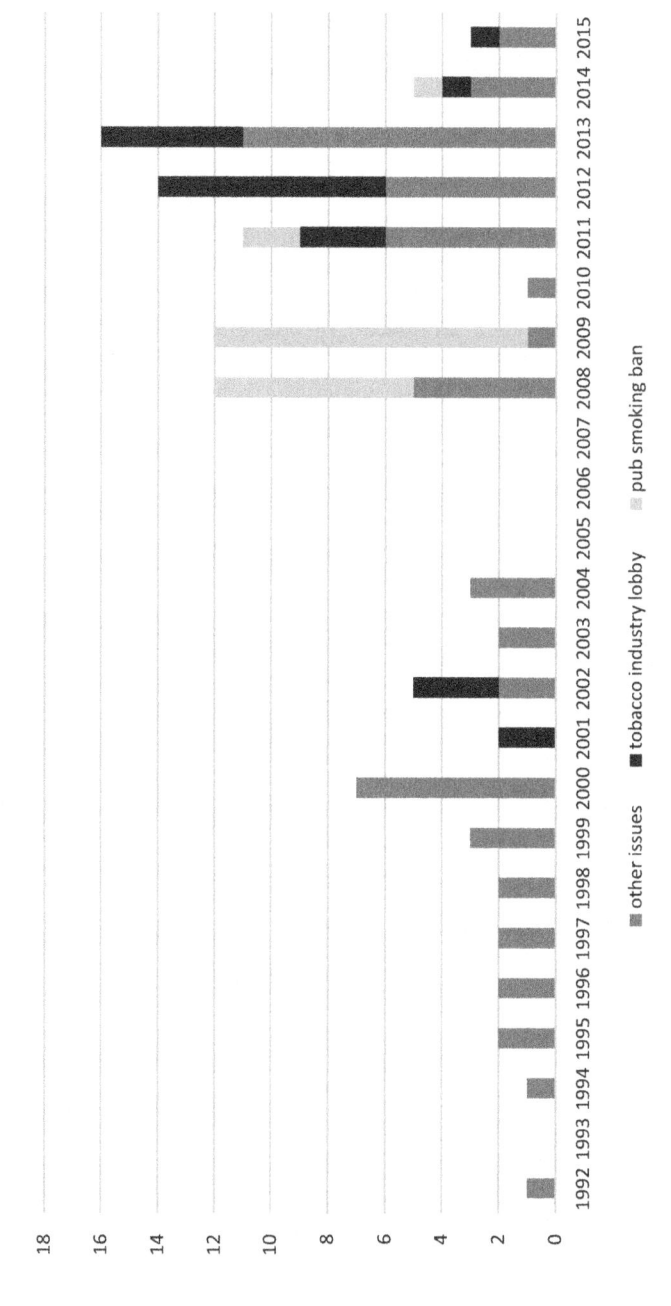

PROBLEM IDENTIFICATION AND AGENDA SETTING 297

Fig. 10.1 Number of parliamentary questions since 1992 on tobacco policy, by year. Source: https://zoek.officielebekendmakingen.nl/zoeken/parlementaire_documenten

Conclusion

According to Kingdon's multiple streams analysis, major tobacco control policy changes will only happen when a window of opportunity opens and three "streams" come together (Kingdon, 2003). There must be increased attention to the tobacco problem, a clear solution must be readily available, and policymakers must have both the motive and opportunity to adopt a new policy. Such moments have rarely occurred in the Netherlands. Dutch governments treated smoking most of the time as a low-level issue, a chronic "condition" and not a pressing political concern. The Dutch political landscape has been dominated by coalitions that executed neoliberal agendas. Conservative governments tend to regard tobacco control legislation and regulation as infringements on citizens' freedom, and tobacco control measures with paternalistic undertones were time and time again bluntly rejected by parliament. Tobacco control remained low on the policy agenda, especially in times of economic hardship. Only once there was a "natural" feeling of urgency, when smoking rates did not go down for several years in a row at the end of the 1990s. During the Kok cabinets (1994–2002), a window of opportunity opened: the ruling coalition was relatively progressive and smoking rates had been going up at an alarming rate—something had to be done. An important beneficial factor was personal commitment to tobacco control by a determined Health Minister Els Borst. The fact that the economy was prospering was important as well, since this made it possible to invest money in education and campaigns, which was crucial in obtaining support from the CDA for the revised Tobacco Act, to which the liberal–conservative VVD was opposed. A particularly strong and consistent public health frame used by the tobacco control coalition supported the government's tobacco control ambitions.

In later years the tobacco control coalition has been less successful in finding frames that strike a chord with political parties. The once effective public health frame used by the coalition to argue for tobacco control in the 1990s did not inspire society and politicians to support tobacco control in the 2000s. When the fourth Balkenende cabinet with Health Minister Ab Klink (2007–2010) came to power, a second window of opportunity opened for tobacco control: the policy intention of banning smoking in bars and restaurants was part of the coalition agreement, and the health minister seemed open to tobacco control. However, the industry was successful in framing tobacco control as contradictory to libertarian values and Klink was portrayed as a moral crusader, which shut the door to further tobacco control initiatives. The tobacco control coalition was less successful in media advocacy and lost its grip on the implementation of the smoking ban in bars. Only very recently, by portraying tobacco control as necessary to protect children against smoking, has the tobacco control coalition found a more effective strategy.

Notes

1. Parliamentary papers II, 1992–1993, 22,894, nr. 1.
2. RVZ is an independent advisory body for government and parliament.
3. Proceedings I, 26 March 2002, 24–1273.
4. IBO stands for *Interdepartementaal Beleidsonderzoek* (Interdepartmental Policy Research). IBO reports are mandatory for all ministries and have the explicit aim of finding cost reductions and concrete proposals to increase the efficiency of governmental policy. On average, ten IBO reports are written each year and they cut across all branches of government (Van den Berg & Kabel, 2010).
5. The economic left–right dimension as the main aspect of "ideology" is outdated. For the Netherlands, other important dimensions have to do with cultural orientation, economic equality, libertarianism, self-determination, and populism (Laméris, Jong-A-Pin, & Garretsen, 2017).
6. The CDA did not yet exist in 1972. The 1972 government included two Christian parties (KVP, ARP) that would merge in 1977 into the CDA.
7. Parliamentary papers II, 1990–1991, 19,243, nr. 14.
8. Proceedings II, 1991–1992, 22,300 XVI, nr. 7.
9. Proceedings II, 1998–1999, 26,472, nr. 3; Proceedings I, 26 maart 2002, 24–1257; Proceedings II, 1999–2000, Aanhangsel 3301; Proceedings II, 2000–2001, Aanhangsel 1696.
10. Proceedings II, Tabakswet 31 mei 2001 TK 82-5210.
11. Proceedings I, 26 March 2002, 24–1257.
12. Proceedings II, 31 May 2001.
13. Proceedings II, 14 May 2009, 84–6613.
14. Proceedings II, 2014–2015, 32,011, nr. 46.
15. Parliamentary papers II, 2007–2008, 22,894, nr. 176.
16. Parliamentary papers II, 2007–2008, 22,894, nr. 176.
17. The data were generated by searching the parliament database, using search terms such as tabak*, sigaret*, and roke*.

References

Asare, B., Cairney, P., & Studlar, D. T. (2009). Federalism and multilevel governance in tobacco policy: The European Union, the United Kingdom, and devolved UK institutions. *Journal of Public Policy, 29*, 79. https://doi.org/10.1017/s0143814x09000993

Bosdriesz, J. R., Willemsen, M. C., Stronks, K., & Kunst, A. E. (2014). Tobacco control policy development in the European Union—Do political factors matter? *European Journal of Public Health, 25*(2), 190–194. https://doi.org/10.1093/eurpub/cku197

Bosdriesz, J. R., Willemsen, M. C., Stronks, K., & Kunst, A. E. (2015). Socioeconomic inequalities in smoking cessation in 11 European countries from 1987 through 2012. *Journal of Epidemiology Community Health, 69*, 886–892. https://doi.org/10.1136/jech-2014-205171

Britton, J., Bates, C., Channer, K., Cuthbertson, L., Godfrey, C., Jarvis, M., & McNeill, A. (2000). *Nicotine addiction in Britain: A report of the Tobacco Advisory Group of the Royal College of Physicians*. London: Royal College of Physicians of London.

Brown, T., Platt, S., & Amos, A. (2014). Equity impact of population-level interventions and policies to reduce smoking in adults: A systematic review. *Drug Alcohol Depend, 138*, 7–16. https://doi.org/10.1016/j.drugalcdep.2014.03.001

Buse, K., Mays, N., & Walt, G. (2012). *Making health policy* (2nd ed.). Berkshire: Open University Press.

Cairney, P. (2012). *Understanding public policy: Theories and issues*. Basingstoke: Palgrave Macmillan.

CBO. (2006). *Guideline treatment of tobacco dependence*. Utrecht: CBO/Partnership Stoppen met Roken.

Cobb, R. W., Ross, J.-K., & Ross, M. H. (1976). Agenda building as a comparative political process. *American Political Science Review, 70*, 126–138. https://doi.org/10.2307/1960328

Cohen, J. E., Milio, N., Rozier, R. G., Ferrence, R., Ashley, M. J., & Goldstein, A. O. (2000). Political ideology and tobacco control. *Tobacco Control, 9*(3), 263–267. https://doi.org/10.1136/tc.9.3.263

Department of Health. (2011). *Health lives, healthy people: A tobacco control plan for England*. London: Department of Health.

Flynn, B. S., Goldstein, A. O., Solomon, L. J., Bauman, K. E., Gottlieb, N. H., Cohen, J. E., ... Dana, G. S. (1998). Predictors of state legislators' intentions to vote for cigarette tax increases. *Preventive Medicine, 27*, 157–165. https://doi.org/10.1006/pmed.1998.0308

Fox, B. (2005). Framing tobacco control efforts within an ethical context. *Tobacco Control, 14*(Suppl II), ii38–ii44.

Grüning, T., Strünk, C., & Gilmore, A. B. (2008). Puffing away? Explaining the politics of tobacco control in Germany. *German Politics, 17*, 140–164.

Hall, P., Land, H., Parker, R., & Webb, A. (1975). *Change, choice and conflict in social policy.* London: Heinemann.
Hoogervorst, H. (2005). Brief Evaluatie tabaksontmoedigingsbeleid. *Kamerstuk 22894-55-b2.*
Jacobson, P. D., & Banerjee, A. (2005). Social movements and human rights rhetoric in tobacco control. *Tobacco Control, 14*(Suppl II), ii45–ii49.
Katz, J. E. (2005). Individual rights advocacy in tobacco control policies: An assessment and recommendation. *Tobacco Control, 14*(Suppl II), ii31–ii37. https://doi.org/10.1136/tc.2004.008060
Kingdon, J. W. (2003). *Agendas, alternatives and public policies* (2nd ed.). New York: Addison-Wesley.
Klaver, J. (2015). *De mythe van het economisme. Pleidooi voor een nieuw idealisme.* Amsterdam: De Bezige Bij.
Klink, A. (2008). Preventiebeleid voor de volksgezondheid. *kamerstuk 22894 nr. 154.*
Knopick, P. (1980). Confidential memorandum: Minnesota tobacco litigation. *Tobacco Institute Records,* Bates No. TIMN0107822–TIMN0107823. Retrieved from https://www.industrydocumentslibrary.ucsf.edu/tobacco/docs/lqnn0146
Krasnegor, N. A. (Ed.). (1979). *Cigarette smoking as a dependence process.* Rockville, MD: Department of Health, Education, and Welfare.
Laméris, M., Jong-A-Pin, R., & Garretsen, H. (2017, maart 9). Kiezersvoorkeuren: links en rechts ingehaald. *Economie & Samenleving ESB, 102* (4747), 140-143.
Leshner, A. L. (1997). Addiction is a brain disease, and it matters. *Science, 278,* 45–47. https://doi.org/10.1126/science.278.5335.45
Lynch, B. S., & Bonnie, R. J. (1994). *Growing up tobacco free: Preventing nicotine addiction in children and youths.* Washington, DC: National Academy Press.
Maarse, J. A. M. (2011). *Sturing op gezondheidsdoeleinden en gezondheidswinst op macroniveau. Achtergrondstudie bij RVZ-rapport: Sturen op gezondheid.* Den Haag: RVZ.
Malone, R. E. (2014). The symbolic and the material in tobacco control: Both matter. *Tobacco Control, 23*(1), 1–2. https://doi.org/10.1136/tobaccocontrol-2013-051442
McCombs, M. (2005). A look at agenda-setting: Past, present and future. *Journalism Studies, 6,* 543–557.
McDaniel, P. A., Cadman, B., & Malone, R. E. (2016). Shared vision, shared vulnerability: A content analysis of corporate social responsibility information on tobacco industry websites. *Preventive Medicine, 89,* 337–344. https://doi.org/10.1016/j.ypmed.2016.05.033
Meijer, J. W., & Tjioe, B. K. (1990). *Maatschappelijke kosten alcoholmisbruik en tabaksgebruik.* Rotterdam: Nederlands Economisch Instituut (NEI).
Meijerink, R., & Vos, P. (2011). *Preventie van welvaartsziekten effectief en efficiënt georganiseerd.* The Hague: Raad voor de Volksgezondheid en Zorg.

Morley, C. P., & Pratte, M. A. (2013). State-level tobacco control and adult smoking rate in the United States: An ecological analysis of structural factors. *Journal of Public Health Management Practice, 19*, E20–E27. https://doi.org/10.1097/PHH.0b013e31828000de

Nagelhout, G. E., Van den Putte, B., De Vries, H., Crone, M., Fong, G. T., & Willemsen, M. C. (2012). The influence of newspaper coverage and a media campaign on smokers' support for smoke-free bars and restaurants and on secondhand smoke harm awareness: Findings from the International Tobacco Control (ITC) Netherlands Survey. *Tobacco Control, 21*(1), 24–29. https://doi.org/10.1136/tc.2010.040477

Nuffield Council on Bioethics. (2007). *Public health: Ethical issues*. Cambridge: Cambridge Publishers Ltd.

Raw, M., McNeill, A., & West, R. (1998). Smoking cessation guidelines for health professionals. *Thorax, 53*(Suppl 5, Part 1), S1–S18.

RIVM. (1993). *Volksgezondheid Toekomst Verkenning: De gezondheidstoestand van de Nederlandse bevolking in de periode 1950–2010. Kernboodschappen*. Den Haag: SdU Uitgeverij.

RIVM. (1997). *Volksgezondheids Toekomst Verkenning 1991: De som der delen*. Bilthoven: Rijksinstituut voor Volksgezondheid en Milieu.

RIVM. (2002). *Gezondheid op koers? Volksgezondheid Toekomst Verkenning 2002*. Bilthoven: Rijksinstituut voor Volksgezondheid en Milieu.

RIVM. (2006). *Zorg voor gezondheid—Volksgezondheid Toekomst Verkenning 2006*. Bilthoven: Rijksinstituut voor Volksgezondheid en Milieu.

RIVM. (2010). *Van gezond naar beter. Volksgezondheid Toekomst Verkenning 2010*. Bilthoven: Rijksinstituut voor Volksgezondheid en Milieu.

RIVM. (2014). *A healthier Netherlands: Key findings from the Dutch 2014 Public Health Status and Foresight Report*. Bilthoven: Rijksinstituut voor Volksgezondheid en Milieu.

RVZ. (2010). *Perspectief op gezondheid 20/20*. Den Haag: Raad voor de Volksgezondheid en Zorg.

RVZ. (2011). *Sturen op gezondheidsdoelen*. Den Haag: Raad voor de Volksgezondheid en Zorg.

Shiffman, J., Quissell, K., Schmitz, H., Pelletier, D., Smith, S., Berlan, D., ... Walt, G. (2015). A framework on the emergence and effectiveness of global health networks. *Health Policy Plan, 31*, i3–i16. https://doi.org/10.1093/heapol/czu046

Smith, K. (2013). *Beyond evidence-based policy in public health: The interplay of ideas*. London: Palgrave Macmillan.

Smith, K. E. (2013). Understanding the influence of evidence in public health policy: What can we learn from the 'Tobacco Wars'? *Social Policy & Administration, 47*(4), 382–398. https://doi.org/10.1111/spol.12025

Studlar, D. T. (2007a). Ideas, institutions and diffusion: What explains tobacco control policy in Australia, Canada and New Zealand? *Commonwealth &*

Comparative Politics, 45(2), 164–184. https://doi.org/10.1080/14662040701317493

Studlar, D. T. (2007b). *What explains policy change in tobacco control policy in advanced industrial democracies?* Paper presented at the European Consortium of Political Research, Helsinki.

Thieme, M., & Engelen, E. (2016). *De kanarie in de kolenmijn.* Amsterdam: Prometheus.

Tobacco Free Initiative. (2003). *Tobacco industry and corporate responsibility…an inherent contradiction.* Geneva: WHO.

U.S. Department of Health and Human Services. (1988). *The health consequences of smoking: Nicotine Addiction.* Washington: Public Health Service, Centers for Disease Control, Center for Chronic Disease Prevention and Health Promotion, Office on Smoking and Health.

Van Aelst, P., & Vliegenthart, R. (2013). Studying the tango. *Journalism Studies,* 15(4), 392–410. https://doi.org/10.1080/1461670X.2013.831228

Van Berkum, M. (2016). Pionieren met nieuwe filosofie. Retrieved April 29, 2017, from https://www.gezondin.nu/thema/roken/blog/43-pionieren-met-nieuwe-filosofie

Van den Berg, P. J. C. M., & Kabel, D. L. (2010). Achtergrond en opzet van de brede heroverwegingen. *Tijdschrift voor Openbare Financieën,* 42(2), 69–75.

Van den Braak, B. H., & Van den Berg, J. T. J. (2017). Historisch overzicht cijfers kabinetten. *Parlement & Politiek.* Retrieved July 20, 2017, from https://www.parlement.com/id/vht7jba3jsy6/historisch_overzicht_cijfers_kabinetten

Van Noije, L., Kleinnijenhuis, J., & Oegema, D. (2008). Loss of parliamentary control due to mediatization and Europeanization: A longitudinal and cross-sectional analysis of agenda building in the United Kingdom and the Netherlands. *British Journal of Political Science,* 38, 455–478.

Van Weel, C. (2004). *Richtlijn Behandeling van tabaksverslaving.* Alphen aan den Rijn: van Zuiden Communications BV.

VARA. (2011). Minister of Tobacco [TV documentary]. *Zembla.* Retrieved July 26, 2017, from https://zembla.vara.nl/nieuws/minister-of-tobacco

VWS. (1995). Volkgezondheidsbeleid 1995-1998 (Nota "Gezond en Wel"). *Handelingen II, 1994–1995,* 24126, nr.2.

VWS. (2002). Jaarverslag van het ministerie van VWS over het jaar 2001. *Kamerstuk 28380, nr. 38.*

VWS. (2003). *Langer Gezond Leven: Ook een kwestie van gezond gedrag.* Den Haag: Ministerie van VWS.

VWS. (2005). *Evaluatie Tabaksontmoediging.* Den Haag: Ministerie van VWS.

VWS. (2006a). *Nationaal Programma Tabaksontmoediging.* Den Haag: Ministerie van VWS.

VWS. (2006b). *Preventienota Kiezen voor gezond leven. [Prevention Nota Choosing healthy life style].* Den Haag: Ministerie van VWS.

VWS. (2007a). *Gezond zijn, gezond blijven. Een visie op gezondheid en preventie.* Den Haag: Ministerie van VWS.

VWS. (2007b). Kaderbrief 2007–2011 visie op gezondheid en preventie. *Kamerstuk 22894, nr. 134.*
VWS. (2008). *Naar een weerbare samenleving: Beleidsplan aanpak gezondheidsverschillen op basis van sociaaleconomische achtergronden.* Den Haag: Ministerie van VWS.
VWS. (2011). *Gezondheid dichtbij. Landelijke nota gezondheidsbeleid.* Den Haag: Ministerie van VWS.
VWS. (2013). *Alles is gezondheid: Het Nationaal Programma Preventie 2014–2016.* Den Haag: Ministerie van VWS.
Walt, G. (1994). *Health policy: An introduction to process and power.* London: Zed Books.
Weiss, J. A. (1989). The powers of problem definition: The case of government paperwork. *Policy Sciences, 22*(2), 97–121.
Werkgroep IBO preventie. (2007). Gezond gedrag bevorderd. Eindrapportage van de werkgroep IBO preventie *Interdepartementaal beleidsonderzoek, 2006–2007.* Den Haag: Ministerie van VWS.
WHO. (2001). *Evidence based recommendations on the treatment of tobacco dependence.* Geneva: World Health Organization.
WHO. (2013). *Draft comprehensive global monitoring framework and targets for the prevention and control of noncommunicable diseases.* Geneva: World Health Organisation.
Willemsen, M. C. (2010). Tabaksverslaving: de impact van gezondheidsvoorlichting en hulpverlening op de totale populatie rokers. *Psychologie en Gezondheid, 38*, 119–130.
WRR. (2017). *Weten is nog geen doen. Een realistisch perspectief op redzaamheid.* Den Haag: Wetenschappelijke Raad voor het Regeringsbeleid.
WVC. (1986). Over de ontwikkeling van gezondheidsbeleid: feiten, beschouwingen en beleidsvoornemens (Nota 2000). *Handelingen II, 1985–1986, 19500, nr 1–2.*
WVC. (1991). Gezondheid met beleid. *Handelingen II, 1991–1992, 22459, nr 2.*

Open Access This chapter is licensed under the terms of the Creative Commons Attribution 4.0 International License (http://creativecommons.org/licenses/by/4.0/), which permits use, sharing, adaptation, distribution and reproduction in any medium or format, as long as you give appropriate credit to the original author(s) and the source, provide a link to the Creative Commons license and indicate if changes were made.

The images or other third party material in this chapter are included in the chapter's Creative Commons license, unless indicated otherwise in a credit line to the material. If material is not included in the chapter's Creative Commons license and your intended use is not permitted by statutory regulation or exceeds the permitted use, you will need to obtain permission directly from the copyright holder.

CHAPTER 11

Conclusions

Public policy scholars propose that policy change emerges from the interaction of five elements: (1) the policy context, which can be more or less conducive to tobacco control policy change; (2) the workings of the institutions involved in the process of policymaking; (3) the diffusion of knowledge and ideas which highlight the urgency of a problem and inspire policy solutions; (4) the organisation and advocacy potential of coalitions; and (5) the relative success of opposing coalitions in setting the agenda of policymaking through issue framing (Cairney, Studlar, & Mamudu, 2012; John, 2012). I presented a general framework in Chap. 1 to illustrate how these elements are related and influence each other over time (Fig. 1.1). The reader may want to occasionally consult the framework while reading this concluding chapter.

CONTEXT AND INSTITUTIONS

Stable environmental factors rarely change within periods of a decade or less, and directly or indirectly influence all aspects and stages of the policymaking process. The dominant type of governance system is one such all-encompassing stable environmental characteristic. The preference for self-regulation can be explained by the Dutch corporatist tradition of policymaking, where the business community is allowed to deal with a problem before the state intervenes. This means that interest groups are

© The Author(s) 2018
M. C. Willemsen, *Tobacco Control Policy in the Netherlands*,
Palgrave Studies in Public Health Policy Research,
https://doi.org/10.1007/978-3-319-72368-6_11

integrated into the policymaking process itself and need to rely less on outside pressure strategies. Most often, negotiations with the industry over self-regulation pre-empt formal regulation by the state. Dutch policymakers are content with this arrangement because they want to avoid polarisation and conflicts between groups by trying the least controversial option first. As a consequence, most of the time tobacco control has advanced in small incremental steps, to prevent clashes with tobacco interest groups defending the status quo and at the same time trying to pacify groups that want to advance tobacco control. This preference for seeking compromise (*polderen*) explains why it has been difficult in the Netherlands to move from an entrenched system of corporatism, with tobacco companies close to policymakers, to a system that no longer allows tobacco industry representatives to be consulted.

Although corporatism is considered a relatively stable characteristic, over a long period of time its importance in the Netherlands is believed to decline. With the increasing fragmentation of parliament, cabinets can no longer rely on comfortable majorities, and the influence of opposition parties in parliament has grown. This is seen in other corporatist countries in Europe as well (Christiansen et al., 2010; Kurzer & Cooper, 2016; Rommetvedt, Thesen, Christiansen, & Nørgaard, 2012). In the Netherlands there is increased lobbying at the expense of corporatism, evidenced by more frequent, more intense contact between interest groups and parliamentarians, a greater use of the legislative arena, and a reduced role for institutionalised "old school" corporatist policymaking practices where civil servants act as policy brokers between competing coalitions. The judicial venue (taking the industry or the government to court) is increasingly used to enforce breakthroughs when policymaking is slow. The pressure on the government (including the use of legal action) to adhere to Article 5.3 of the Framework Convention on Tobacco Control in the Netherlands fits in perfectly with these developments. Political parties have become more central to policy change and the influence of public opinion and media advocacy has grown. Tobacco control policymaking has moved from closed meetings and the internal workings of governmental bureaucracy to parliament and the wider society, benefiting tobacco control groups.

A second important stable environmental factor is cultural values, which permeated tobacco control policymaking in many ways. Christian and liberal principles that have had a profound mark on Dutch tobacco control policymaking are rooted in the unique combination of individualistic and "feminine" (egalitarian) values. There is less societal, and hence less political support, for measures with paternalistic overtones or that are considered particularly harsh for smokers. Such values explained why Dutch governments were reluctant to initiate hard-hitting risk awareness campaigns.

Various important relatively dynamic context factors have also been identified. The Advocacy Coalition Framework (ACF) defines major policy change as an alternation in "policy core beliefs", provoked by external events (Sabatier & Weible, 2007; Weible, Sabatier, & McQueen, 2009). The most important external event is a change of government, when opportunities for policy change arise (advocates may get tobacco control into a coalition agreement) and any change of ideology may be more advantageous to one interest group than another—it may favour tobacco control, or favour a laissez-faire approach. The Dutch case presented three examples of major policy change following a regime change. The first was when the Purple cabinet came to power. For the first time in history, Christian Democrats were no longer part of the ruling coalition. This shattered the tobacco industry coalition's decade-long grip on tobacco control policymaking. The new government appointed a health minister (Els Borst) dedicated to a strong tobacco control agenda and achieved a major focal shift by removing tobacco control from the supervision of the Ministry of Economic Affairs and handing it over to the Ministry of Health. Economic considerations were superseded by a public health frame of reference. A second window opened in 2007 when the tobacco control coalition succeeded in getting the idea of a smoking ban in pubs into the coalition agreement. However, when Minister of Health Ab Klink attempted to implement this, the health coalition failed to use media advocacy in a way that would consolidate the ban and prevent the industry from hijacking the issue. A few years later in 2010 a window of opportunity opened for the tobacco industry to frustrate tobacco control, when Edith Schippers of the *Volkspartij voor Vrijheid en Democratie* (People's Party for Freedom and Democracy) (VVD) was appointed minister of health in 2010. She had opposed most tobacco control proposals as a VVD parliamentarian. This led to chaos and a weakening of the tobacco control coalition, and gave the tobacco industry's policy agenda a temporary advantage.

The Dutch example testifies to the fundamentally ideological nature of decision-making concerning smoking, which is regarded as a difficult, politically contested subject matter, and illustrates how outcomes very much depend on the prevailing ideology of politicians and policymakers.

Dutch policymakers always had to find compromises between economy, public health, and ideology. Dutch governments have almost always been centre-right oriented with a majority backing in parliament. Politicians and policymakers were preoccupied with promoting a strong economy, alongside a trust in the power of the free market. This made it difficult to advance a tobacco control agenda. Even when ministers had personal motives to combat smoking, as did liberal–conservative Minister Hoogervorst (2003–2007), a non-smoker who was inspired by the fight against smoking when he went to university in the United States, they were unable to accomplish much without support from parliament.

Policy was for the main part determined by what is written in coalition agreements, which are the basis for state governance. Tobacco control was mentioned only three times in the coalition agreements of the 15 cabinets since 1972, and on only two occasions was it a positive statement for tobacco control. The importance of getting the topic in a coalition agreement was paramount: one resulted in the important 2002 Tobacco Act and the other led to a smoking ban in bars and restaurants. That tobacco control had not been included in more coalition agreements might suggest that the tobacco control lobby has been weak, but it also reflects a political environment not open to legislative tobacco control, with few windows of opportunity for control advocates.

Other relatively dynamic factors that followed from the ideological preferences of governments and have come to define the Dutch policy context are retreating government and the accompanying process of decentralisation and the sharing of responsibility with lower levels of governance and civil society. These processes have inhibited state-led tobacco control ambitions and leadership. Subsequent cabinets increasingly shared responsibility for disease prevention with local governments, the private sector, and civil society—and when health promotion was decentralised, it no longer was only a national priority. These ideological trends went against the need for a strong and well-coordinated strategy from the state to combat national smoking rates, as was emphasised by the FCTC. The process of handing over the responsibility for tobacco control to non-governmental organisations has already reached a point where central oversight over tobacco control has become scant and increasingly complex.

Much of tobacco control has become a Brussels affair. European Union (EU) governance became increasingly important, since EU directives cannot be ignored by the government. Tobacco industry lobbying has also focused more and more on the EU level: much of the national industry lobby is directly or indirectly aimed at influencing EU policymaking. In contrast with EU tobacco control initiatives, the FCTC treaty is more easily ignored by the government, and as the Dutch example demonstrates, signing the treaty does not mean much unless there is a policy environment conducive to its implementation. Although FCTC requirements are legally binding, in practice they were more or less ignored since there are no sanctions for non-compliance and much room for discussion about implementation, despite detailed WHO guidelines. While the FCTC was ratified in 2005 by the Dutch government, it took another five years before representatives from the tobacco control network began to give it the attention it deserved (Heijndijk & Willemsen, 2015; Rennen & Willemsen, 2012; STIVORO, 2010), indicating that proper implementation of FCTC in the spirit of WHO intentions must be enforced by civil society. Clean Air Netherlands (CAN) took the government to court over the proper interpretation of FCTC's Article 8.2 (about smoke-free bars), and the Youth Smoking Prevention Foundation prompted the government to a better and more extensive implementation of Article 5.3 of the FCTC, making it more difficult for tobacco industry representatives to contact Dutch government officials.

Diffusion of Knowledge and Ideas

The final acceptance of the health risks of active and passive smoking as scientific fact occurred later in the Netherlands than in leading tobacco control countries such as the United States and the United Kingdom. The Health Council was over-cautious and slow in acknowledging and warning against the public health risks. The government did not publicise the scientific evidence with clear statements about the damage of smoking, and failed to produce authoritative reviews of the literature on the health risks of smoking like the UK and US reports. In addition, there were few leading scientists who publicly spoke out against tobacco and the medical community remained reticent and did not involve itself in the fight against tobacco. Perhaps even more important was the fact that the authorities hid behind the health charities and the *Stichting Volksgezondheid en Roken* (Dutch Smoking or Health Foundation) (STIVORO) to communicate with the public about health risks, giving the false impression that the matter was not to be taken too seriously, and giving the industry leeway to cast doubt on links between smoking and health, whittling away at any political support for tobacco control. STIVORO was not permitted to communicate in a confrontational and clear-cut manner about the health risks of smoking, in line with Dutch "feminine" (egalitarian) cultural values mentioned before. All of these factors might have contributed to the slower start to regulate tobacco, compared to many other countries, until the mid-1990s.

Dutch government officials had an adequate understanding of evidence-based tobacco control policy measures. The government was already familiar with most options in the 1970s, and the evidence concerning effectiveness has accumulated since then. Dutch civil servants were generally well informed through their contacts with the national and international tobacco control epistemic community, and had organisations such as the *Rijksinstituut voor Volksgezondheid en Milieu* (National Institute for Public Health and the Environment) (RIVM) and STIVORO at its disposal to quickly provide up-to-date information about aspects of tobacco control. The government looked at what the effective measures were, but chose which to implement mainly on ideological grounds. Most Dutch health ministers lacked a public health or medical background, which may have further contributed to the inclination to give more weight to ideological and political considerations such as reducing the role of government through deregulation and decentralisation.

Governments need basic national tobacco control capacity to be able to develop and deliver a comprehensive tobacco control programme in accordance with the FCTC. Such capacity rests on three pillars: a good infrastructure, access to empirical evidence and expertise, and leadership (Wipfli et al., 2004). The Dutch government has abundant access to evidence, and the necessary infrastructure to build tobacco control interventions is generally well developed. The weak pillar is undoubtedly leadership and coordination by the government. The government left it to charities and STIVORO to communicate about health risks, but these organisations were not in the same strong position to put the issue firmly and authoritatively on the societal, let alone the political, agenda. Remarkably, given the relatively high contribution of smoking to the national burden of disease, there has never been a distinctly identifiable tobacco control unit at the Ministry of Health—it has always been part of a larger department that deals with lifestyle and addiction. Before 2000 the unit was understaffed and not sufficiently equipped to negotiate with the tobacco industry, leading to delays in the drafting of regulations. Changing jobs within the government's bureaucracy further hampered a continuous development of a coherent tobacco control policy, while industry lobbyists remained at their post for decades.

Problem Identification

Most of the time Dutch politicians and policymakers regarded smoking as a chronic condition that did not involve a crisis or present itself as a pressing concern. Each new government recognised that it remained a serious public health problem, evidenced by Public Health Status and Foresight (VTV) reports which it could not ignore, but the lack of a feeling of urgency made it less likely that a government put it high on the agenda. This caused difficulties for tobacco control coalitions, who had to flog a dead horse, while the industry exploited direct contacts with government and politicians to obstruct any inclination for tobacco control progress.

The interest of policymakers in tobacco control was weakened by several factors. First, the impact of governmental interference with smoking takes many years to appear in national statistics, so it gains policymakers no political credit. Second, smoking kills quietly, so that the direct consequences are not always visible to everyone. Third, smoking is increasingly marginalised in the public domain, reducing the chance that politicians and policymakers will personally experience problems with tobacco smoke and feel a need to take action. Fourth, the VTV reports after 2002 characterised trends in adults and youth in a less alarming manner than before, although smoking rates were still regarded as too high. In the national prevention policy documents tobacco control had to compete with other issues such as alcohol, depression, obesity, and diabetes, and since 2007 the government did not want to commit to a quantifiable target, further reducing the feeling of urgency about tighter tobacco control. This is despite the fact that the number of people in the Netherlands who are chronically ill or die prematurely because of smoking remains high, and tobacco continues to be the largest cause of preventable death in the Netherlands (RIVM, 2017). These factors combined to lead politicians to believe that there is no great urgency, either politically or medically, to deal with smoking and undermined the tobacco control coalition's abilities to convincingly frame smoking as an important health problem.

Coalitions, Issue Expansion, and Framing

The Dutch tobacco control subsystem brought forward two separate coalitions: one of the three health charities (cancer, heart, lung) (coordinated first by STIVORO, more recently by the *Alliantie Nederland Rookvrij* (Dutch Alliance for a Smokefree Society; ANR)), and one led by the tobacco manufacturers. In later years a third tobacco control coalition emerged, instigated by two lung physicians Wanda de Kanter and Pauline Dekker (the *Stichting Rookpreventie Jeugd* or Youth Smoking Prevention Foundation: SRJ), with somewhat different core values and preferred strategies than those of the main tobacco control coalition. The main difference is that the SRJ coalition remained an outsider group, whereas STIVORO and ANR are insider groups. Insider groups are not part of the formal governmental bureaucracy but are nevertheless regarded as legitimate stakeholders, are consulted regularly by the government, and are expected to play by the "rules of the game" (Buse, Mays, & Walt, 2012, pp. 114–115). Insider groups are generally considered to be more effective than outsider groups in corporatist political environments.

What constitutes a successful coalition? Scholars have identified several important characteristics. Shiffman et al. (2015) list distinguished leadership, governance, composition, and framing strategies: a network is more effective when it has capable, well-connected and widely respected leaders, when there is a governing structure in place that is able to organise collective action, can resolve disputes, and links a diversity of actors. Such diversity, which facilitates access to scientific knowledge, also increases the likelihood that solutions to problems will be found. Finally, the network is more likely to be effective if its members know how they can frame an issue in such a way that it resonates well with society and politicians. These factors are congruent with the strategies of ACF theory, which identifies similar necessary conditions for success: having the right allies, having shared resources, and being able to develop a common lobby and advocacy strategy (Sabatier & Weible, 2007).

"Public policy and management scholars have long recognized the importance of effective leaders in agenda setting and organizational effectiveness, as well as their rarity" (Shiffman et al., 2015) and for most of the time, the Netherlands has had no such clearly identifiable effective tobacco control leaders, which have a claim to being heard, are well connected with coalition building, have great rhetorical skills, and are able "to articulate vision amidst complexity" (Shiffman et al., 2015). Leaders must be able to operate effectively within the particular Dutch policy environment, with its corporatist features and emphasises on compromise seeking. The relatively effective leaders were those who organised and lobbied behind the scenes, such as STIVORO's director Boudewijn de Blij.

With respect to governance structure: the decision in 1974 to locate tobacco control in the one organisation, STIVORO, controlled by three charities and the government, thwarted the emergence of a broad nationwide tobacco control coalition. STIVORO was a semi-governmental organisation responsible for executing the lion's share of the government's tobacco policy. In its 40 years of existence, it tried to balance the competing interests of its three "mothers" and the government. While the government and parliament regarded health education as its sole task, the charities expected STIVORO to lobby against the tobacco industry, but also in parliament and against the government, for better tobacco control policy. Only STIVORO's directors were responsible for lobbying and advocacy, which they had to combine with many other demanding tasks. This made the tobacco control coalition vulnerable. Only since 2006 has lobbying been carried out with support from a professional bureau, while the tobacco manufacturers have been employing professional dedicated lobbyists since the 1970s. I noted the few mentions of tobacco control in coalition agreements, which suggests that the tobacco control coalition might have been more successful if it had professionalised its lobbying sooner.

A tobacco control coalition is stronger if it incorporates scientists who are quickly able to deliver evidence that counters industry arguments, and who can convincingly speak with politicians and policymakers. In the Dutch culture of consensus seeking, experts, both scientists and doctors, were not as inclined to become involved with tobacco control advocacy in the same way as their counterparts in countries with more pluralistic traditions, where interest groups are experienced and may be more comfortable in challenging policymakers directly.

In Chap. 10 I tried to capture how tobacco was framed by the two opposing coalitions, and how these frames resonated with those used by the government. The tobacco industry has been successful in framing tobacco control as an infringement on individual liberty and attracting libertarians to its arguments, from individuals fighting for the right to enjoy smoking to organisations that oppose government regulation. Dutch tobacco control advocates have been only moderately successful in setting the agenda, struggling to find the one frame that resonates with policymakers, politicians, and the various tobacco control organisations.

Until the 1970s they used a medical frame, but replaced it with a broader public health frame in the 1980s that remained the dominant frame of reference for many years. In the 2000s smoking as an addiction was added to the repertoire of arguments once science had showed convincingly that nicotine is a highly addictive substance. This stimulated activism among tobacco victims and health professionals and neutralised the industry's frame of smoking as an individual lifestyle choice. It also contributed to finally getting the medical community on board. The public health frame that was effective in the 1990s, when smoking rates were high and the issue of passive smoking was still a noticeable problem for wide segments of society, has now lost most of its appeal. An attempt was made around 2010 to use the frame of an immoral and evil tobacco industry, but this resulted in confrontation and STIVORO lost its insider status with the government's bureaucracy. Most recently, around 2013, the tobacco control organisations reorganised and found a more successful frame in the image of the need to protect vulnerable children from exposure to tobacco smoke and from the seduction of tobacco products. This resulted in the appealing concept of a smoke-free generation, and made tobacco control a just and legitimate cause for a broad range of societal organisations. The preceding illustrates what is sometimes called "issue expansion," which is an important contributing factor for policy change (Baumgartner & Jones, 1993). A coalition can expand an issue by reframing so that groups in society, previously uninvolved, become champions of the cause.

Further Study and Food for Thought

The aim of this book was to understand tobacco control policymaking from the point of view of the government, in the specific context of the Netherlands. However, while much has been uncovered and explained, new questions arose during the process of writing. The role of coalition building received sparse attention here, and it would be worthwhile to examine the characteristics of effective tobacco control coalitions, including the role of leadership, in more detail. A related issue is the role of the scientific and the medical community in tobacco control advocacy in the Netherlands. Other interesting lines of scientific inquiry relate to the success of issue framing by the two opposing coalitions (tobacco control and tobacco industry) over time, and the role of media advocacy in this. Another issue, alluded to in the book but not extensively explored, is the transition from a dominant corporatist policy system to a system with more lobbyist characteristics, and how this influences the effectiveness of pro- and anti-tobacco coalitions. The role that national cultural values and ideology play in tobacco control policymaking is another under-explored area. A final intriguing question is whether the process of decentralising tobacco control responsibilities and the increased dispersion of tobacco control tasks among governmental and civil society contributes to controlling the tobacco epidemic or might be counterproductive.

Closing Remarks

Despite worldwide convergence of tobacco control policies, accelerated by the ratification of the FCTC treaty by most nations, governments develop approaches to tobacco control in line with cultural values and ideological and political preferences. There is no one-size-fits-all approach. The main message in this book is that what works in any one country is contingent on its specific policy environment and the specific cultural values at its core. This book has recounted how the Dutch used various universal tobacco control building blocks to create a unique blend of tobacco control measures. Especially in the beginning of the 2000s, tobacco control was well financed and comprehensive, revolving around yearly smoking cessation mass media campaigns in combination with evidence-based youth prevention programmes, supported by a broad range of smoking cessation counselling options from which smokers could choose. It combined education with a soft, non-patronising and non-confrontational advocacy approach. This was fairly effective, with smoking rates after 2002 in line with the downward trend of other Organisation for Economic Co-operation and Development (OECD) countries. The period between 2002 and 2013 were golden years for Dutch tobacco control, when STIVORO became an example for other countries in Europe. However, the model only worked as long as there was sufficient moral and financial support from the Ministry of Health and political support from parliament. With a retreating government, the model could no longer be sustained.

Another major lesson from the Dutch example is that the process of policy change in the Netherlands was subject to a policy environment not conducive to tobacco control, rooted in values of individual freedom and corporatist traditions where policymakers felt most comfortable when they involved all stakeholders in policymaking. Policymakers in the Netherlands do not march ahead of the troops. In such an environment, securing sufficient, and broad, support in society for policy proposals is crucial for tobacco control advocates. The battle is ultimately fought in society, where hearts and minds must be won, and is no top-down affair controlled solely by the state. When civil organisations are able to show convincingly that society wants to be smoke-free, policymakers will follow.

Around 2013 the three charities aligned and professionalised their tobacco control advocacy capacity, forming a powerful and much broader tobacco control coalition than had existed before. A new issue frame was found in the protection of young people from tobacco, and this resonates better with politicians and society than the worn-out public health frame of death and disease. It ignited an unprecedented number of tobacco control activities at the local level, and civil organisations such as the major health charities have become increasingly important as catalysts for Dutch tobacco control, boosting both local and national efforts. However, the health ministry continues to face major challenges. Most importantly, a quarter of all adults still smoked at the time that this book was completed. The Netherlands still has many places where smoking is condoned, tobacco products are still on display in most shops, and tobacco taxation is rarely deployed as a control instrument. Ever since the adoption of the revised Tobacco Act in 2002 the government has not formulated inspiring prospects or new concrete ambitions. Time will tell whether civil society and the government will find new ways of collaboration which will bring the Dutch closer to a smoke-free Netherlands.

References

Baumgartner, F., & Jones, B. D. (1993). *Agendas and instability in American politics.* Chicago, IL: University of Chicago Press.

Buse, K., Mays, N., & Walt, G. (2012). *Making health policy* (2nd ed.). Berkshire: Open University Press.

Cairney, P., Studlar, D. T., & Mamudu, H. M. (2012). *Global tobacco control: Power, policy, governance and transfer.* New York: Palgrave Macmillan.

Christiansen, P. M., Norgaard, A. S., Rommetvedt, H., Svensson, T., Thesen, G., & Oberg, P. (2010). Varieties of democracy: Interest groups and corporatist committees in Scandinavian policy making. *Voluntas, 21*(1), 22–40. https://doi.org/10.1007/s11266-009-9105-0

Heijndijk, S. M., & Willemsen, M. C. (2015). *Dutch tobacco control: Moving towards the right track?* FCTC Shadow Report 2014. Den Haag: Alliantie Nederland Rookvrij.

John, P. (2012). *Analyzing public policy* (2nd ed.). London: Routledge.
Kurzer, P., & Cooper, A. (2016). The dog that didn't bark: Explaining change in Germany's tobacco control policy at home and in the EU. *German Politics, 25*(4), 541–560. https://doi.org/10.1080/09644008.2016.1196664
Rennen, E., & Willemsen, M. C. (2012). *Dutch tobacco control: Out of control? FCTC shadow report 2011.* Amsterdam: KWF Kankerbestrijding.
RIVM. (2017). Sterfgevallen door ziekten als gevolg van roken, 2013. Retrieved April 28, 2017, from https://www.volksgezondheidenzorg.info/onderwerp/roken/cijfers-context/oorzaken-en-gevolgen#node-sterfte-en-verloren-levensjaren-door-roken
Rommetvedt, H., Thesen, G., Christiansen, P. M., & Nørgaard, A. S. (2012). Coping with corporatism in decline and the revival of parliament: Interest group lobbyism in Denmark and Norway, 1980–2005. *Comparative Political Studies, 46*, 457–485.
Sabatier, P. A., & Weible, C. M. (2007). The advocacy coalition framework: Innovations and clarifications. In P. A. Sabatier (Ed.), *Theories of the policy process* (2nd ed.). Cambridge, MA: Westview Press.
Shiffman, J., Quissell, K., Schmitz, H., Pelletier, D., Smith, S., Berlan, D., … Walt, G. (2015). A framework on the emergence and effectiveness of global health networks. *Health Policy Plan, 31*, i3–i16. https://doi.org/10.1093/heapol/czu046
STIVORO. (2010). *Van onderop en van bovenaf: De toekomst van tabaksontmoediging in Nederland 2011–2020.* Den Haag: STIVORO.
Weible, C. M., Sabatier, P. A., & McQueen, K. (2009). Themes and variations: Taking stock of the advocacy coalition framework. *Policy Studies Journal, 37*(1), 121–140. https://doi.org/10.1111/j.1541-0072.2008.00299.x
Wipfli, H., Stillman, F., Tamplin, S., e Silva, L. d. C. V., Yach, D., & Samet, J. (2004). Achieving the Framework Convention on Tobacco Control's potential by investing in national capacity. *Tobacco Control, 13*, 433–437.

Open Access This chapter is licensed under the terms of the Creative Commons Attribution 4.0 International License (http://creativecommons.org/licenses/by/4.0/), which permits use, sharing, adaptation, distribution and reproduction in any medium or format, as long as you give appropriate credit to the original author(s) and the source, provide a link to the Creative Commons license and indicate if changes were made.

The images or other third party material in this chapter are included in the chapter's Creative Commons license, unless indicated otherwise in a credit line to the material. If material is not included in the chapter's Creative Commons license and your intended use is not permitted by statutory regulation or exceeds the permitted use, you will need to obtain permission directly from the copyright holder.

References

Adriaanse, H., Van Reek, J., & Metsemakers, J. (1986). Smoking behaviour of Dutch general practitioners in the period 1977–1983. *Scandinavian Journal of Primary Health Care, 4*, 151–156.

Adriaanse, H., Van Reek, J., & Van Zutphen, W. (1986). Rookgewoonten van artsen wereldwijd: Een overzicht van 100 onderzoekingen naar tabaksgebruik onder artsen in 31 landen in de periode 1951–1985. *Nederlands Tijdschrift voor Geneeskunde, 130*, 2224–2229.

Alamar, B., & Glantz, S. (2006). Effect of increased social unacceptability of cigarette smoking on reduction in cigarette consumption. *American Journal of Public Health, 97*, 1359–1362.

Albæk, E., Green-Pedersen, C., & Nielsen, L. B. (2007). Making tobacco consumption a political issue in the United States and Denmark: The dynamics of issue expansion in comparative perspective. *Journal of Comparative Policy Analysis: Research and Practice, 9*, 1–20.

Algemene Rekenkamer. (1982). Verslag van een onderzoek naar de gesubsidieerde activiteiten verband houdend met het tegengaan van het roken en daarmee samenhangende aangelegenheden. *Truth Tobacco Industry Documents*, Bates No. JB2303. Retrieved from https://industrydocuments.library.ucsf.edu/tobacco/docs/#id=kpdp0219

Algemene Rekenkamer. (1991). *Voorlichtingscampagnes van het Rijk*. Den Haag: SDU.

Algemene Rekenkamer. (2012). *Bestrijding van accijnsfraude bij alcohol en tabak. EU-beleid: naleving en effecten*. Den Haag: Sdu Uitgevers.

American Cancer Society. (2003). *Tobacco control strategy planning guide #1. Strategy planning for tobacco control advocacy*. Atlanta, GA: American Cancer Society.

Andeweg, R. B., & Irwin, G. A. (2009). *Governance and politics of the Netherlands* (3rd ed.). Hampshire: Palgrave Macmillan.

ARISE. (1995a). Living is more than surviving: The contribution of pleasure to everyday life—International media coverage 1995/96. *British American Tobacco Records*, Bates No. 500853324–500853394. Retrieved from https://www.industrydocumentslibrary.ucsf.edu/tobacco/docs/spmv0211

ARISE. (1995b). A summary of the workshop held in April 1995. Living is more than surviving. *RJ Reynolds Records*, Bates No. 511818234–511818241. Retrieved from https://www.industrydocumentslibrary.ucsf.edu/tobacco/docs/ppnm0089

Arnott, D., Berteletti, F., Britton, J., Cardone, A., Clancy, L., Craig, L., … Willemsen, M. C. (2011). Can the Dutch Government really be abandoning smokers to their fate? *The Lancet, 379*, 121–122. https://doi.org/10.1016/S0140-6736(11)61855-2

Asare, B., Cairney, P., & Studlar, D. T. (2009). Federalism and multilevel governance in tobacco policy: The European Union, the United Kingdom, and devolved UK institutions. *Journal of Public Policy, 29*, 79. https://doi.org/10.1017/s0143814x09000993

Asbridge, M. (2004). Public place restrictions on smoking in Canada: Assessing the role of the state, media, science and public health advocacy. *Social Science & Medicine, 58*, 13–24. https://doi.org/10.1016/S0277-9536(03)00154-0

ASH. (2013). Key dates in the history of anti-tobacco campaigning. Retrieved August 29, 2014, from http://www.ash.org.uk/files/documents/ASH_741.pdf

ASPECT Consortium. (2004). *Tobacco or health in the European Union: Past, present and future*. Luxembourg: European Commission.

Baan, B. (1986). Strategieen ter bevordering van het niet-roken. *Nederlands Tijdschrift voor Geneeskunde, 130*, 1232–1139.

Baba, A., Cook, D. M., McGarity, T. O., & Bero, L. A. (2005). Legislating "Sound Science": The role of the tobacco industry. *American Journal of Public Health, 95*, S20–S27. https://doi.org/10.2105/AJPH.2004.050963

Baha, M., & Le Faou, A. L. (2010). Smokers' reasons for quitting in an antismoking social context. *Public Health, 124*(4), 225–231. https://doi.org/10.1016/j.puhe.2010.02.011

Bala, M. M., Strzeszynski, L., Topor-Madry, R., & Cahill, K. (2013). Mass media interventions for smoking cessation in adults. *Cochrane Database of Systematic Reviews, 6*, CD004704.

Baltesen, F., & Rosenberg, E. (2009, June 22). Big tobacco pays Dutch opposition to smoking ban. *NRC Handelsblad*. Retrieved from http://vorige.nrc.nl/

international/article2278646.ece/Big_tobacco_pays_Dutch_opposition_to_smoking_ban

Barneveld, J. T. A., Dalesio, O. B., & Van Leeuwen, F. E. (1992). Een ontmoedigend tabaksontmoedigingsbeleid: Pleidooi voor een integrale aanpak. *Medisch Contact, 47,* 943–944.

Barnsley, K., Walters, H., & Wood-Baker, R. (2015). Bureaucratic barriers to evidence-based tobacco control policy: A Tasmanian case study. *Universal Journal of Public Health, 3,* 6–15.

BAT. (1996). EU issues. *British American Tobacco Records,* Bates No. 322122073–322122107. Retrieved from https://www.industrydocumentslibrary.ucsf.edu/tobacco/docs/rkyb0207

BAT. (n.d.). Shaping the regulatory environment: Advertising and public smoking. *British American Tobacco Records,* Bates No. 322121140–322121143. Retrieved from https://www.industrydocumentslibrary.ucsf.edu/tobacco/docs/jpcd0211

Baumgartner, F., & Jones, B. D. (1993). *Agendas and instability in American politics.* Chicago, IL: University of Chicago Press.

Beernink, J. F., & Plokker, J. H. (1975). Maatregelen tot beperking van het roken. Advies van de Gezondheidsraad. *Verslagen, Adviezen, Rapporten* (Vol. 23). Leidschendam: Ministerie van Volksgezondheid en Milieuhygiëne.

Bekker, R. (2007). *Introductiedossier nieuwe bewindspersonen Ministeries van VWS.* Den Haag: VWS.

Bensing, J., Brand, P., & Borst, E. (2010). Brief aan de informateurs [letter to the inquirers]. Retrieved from http://www.ggdghor.nl/media/filebank/557bea2639e542e8843db5db9797445c/stivorobrief.pdf

Berridge, V., & Loughlin, K. (2005). Smoking and the new health education in Britain 1950s–1970s. *American Journal of Public Health, 95,* 956–964. https://doi.org/10.2105/AJPH.2004.037887

Best, A., Clark, P., Leichow, S. J., & Trochim, W. M. K. (2007). *Greater than the sum: Systems thinking in tobacco control.* Tobacco control monograph. Bethesda, MD: U.S. Department of Health and Human Services, National Institutes of Health, National Cancer Institute.

Betzner, A. E., Boyle, R. G., Luxenberg, M. G., Schillo, B. A., Keller, P. A., Rainey, J., ... Saul, J. E. (2012). Experience of smokers and recent quitters with smoke-free regulations and quitting. *American Journal of Preventive Medicine, 43,* S163–S170. https://doi.org/10.1016/j.amepre.2012.08.005

Biener, L., Hamilton, W. L., Siegel, M., & Sullivan, E. M. (2010). Individual, social-normative, and policy predictors of smoking cessation: A multilevel longitudinal analysis. *American Journal of Public Health, 100,* 547–554. https://doi.org/10.2105/ajph.2008

Biener, L., Reimer, R., Wakefield, M., Szczypka, G., Rigotti, N. A., & Connolly, G. (2006). Impact of smoking cessation aids and mass media among recent quitters. *American Journal of Preventive Medicine, 30,* 217–224.

Birkland, T. (2011). *An introduction to the policy process: Theories, concepts, and models of public policy making* (3rd ed.). Armonk, NY: M.E. Sharpe.

Bitton, A., Neuman, M. D., & Glantz, S. A. (2002). *Tobacco industry attempts to subvert European Union tobacco advertising legislation*. San Francisco, CA: Center for Tobacco Control Research and Education University of California.

Blackman, V. S. (2005). Putting policy theory to work: Tobacco control in California. *Policy, Politics, & Nursing Practice, 6*, 148–155. https://doi.org/10.1177/1527154405276289

Blankert, J. (1997). Wijzigingen tabakswet. *Dutch Tobacco Industry Collection*, Bates No. JB2074. Retrieved from https://www.industrydocumentslibrary.ucsf.edu/tobacco/docs/xjdp0219

Blankert, J. (1999). [Letter to Jorritsma]. *Dutch Tobacco Industry Collection*, Bates No. JB2377. Retrieved from https://www.industrydocumentslibrary.ucsf.edu/tobacco/docs/fsdp0219

Blecher, E., Ross, H., & Leon, M. E. (2013). Cigarette affordability in Europe. *Tobacco Control, 22*, e6. https://doi.org/10.1136/tobaccocontrol-2012-050575

BMA. (1986). *Smoking out the barons: The campaign against the tobacco industry. A report of the British Medical Association Public Affairs Division*. Chichester: Wiley & Sons.

Board of Appeal. (1982). Decision in the case of Dijkstra/Public Health and Smoking Foundation. *Dutch Tobacco Industry Collection*, Bates No. JB1457. Retrieved from https://www.industrydocumentslibrary.ucsf.edu/tobacco/docs/#id=zkgp0219

Boessen, S. (2008). *The politics of European health policy-making: An actor-centred institutionalist analysis* (Doctoral dissertation), Maastricht University, Maastricht.

Boessen, S., & Maarse, H. (2008). The impact of the treaty basis on health policy legislation in the European Union: A case study on the tobacco advertising directive. [20]. *BMC Health Services Research, 8*, 77. https://doi.org/10.1186/1472-6963-8-77

Bogdanovica, I., Murray, R., McNeill, A., & Britton, J. (2012). Cigarette price, affordability and smoking prevalence in the European Union. *Addiction, 107*, 188–196. https://doi.org/10.1111/j.1360-0443.2011.03588.x

Bonhoff, E. J. (2002). Brief van het ministerie van VWS aan de Stichting Sigarettenindustrie over het Tabaksontmoedigingsbeleid. *Dutch Tobacco Industry Collection*, Bates No. JB3527.

Borland, R., & Balmford, J. (2003). Understanding how mass media campaigns impact on smokers. *Tobacco Control, 12*(Suppl 2), ii45–ii52. https://doi.org/10.1136/tc.12.suppl_2.ii45

Bornhauser, A., McCarthy, J., & Glantz, S. A. (2006). German tobacco industry's successful efforts to maintain scientific and political respectability to prevent regulation of secondhand smoke. *Tobacco Control,* 15, e1. https://doi.org/10.1136/tc.2005.012336

Borst-Eilers, E. (1996). Verslag overleg tabaksontmoedigingsbeleid. *Dutch Tobacco Industry Collection,* Bates No. JB2069. Retrieved from https://www.industrydocumentslibrary.ucsf.edu/tobacco/docs/txdp0219

Bosdriesz, J. R., Kunst, A., Muntaner, C., Willemsen, M. C., & O'Campo, P. (2017). The effect of tobacco tax and price increases on smoking cessation or reduction—A scoping realist review. *Article submitted.*

Bosdriesz, J. R., Willemsen, M. C., Stronks, K., & Kunst, A. E. (2014). Tobacco control policy development in the European Union—Do political factors matter? *European Journal of Public Health,* 25(2), 190–194. https://doi.org/10.1093/eurpub/cku197

Bosdriesz, J. R., Willemsen, M. C., Stronks, K., & Kunst, A. E. (2015). Socioeconomic inequalities in smoking cessation in 11 European countries from 1987 through 2012. *Journal of Epidemiology Community Health,* 69, 886–892. https://doi.org/10.1136/jech-2014-205171

Boucher, P. (2000). Rendez-vous with Trudy Prins. Retrieved from http://archive.tobacco.org/News/rendezvous/prins.html

Bouma, J. (1999). De overheid werd te laat actief. *Trouw.*

Bouma, J. (2000). Echo's uit de prairie. *Dossiers Onderzoeksjournalistiek.* Retrieved 29 July, 2017, from https://www.villamedia.nl/journalist/n/dossiers/onderzoekphilipmorris.shtm

Bouma, J. (2001). *Het rookgordijn: De macht van de Nederlandse tabaksindustrie.* Amsterdam: Veen.

Bouma, J. (2012, February 21). Tabakslobby op schoot bij minister Schippers. *Trouw.* Retrieved from http://www.trouw.nl/tr/nl/4516/Gezondheid/article/detail/3193743/2012/02/21/Tabakslobby-op-schoot-bij-minister-Schippers.dhtml

Braam, S., & Van Woerden, I. (2013, juni 27). De laatste vriend van de sigaret. *Vrij Nederland.*

Breton, E., Richard, L., Gagnon, F., Jacques, M., & Bergeron, P. (2008). Health promotion research and practice require sound policy analysis models: The case of Quebec's tobacco act. *Social Sciences & Medicine,* 67(11), 1679–1689. https://doi.org/10.1016/j.socscimed.2008.07.028

Britton, J., Bates, C., Channer, K., Cuthbertson, L., Godfrey, C., Jarvis, M., & McNeill, A. (2000). *Nicotine addiction in Britain: A report of the Tobacco Advisory Group of the Royal College of Physicians.* London: Royal College of Physicians of London.

Brown, T., Platt, S., & Amos, A. (2014). Equity impact of population-level interventions and policies to reduce smoking in adults: A systematic review. *Drug Alcohol Depend,* 138, 7–16. https://doi.org/10.1016/j.drugalcdep.2014.03.001

Bruggink, J.-W. (2013). Ontwikkelingen in het aandeel rokers in Nederland sinds 1989. *Tijdschrift voor Gezondheidswetenschappen,* 91(4), 234–240.

Bruinsma, J. (1996, October 30). Alleen Jet Nijpels wijzigde standpunt na bezoek tabaksindustrie. Kamerleden ontkennen invloed lobby, *de Volkskrant*, p. 7. Retrieved from https://www.industrydocumentslibrary.ucsf.edu/tobacco/docs/thcp0219

Bryan-Jones, K., & Chapman, S. (2008). Political dynamics promoting the incremental regulation of secondhand smoke: A case study of New South Wales, Australia. *BMC Public Health, 6*, 192.

Burson-Marstellar. (1990). An accommodation strategy in EEMA: A strategic brief. *Philip Morris Collection*, Bates No. 2021181862–2021181887. Retrieved from https://www.industrydocumentslibrary.ucsf.edu/tobacco/docs/nppf0117

Buse, K., Mays, N., & Walt, G. (2012). *Making health policy* (2nd ed.). Berkshire: Open University Press.

Cairney, P. (2007). A 'Multiple Lenses' approach to policy change: The case of tobacco policy in the UK. *British Politics, 2*(2), 295–295.

Cairney, P. (2009). The role of ideas in policy transfer: The case of UK smoking bans since devolution. *Journal of European Public Policy, 16*(3), 471–488. https://doi.org/10.1080/13501760802684718

Cairney, P. (2012). *Understanding public policy: Theories and issues*. Basingstoke: Palgrave Macmillan.

Cairney, P. (2013). Policy concepts in 1000 words: The Advocacy Coalition Framework. Retrieved 20 July, 2017, from https://paulcairney.wordpress.com/2013/10/30/policy-concepts-in-1000-words-the-advocacy-coalition-framework/

Cairney, P., & Mamudu, H. (2014). The global tobacco control 'endgame': Change the policy environment to implement the FCTC. *Journal of Public Health Policy, 35*, 506–517. https://doi.org/10.1057/jphp.2014.18

Cairney, P., & Oliver, K. (2017). Evidence-based policymaking is not like evidence-based medicine, so how far should you go to bridge the divide between evidence and policy? *Health Research Policy and Systems, 15*, 35. https://doi.org/10.1186/s12961-017-0192-x

Cairney, P., Oliver, K., & Wellstead, A. (2016). To bridge the divide between evidence and policy: Reduce ambiguity as much as uncertainty. *Public Administration Review, 76*, 399–402.

Cairney, P., Studlar, D. T., & Mamudu, H. M. (2012). *Global tobacco control: Power, policy, governance and transfer*. New York: Palgrave Macmillan.

Campaign for smoke-free kids. (2014). Dutch Association of CAN v. Netherlands. Retrieved October 30, 2013, from http://www.tobaccocontrollaws.org/litigation/decisions/nl-20141010-dutch-association-of-can-v.-ne

Castles, F. G., & Obinger, H. (2008). Worlds, families, regimes: Country clusters in European and OECD area public policy. *West European Politics, 31*, 321–344. https://doi.org/10.1080/01402380701835140

CBO. (2004). *Richtlijn Behandeling van tabaksverslaving*. Alphen aan den Rijn: van Zuiden Communications BV.

CBO. (2006). *Guideline treatment of tobacco dependence*. Utrecht: CBO/Partnership Stoppen met Roken.

CDC. (1999). *Best practices for comprehensive tobacco control programs*. Atlanta: U.S. Department of Health and Human Services, Centers for Disease Control and Prevention, National Center for Chronic Disease Prevention and Health Promotion, Office on Smoking and Health.

Chaiton, M. O., Cohen, J. E., & Frank, J. (2003). Population health and the hardcore smoker: Geoffrey Rose revisited. *Journal of Public Health, 307*, 429–432.

Chaloupka, F. J., Straif, K., & Leon, M. E. (2011). Effectiveness of tax and price policies in tobacco control. *Tobacco Control, 20*(3), 235–238. https://doi.org/10.1136/tc.2010.039982

Chaloupka, F. J., Yurekli, A., & Fong, G. T. (2012). Tobacco taxes as a tobacco control strategy. *Tobacco Control, 21*(2), 172–180. https://doi.org/10.1136/tobaccocontrol-2011-050417

Chapman, S. (2007). *Public health advocacy and tobacco control: Making smoking history*. Oxford: Blackwell Publishing.

Chapman, S. (2017). Why researchers have a duty to try and influence policy. Retrieved from The Conversation website: https://theconversation.com/why-researchers-have-a-duty-to-try-and-influence-policy-71081

Christiansen, P. M., Norgaard, A. S., Rommetvedt, H., Svensson, T., Thesen, G., & Oberg, P. (2010). Varieties of democracy: Interest groups and corporatist committees in Scandinavian policy making. *Voluntas, 21*(1), 22–40. https://doi.org/10.1007/s11266-009-9105-0

CHRODIS. (2015). *Health promotion and primary prevention in 14 European countries: A comparative overview of key policies, approaches, gaps and needs*. Brussels: CHRODIS.

Cigarette shag information bureau. (1991). STIVORO trial ended: Tobacco Industry satisfied with court verdict. *Dutch Tobacco Industry Collection*, Bates No. JB1025. Retrieved from https://www.industrydocumentslibrary.ucsf.edu/tobacco/docs/xqfp0219

Clairmonte, F. F. (1983, December). The transnational tobacco and alcohol conglomerates: A world oligolopy. *New York State Journal of Medicine, 83*, 1322–1323.

Clavier, C., & De Leeuw, E. (Eds.). (2013). *Framing public policy in health promotion: Ubiquitous, yet elusive*. London: Oxford University Press.

Cobb, R. W., Ross, J.-K., & Ross, M. H. (1976). Agenda building as a comparative political process. *American Political Science Review, 70*, 126–138. https://doi.org/10.2307/1960328

Coglianese, C., Zeckhauser, R., & Parson, E. (2004). Seeking truth for power: Informational strategy and regulatory policy making. *Faculty Research Working*

Papers Series Harvard University, John F. Kennedy School of Government, RWP04-021.

Cohen, J. E., Milio, N., Rozier, R. G., Ferrence, R., Ashley, M. J., & Goldstein, A. O. (2000). Political ideology and tobacco control. *Tobacco Control, 9*(3), 263–267. https://doi.org/10.1136/tc.9.3.263

Colby, F. G. (1979). Summary of the PR program of the Dutch Cigarette Manufactures Association. *RJ Reynolds Records Collection*, Bates No. 500877429–500877431. Retrieved from https://industrydocuments.library.ucsf.edu/tobacco/docs/#id=jrpj0096

Costa, H., Gilmore, A. B., Peeters, S., McKee, M., & Stuckler, D. (2014). Quantifying the influence of the tobacco industry on EU governance: Automated content analysis of the EU Tobacco Products Directive. *Tobacco Control, 23*(6), 473–478. https://doi.org/10.1136/tobaccocontrol-2014-051822

Davies, H. T. O., Nutley, S., & Smith, P. C. (Eds.). (2000). *What works? Evidence-based policy and practice in public services.* Bristol: The Policy Press.

De Blij, B. (1995). [Brieven van Stivoro aan de ministeries van EZ en VWS]. *Dutch Tobacco Industry Collection*, Bates No. JB2574. Retrieved from https://www.industrydocumentslibrary.ucsf.edu/tobacco/docs/nlwp0219

De Blij, B. (1996a). Amendement Tabaksaccijns. *Dutch Tobacco Industry Collection*, Bates No. JB2691. Retrieved from https://www.industrydocumentslibrary.ucsf.edu/tobacco/docs/tqwp0219

De Blij, B. (1996b). Letter to Wijers. *Dutch Tobacco Industry Collection*, Bates No. JB2517. Retrieved from https://www.industrydocumentslibrary.ucsf.edu/tobacco/docs/mxwp0219

De Blij, B. (1996c). Tabaksontmoedigingsbeleid. *Dutch Tobacco Industry Collection*, Bates No. JB2695. Retrieved from https://www.industrydocumentslibrary.ucsf.edu/tobacco/docs/gnfp0219

De Goeij, J. I. M. (2006). [Letter to VNK]. *Dutch Tobacco Industry Collection*, Bates No. JB3059. Retrieved from https://www.industrydocumentslibrary.ucsf.edu/tobacco/docs/jtwn0217

De Goeij, J. I. M. (2007). Kabinetsreactie Groenboek rookvrij Europa. *Dutch Tobacco Industry Collection*, Bates No. JB0441. Retrieved from https://www.industrydocumentslibrary.ucsf.edu/tobacco/docs/tthb0191

De Jager, J. H. (2008). Beleidsvoornemens tabaksontmoediging. *Dutch Tobacco Industry Collection*, Bates No. JB0562. Retrieved from https://www.industrydocumentslibrary.ucsf.edu/tobacco/docs/hkxb0191

De Jong, A. (2000). Complete prohibition on smoking in the workplace. *British American Tobacco Records*, Bates No. 322075711–322075712. Retrieved from http://legacy.library.ucsf.edu/tid/llp14a99

De Jong, R. (1984). Commentaar op de ontwerp tabakswet [letter]. *Dutch Tobacco Industry Collection*, Bates No. JB2104. Retrieved from https://www.industrydocumentslibrary.ucsf.edu/tobacco/docs/hpfp0219

De Jong, R. (1989). Notitie met het oog op de uitvoering van het meerjaren voorlichtingsprogramma niet-roken. *Dutch Tobacco Industry Collection*, Bates No. JB1425. Retrieved from https://www.industrydocumentslibrary.ucsf.edu/tobacco/docs/kzhp0219

De Jong, R., & Nelissen, J. G. M. (1984). [Brief van Stivoro aan de voorzitter en Leden der Staten-Generaal]. *Dutch Tobacco Industry Collection*, Bates No. JB2305. Retrieved from https://www.industrydocumentslibrary.ucsf.edu/tobacco/docs/mpdp0219

De Landsadvocaat. (1995). Verbod tabaksreclame. *Dutch Tobacco Industry Collection*, Bates No. JB1037. Retrieved from https://www.industrydocumentslibrary.ucsf.edu/tobacco/docs/gtcp0219

De Leeuw, E. (2013). Gezondheidsbeleidswetenschap: Tijd voor theorie. *Tijdschrift voor Gezondheidswetenschappen, 91*, 241–242.

De Poorter, J.-P. (1996). [Brief van de Nationale Jongerenraad voor Milieu en Ontwikkeling aad de Tweede kamer fractie van CDA]. *Dutch Tobacco Industry Collection*, Bates No. JB1948. Retrieved from https://www.industrydocumentslibrary.ucsf.edu/tobacco/docs/jjbp0219

De Steur, M. (n.d.). De Nederlandse tabakverwerkende industrie. CBS.

De Vries, M. S. (2000). The rise and fall of decentralization: A comparative analysis of arguments and practices in European countries. *European Journal of Political Research, 38*, 193–224.

De Wolff, F. A. (1994a). Comments on the OSHA proposed rule on indoor air quality, April 5. *Dutch Tobacco Industry Collection*, Bates No. JB1177. Retrieved from https://www.industrydocumentslibrary.ucsf.edu/tobacco/docs/hkxp0219

De Wolff, F. A. (1994b). Risico van longkanker door passief roken nog onbewezen. *Nederlands Tijdschrift voor Geneeskunde, 138*, 503–506.

Dechesne, F., Dignum, V., & Tan, Y.-H. (2011). Understanding compliance differences between legal and social norms: The case of smoking ban. In F. Dechesne, H. Hattori, A. Ter Mors, J. M. Such, D. Weyns, & F. Dignum (Eds.), *Advanced agent technology. AAMAS 2011. Lecture Notes in Computer Science* (Vol. 7068). Berlin: Springer.

Dechesne, F., Di Tosto, G., Dignum, V., & Dignum, F. (2013). No smoking here: Values, norms and culture in multi-agent systems. *Artificial Intelligence and Law, 21*, 79. https://doi.org/10.1007/s10506-012-9128-5

Dekker, E. (1981). De huisarts en het rookpatroon. In STIVORO (Ed.), *Trekt de rook langzaam op? Voordrachten van het symposium*. Den Haag: STIVORO.

Dekker, E., & Saan, H. (1990). Policy papers, papers or policies: HFA under uncertain political conditions. *Health Promotion International, 5*, 279–290.

Dekker, H., Soethout, J., & Tijsmans, N. (2009). *Even uitblazen. Eén jaar rookvrije horeca*. Amsterdam: Regioplan Beleidsonderzoek.

Den Exter Blokland, E. A. W., Engels, R. C. M. E., Hale, W. W., III, Meeus, W., & Willemsen, M. C. (2004). Lifetime parental smoking history and cessation and early adolescent smoking behavior. *Preventive Medicine, 38*(3), 359–368. https://doi.org/10.1016/j.ypmed.2003.11.008

Department of Health. (1998). *Smoking kills. A white paper on tobacco.* London: Department of Health.

Department of Health. (2004). *Choosing health: Making healthy choices easier.* London: UK Department of Health.

Department of Health. (2010). *A smokefree future: A comprehensive tobacco control strategy for England.* London: Department of Health.

Department of Health. (2011). *Health lives, healthy people: A tobacco control plan for England.* London: Department of Health.

Derthick, M. A. (2005). *Up in smoke: From legislation to litigation in tobacco politics* (2nd ed.). Washington, DC: CQ Press.

Doll, R., & Hill, A. B. (1950). Smoking and carcinoma of the lung: Preliminary report. *British Medical Journal, 2,* 739–748.

Dollisson, J. (1990). EEC advertising directive. *Philip Morris Records*, Bates No. 2024671385–2024671388. Retrieved from http://legacy.library.ucsf.edu/tid/box36e00/pdf?search=%222024671385%201388%22

Dortland, R. (2005). Brief van het ministerie van VWS aan de Stichting Sigarettenindustrie betreffende de Tabakswet. *Dutch Tobacco Industry Collection*, Bates No. JB3525. Retrieved from https://www.industrydocumentslibrary.ucsf.edu/tobacco/docs/fswn0217

Dresscher, I., Elzinga, A., & Koldenhof, E. (1991). *Evaluatie tabakswet en zelfregulering tabaksreclame.* Zoetermeer: Research voor Beleid.

Drogendijk, A. C. (1978). *Verstandig roken.* Amsterdam: Buijten & Schipperheijn.

Duina, F., & Kurzer, P. (2004). Smoke in your eyes: The struggle over tobacco control in the European Union. *Journal of European Public Policy, 1,* 57–77. https://doi.org/10.1080/1350176042000164307

Duivenvoorden, E. (2009). *Magiër van een nieuwe tijd: Het leven van Robert Jasper Grootveld.* Amsterdam: De Arbeiderspers.

Durkin, S., Brennan, E., & Wakefield, M. (2012). Mass media campaigns to promote smoking cessation among adults: An integrative review. *Tobacco Control, 21*(2), 127–138. https://doi.org/10.1136/tobaccocontrol-2011-050345

Elsevier. (2010). *Wacht op onze daden: Alle regeringsverklaringen van Lubbers tot en met Rutte.* Amsterdam: Elsevier Boeken.

Emmelot, P. (1979). Wetenschappelijke Adviesraad Roken en Gezondheid (WARG). *Dutch Tobacco Industry Collection*, Bates No. JB1400. Retrieved from https://www.industrydocumentslibrary.ucsf.edu/tobacco/docs/jqgp0219

Engelsman, E. (1992). Mondeling overleg tabaksontmoedigingsbeleid. *Dutch Tobacco Industry Collection*, Bates No. JB2031. Retrieved from https://www.industrydocumentslibrary.ucsf.edu/tobacco/docs/rmfp0219

EPA. (1992). *Respiratory health effects of passive smoking (also known as exposure to secondhand smoke or Environmental Tobacco Smoke—ETS).* Washington, DC: U.S. Environmental Protection Agency (EPA).

EPA. (1994). *Setting the record straight: Secondhand smoke is a preventable health risk.* Washington, DC: U.S. Environmental Protection Agency (EPA).

European Commission. (1984). *Cooperation at community level on health related problems. Communication from the Commission to the Council.* Brussels: European Commission.

European Commission. (1987). *Survey: Europeans and the prevention of cancer. A working document of the services of the European Commission.* Brussels: European Commission.

European Commission. (2007). *Green paper towards a Europe free from tobacco smoke: Policy options at EU level.* Brussels: European Commission, Directorate C—Public Health and Risk Assessment.

European Commission. (2017a). Register of communication expert groups and other similar entities: Group of experts on tobacco policy (E03150). Retrieved April 14, 2017, from http://ec.europa.eu/transparency/regexpert/index.cfm?do=groupDetail.groupDetail&groupID=3150

European Commission. (2017b). Tobacco: All events. Retrieved July 7, 2017, from http://ec.europa.eu/health/tobacco/events/index_en.htm#anchor6

Evenhuis, A. (1988). *Reclamecode sigaretten en shag Dutch Tobacco Industry Collection*, Bates No. JB2182. Retrieved from https://www.industrydocumentslibrary.ucsf.edu/tobacco/docs/fndp0219

Farquhar, J. W., Magnus, P. F., & Maccoby, N. (1981). The role of public information and education in cigarette smoking controls. *Canadian Journal of Public Health, 72*(6), 412–420.

Farquharson, K. (2003). Influencing policy transnationally: Pro-and anti-tobacco global advocacy networks. *Australian Journal of Public Administration, 62*, 80–92. https://doi.org/10.1111/j..2003.00351.x

Feldman, E., & Bayer, R. (2004). *Unfiltered: Conflicts over tobacco policy and public health.* Cambridge, MA: Harvard University Press.

Fenger, F. (2007). Welfare regimes in Central and Eastern Europe: Incorporating post-communist countries in a welfare regime typology. *Contemporary Issues and Ideas in Social Sciences, 3*(2), 1–30.

Flynn, B. S., Goldstein, A. O., Solomon, L. J., Bauman, K. E., Gottlieb, N. H., Cohen, J. E., ... Dana, G. S. (1998). Predictors of state legislators' intentions to vote for cigarette tax increases. *Preventive Medicine, 27*, 157–165. https://doi.org/10.1006/pmed.1998.0308

Forces USA. (1998). The speakers of the 1997 Smokepeace International Conference. *Philip Morris Collection*, Bates No. 2073643759–2073643760. Retrieved from https://www.industrydocumentslibrary.ucsf.edu/tobacco/docs/nhbb0088

Fox, B. (2005). Framing tobacco control efforts within an ethical context. *Tobacco Control, 14*(Suppl II), ii38–ii44.

Framework Convention Alliance. (2017). Latest ratifications of the WHO FCTC. Retrieved July 7, 2017, from http://www.fctc.org/about-fca/tobacco-control-treaty/latest-ratifications

Gadourek, I. (1963). *Riskante gewoonten en zorg voor eigen welzijn*. Groningen: J.B. Wolters.

Gallus, S., Schiaffino, A., La Vecchia, C., Townsend, J., & Fernandez, E. (2006). Price and cigarette consumption in Europe. *Tobacco Control, 15*(2), 114–119. https://doi.org/10.1136/tc.2005.012468

Gemeente Bergen op Zoom. (1996). Accijnsverhoging op tabaksproducten [letter to the prime minister]. *Dutch Tobacco Industry Collection*, Bates No. JB2646. Retrieved from https://www.industrydocumentslibrary.ucsf.edu/tobacco/docs/xywp0219

Geus, M., & Van der Lee, J. (1997). STIVORO/Produktaansprakelijkheid. *Dutch Tobacco Industry Collection*, Bates No. JB1011. Retrieved from https://www.industrydocumentslibrary.ucsf.edu/tobacco/docs/ftcp0219

Gezondheidsraad. (1990). *Passief roken: Beoordeling van de schadelijkheid van omgevingstabaksrook voor de gezondheid*. Den Haag: Gezondheidsraad.

Gezondheidsraad. (2003). *Volksgezondheidsschade door passief roken*. Den Haag: Gezondheidsraad.

Gezondheidsraad. (2006). *Plan de campagne: Bevordering van gezond gedrag door massamediale voorlichting*. The Hague: Health Council of the Netherlands.

GfK Great Britain. (1998). ETS world report Philip Morris 1998. *Philip Morris Records*, Bates No. 2065221475–2065221544. Retrieved from http://legacy.library.ucsf.edu/tid/fnq90g00/pdf

GGD Nederland. (2013). *Gezondheidsbeleid in de groei*. Utrecht: GGD Nederland.

Gielkens-Sijstermans, C. M., Mommers, M. A., Hoogenveen, R. T., Feenstra, T. L., Vreede, J. d., Bovens, F. M., & Schayck, O. C. v. (2009). Reduction of smoking in Dutch adolescents over the past decade and its health gains: A repeated cross-sectional study. *European Journal of Public Health, 20*(3), 146–150.

Gilmore, A., & McKee, M. (2004). Tobacco-control policy in the European Union. In E. A. Feldman & R. Bayer (Eds.), *Unfiltered: Conflicts over tobacco policy and public health* (pp. 219–245). London: Harvard University Press.

Global Tobacco Control Forum. (2010). *Canada's implementation of the Framework Convention on Tobacco Control: A civil society 'shadow report'*. Ottawa: Global Tobacco Control Forum (GTCF).

Gneiting, U., & Schmitz, H. P. (2016). Comparing global alcohol and tobacco control efforts: Network formation and evolution in international health governance. *Health Policy Plan, 31*(Suppl 1), i98–i109. https://doi.org/10.1093/heapol/czv125

Godlee, F. (2000). WHO faces up to its tobacco links. *Report provides compelling evidence for transparency about competing interests. BMJ: British Medical Journal, 321*(7257), 314–315. https://doi.org/10.1136/bmj.321.7257.314

Goldberg, H. (1999a). Accommodation programs. *Philip Morris Collection*, Bates No. 2072577224–2072577238. Retrieved from http://legacy.library.ucsf.edu/tid/otq59h00

Goldberg, H. (1999b). International accommodation programs. *Philip Morris Collection*, Bates No. 2074399542–2074399568. Retrieved from http://legacy.library.ucsf.edu/tid/thp11h00

Gonzalez, M., & Glantz, S. A. (2013). Failure of policy regarding smoke-free bars in the Netherlands. *European Journal of Public Health, 23*(1), 139–145. https://doi.org/10.1093/eurpub/ckr173

Graham, E. R., Shipan, C. R., & Volden, C. (2012). The diffusion of policy diffusion research in political science. *British Journal of Political Science, 43*(3), 673–701. https://doi.org/10.1017/S0007123412000415

Gravely, S., Giovino, G. A., Craig, L., Commar, A., Déspaignet, E. T., Schotte, K., & Fong, G. T. (2017). Implementation of key demand-reduction measures of the WHO Framework Convention on Tobacco Control and change in smoking prevalence in 126 countries: An association study. *The Lancet, 2*, e166–e174. https://doi.org/10.1016/S2468-2667(17)30045-2

Grüning, T., Strünk, C., & Gilmore, A. B. (2008). Puffing away? Explaining the politics of tobacco control in Germany. *German Politics, 17*, 140–164.

Hall, P. (1993). Policy paradigms, social learning, and the state: The case of economic policymaking in Britain. *Comparative Politics, 25*, 257–296.

Hall, P., Land, H., Parker, R., & Webb, A. (1975). *Change, choice and conflict in social policy*. London: Heinemann.

Hamers, J., & Vermeulen, A. (1996). Tabakaccijns [letter to the prime minister]. *Dutch Tobacco Industry Collection*, Bates No. JB2670. Retrieved from https://www.industrydocumentslibrary.ucsf.edu/tobacco/docs/qpwp0219

Hammond, D., Fong, G. T., Zanna, M. P., Thrasher, J. F., & Borland, R. (2006). Tobacco denormalization and industry beliefs among smokers from four countries. *American Journal of Preventive Medicine, 31*(3), 225–232. https://doi.org/10.1016/j.amepre.2006.04.004

Hastings, G., & Angus, K. (2004). The influence of the tobacco industry on European tobacco-control policy. In The ASPECT Consortium (Ed.), *Tobacco or health in the European Union: Past, present and future*. Luxembourg: European Commission.

Heijndijk, S. M., & Willemsen, M. C. (2015). *Dutch tobacco control: Moving towards the right track?* FCTC Shadow Report 2014. Den Haag: Alliantie Nederland Rookvrij.

Helweg-Larsen, M., & Nielsen, G. A. (2009). Smoking cross-culturally: Risk perceptions among young adults in Denmark and the United States. *Psychology & Health, 24*(1), 81–93. https://doi.org/10.1080/08870440801932656

Hill, D. (1999). Why we should tackle adult smoking first. *Tobacco Control, 8*, 333–335.

Hilvering, C., Knol, K., & Wagener, D. J. (1995). Petitie tot strenge beperking tabaksreclame. *Dutch Tobacco Industry Collection*, Bates No. JB2550. Retrieved from https://www.industrydocumentslibrary.ucsf.edu/tobacco/docs/gggp0219

Hoffman, S. J., & Toan, C. (2015). Overview of systematic reviews on the health-related effects of government tobacco control policies. *BMC Public Health, 15*, 744.
Hofstede Centre. (2015). The Netherlands. Retrieved May 4, 2015, from http://geert-hofstede.com/netherlands.html
Hofstede, G. J. (1980). *Culture's consequences. International differences in work-related values.* Beverly Hills, CA: Sage.
Hoogervorst, H. (2003a). Regeling lijsten tabaksingrediënten [letter to SSI]. *Dutch Tobacco Industry Collection*, Bates No. JB3259. Retrieved from https://www.industrydocumentslibrary.ucsf.edu/tobacco/docs/nybn0217
Hoogervorst, H. (2003b). Regulier overleg tabaksontmoedigingsbeleid. *Dutch Tobacco Industry Collection*, Bates No. JB0278. Retrieved from https://www.industrydocumentslibrary.ucsf.edu/tobacco/docs/sjhb0191
Hoogervorst, H. (2005). Brief Evaluatie tabaksontmoedigingsbeleid. *Kamerstuk 22894-55-b2.*
Hoogervorst, H. (2006a). Antwoordbrief aan VNK en SSI. *Dutch Tobacco Industry Collection*, Bates No. JB0412.
Hoogervorst, H. (2006b). Brief van het ministerie van VWS aan de Vereniging Nederlandse Kerftabakindustrie. *Dutch Tobacco Industry Collection*, Bates No. JB3333. Retrieved from https://www.industrydocumentslibrary.ucsf.edu/tobacco/docs/ftwn0217
Hoogervorst, H., Zoun, J. P. M., De Blij, B. A. J. M., & Hanselaar, A. G. J. M. (2005). Intentieverklaring tabaksontmoediging. *Dutch Tobacco Industry Collection*, Bates No. JB3189. Retrieved from https://www.industrydocumentslibrary.ucsf.edu/tobacco/docs/kgdn0217
Hoppe, R., Woldendorp, J., & Bandelow, N. (2015). *2015 Netherlands report.* Gütersloh: Bertelsmann Stiftung.
Horeca Nederland. (2002). Overleg Tabakswet [letter to Borst]. *Dutch Tobacco Industry Collection*, Bates No. JB3517. Retrieved from https://www.industrydocumentslibrary.ucsf.edu/tobacco/docs/flwn0217
Hosking, W., Borland, R., Yong, H. H., Fong, G., Zanna, M., Laux, F., ... Omar, M. (2009). The effects of smoking norms and attitudes on quitting intentions in Malaysia, Thailand and four western nations: A cross-cultural comparison. *Psychology & Health, 24*, 95–107. https://doi.org/10.1080/08870440802385854
Huijsman, F., van der Meer, R. M., de Beer, M. A. M., van Emst, A. J., & Willemsen, M. C. (2013). Decentralisation of tobacco control: Smoking policy falls through the cracks. *Tijdschrift voor Gezondheidswetenschappen, 91*, 52–59.
Huijts, P. H. A. M. (2009). Gesprek 24 Augsutus jl. *Dutch Tobacco Industry Collection*, Bates No. JB0611. Retrieved from https://www.industrydocumentslibrary.ucsf.edu/tobacco/docs/hnxb0191
Huisman, C. (2005). Uit de walm. *Volkskrant.* Retrieved from http://www.volkskrant.nl/archief/uit-de-walm~a643849/

Huisman, E., Kooistra, S., & Korteweg, A. (2016). Kwart oud-politici wordt lobbyist. Retrieved May 18, 2017, from http://www.volkskrant.nl/politiek/kwart-oud-politici-wordt-lobbyist~a4234963/

Hummel, K., Willemsen, M. C., Monshouwer, K., De Vries, H., & Nagelhout, G. E. (2016). Social acceptance of smoking restrictions during 10 years of policy implementation, reversal, and reenactment in the Netherlands: Findings from a national population survey. *Nicotine & Tobacco Research, 19*, 1–8. https://doi.org/10.1093/ntr/ntw169

IARC. (1986). Tobacco smoking. IARC monographs on the evaluation of carcinogenic risks of chemicals to humans. In *IARC monographs no 38* (Vol. 38). Lyon: International Agency for Research on Cancer (IARC).

IARC. (2011). *Effectiveness of tax and price policies for tobacco control. IARC handbooks of cancer prevention: Tobacco control* (Vol. 14). Lyon: International Agency for Research on Cancer (IARC).

ICBT. (1981). *Advies inzake maatregelen ter beperking van het tabaksgebruik*. Den Haag: Interdepartementale Commissie Beperking Tabaksgebruik (ICBT), Ministerie van Volksgezondheid en Milieu.

Inspectie van de Gezondheidszorg. (2010). *De staat van de gezondheidszorg: Meer effect mogelijk van publieke gezondheidszorg*. Utrecht: IGZ.

Interdepartementale Commissie Tabaksreclame. (1972a). Verslag van een Hearing op 24 januari 1972 over het onderwerp reklame voor tabaksprodukten, gehouden door de Interdepartementale Commissie. *Dutch Tobacco Industry Collection*, Bates No. JB1936. Retrieved from https://industrydocuments.library.ucsf.edu/tobacco/docs/mhbp0219

Interdepartementale Commissie Tabaksreclame. (1972b). Verslag vergadering Interdepartementale Werkgroep Tabaksreclame 13 juli 1972. *Dutch Tobacco Industry Collection*, Bates No. JB1858. Retrieved from https://www.industrydocumentslibrary.ucsf.edu/tobacco/docs/hkgp0219

Intraval. (2010). *Inventarisatie naleefniveau rookvrije horeca najaar 2010*. Groningen: Intraval.

IOM (Institute of Medicine). (2007). *Ending the tobacco problem: A blue-print for the nation*. Washington, DC: The National Academies Press.

Isett, K. (2013). In and across bureaucracy: Structural and administrative issues for the tobacco endgame. *Tobacco Control, 22*, i58–i60. https://doi.org/10.1136/tobaccocontrol-2012-050828

ITC Project. (2010). *The International Tobacco Control Policy Evaluation Project: ITC Netherlands National Report*. Ontario, The Hague: ITC Project, University of Waterloo, Canada.

ITC Project. (2015). ITC Netherlands National Report. Findings from the Wave 1 to 8 Surveys (2008–2014). Waterloo, ON, Canada: University of Waterloo.

Jacobson, P. D., & Banerjee, A. (2005). Social movements and human rights rhetoric in tobacco control. *Tobacco Control, 14*(Suppl II), ii45–ii49.

Jansen, D. F., Van Barneveld, T. A., & Van Leeuwen, F. E. (1993). *Passief roken en longkanker: Het EPA rapport.* Amsterdam: Nederlands Kanker Instituut.

Jha, P., & Chaloupka, F. J. (2000). The economics of global tobacco control. *BMJ: British Medical Journal, 321*(7257), 358–361.

John, P. (2012). *Analyzing public policy* (2nd ed.). London: Routledge.

Jongejan, B. A. J., Hummel, H., Roelants, H. J., Lugtenberg, G., & Hoekstra, G. A. (2003). *National Cancer Control Programme. Part I—NPK vision and summary 2005–2010.* Den Haag: NPK Steering Group.

Joossens, L. (2004). *Effective tobacco control policies in 28 European countries.* Brussels: ENSP.

Joossens, L., & Raw, M. (2006). The tobacco control scale: A new scale to measure country activity. *Tobacco Control, 15*(3), 247–253. https://doi.org/10.1136/tc.2005.015347

Joossens, L., & Raw, M. (2011). *The tobacco control scale 2010 in Europe.* Brussels: Association of European Cancer Leagues.

Joossens, L., & Raw, M. (2017). *The tobacco control scale 2016 in Europe.* Brussels: Association of European Cancer Leagues.

Kagan, R. A., & Nelson, W. P. (2001). The politics of tobacco regulation in the United States. In R. Rabin & S. Sugarman (Eds.), *Regulating tobacco* (pp. 11–38). New York: Oxford University Press.

Kalis, A. W. (2000a). Tabaksaccijns. *Dutch Tobacco Industry Collection*, Bates No. JB2028. Retrieved from https://www.industrydocumentslibrary.ucsf.edu/tobacco/docs/lpfp0219

Kalis, A. W. (2000b). Tabakseditie British Medical Journal. *Dutch Tobacco Industry Collection*, Bates No. JB2030. Retrieved from https://www.industrydocumentslibrary.ucsf.edu/tobacco/docs/hmfp0219

Kalis, A. W. (2002). Consultatie inzake inwerkingtreding van gewijzigde Tabakswet. *Dutch Tobacco Industry Collection*, Bates No. JB3519. Retrieved from https://www.industrydocumentslibrary.ucsf.edu/tobacco/docs/jkcn0217

Kalis, A. W. (2003). Regulier overleg tabaksontmoedigingsbeleid. *Dutch Tobacco Industry Collection*, Bates No. JB0272. Retrieved from https://www.industrydocumentslibrary.ucsf.edu/tobacco/docs/mjhb0191

Kalra, A., Bansal, P., Wilson, D., & Lasseter, T. (2017). Inside Philip Morris' campaign to subvert the global anti-smoking treaty. Retrieved July 15, 2017, from https://www.reuters.com/investigates/special-report/pmi-who-fctc/

Kaper, J., Wagena, E. J., & Van Schaijck, O. (2003). *Het effect van het vergoeden van ondersteuning voor stoppen met roken: Resultaten van een gerandomiseerd experiment.* Maastricht: Universiteit van Maastricht.

Katz, J. E. (2005). Individual rights advocacy in tobacco control policies: An assessment and recommendation. *Tobacco Control, 14*(Suppl II), ii31–ii37. https://doi.org/10.1136/tc.2004.008060

Kim, S.-H., & Shanahan, J. (2003). Stigmatizing smokers: Public sentiment toward cigarette smoking and its relationship to smoking behaviors. *Journal of Health Communication*, 8, 343–367. https://doi.org/10.1080/10810730305723

Kingdon, J. W. (2003). *Agendas, alternatives and public policies* (2nd ed.). New York: Addison-Wesley.

Klaver, J. (2015). *De mythe van het economisme. Pleidooi voor een nieuw idealisme*. Amsterdam: De Bezige Bij.

Klijn, W., & Toet, R. L. J. (1991). [Letter to Ministry of Finance]. *Dutch Tobacco Industry Collection*, Bates No. JB2781. Retrieved from https://www.industrydocumentslibrary.ucsf.edu/tobacco/docs/mtwp0219

Klink, A. (2007a). *Kaderbrief 2007–2011 visie op gezondheid en preventie*. Den Haag: Ministry of Health.

Klink, A. (2007b). Tabaksontmoedigingsbeleid (letter to SSI). *Dutch Tobacco Industry Collection*, Bates No. JB0454. Retrieved from https://www.industrydocumentslibrary.ucsf.edu/tobacco/docs/qzhb0191

Klink, A. (2008). Preventiebeleid voor de volkgsgezondheid. *kamerstuk 22894 nr. 154*.

KNMG. (2007). *Volksgezondheid en Preventie De visie van de KNMG*. Utrecht: KNMG.

KNMG. (2016). *Tobacco discouragement: Towards a smoke-free society*. Utrecht: Royal Dutch Medical Association.

Knol, K. (1995, January 11). Kinderen doelwit van tabaksreclame. *Trouw*. Retrieved August 19, 2017, from http://www.trouw.nl/tr/nl/5009/Archief/article/detail/2663243/1995/01/11/Kinderen-doelwit-van-tabaksreclame.dhtml

Knol, K. (1996a). [Brief van Knol aan Borst]. *Dutch Tobacco Industry Collection*, Bates No. JB1947. Retrieved from https://www.industrydocumentslibrary.ucsf.edu/tobacco/docs/ytvp0219

Knol, K. (1996b). Medische Alliantie tegen het roken. *Dutch Tobacco Industry Collection*, Bates No. JB2673. Retrieved from https://www.industrydocumentslibrary.ucsf.edu/tobacco/docs/spwp0219

Knol, K. (1997). De toekomst van de strijd tegen het roken. *Medisch Contact*, 52(25), 803–804.

Knopick, P. (1980). Confidential memorandom: Minnesota tobacco litigation. *Tobacco Institute Records*, Bates No. TIMN0107822–TIMN0107823. Retrieved from https://www.industrydocumentslibrary.ucsf.edu/tobacco/docs/lqnn0146

Kok, W. (1996, September 2). Verhoging tabakaccijns. Retrieved from https://www.industrydocumentslibrary.ucsf.edu/tobacco/docs/rywp0219

Koopmans, F. S. L. (2011). Going Dutch: Recent drug policy developments in the Netherlands. *Journal of Global Drug Policy and Practice, 5*(3), 1–9.

Korteweg, A., & Huisman, E. (2016). *Lobbyland: De geheime krachten in Den Haag.* Amsterdam: De Geus.

Krasnegor, N. A. (Ed.). (1979). *Cigarette smoking as a dependence process.* Rockville, MD: Department of Health, Education, and Welfare.

Kroes, M. E., & Lock, A. J. J. (2003). *Stoppen met roken ondersteuning: Zeker weten!* Diemen: College voor Zorgverzekeringen (CVZ).

Kurzer, P., & Cooper, A. (2016). The dog that didn't bark: Explaining change in Germany's tobacco control policy at home and in the EU. *German Politics, 25*(4), 541–560. https://doi.org/10.1080/09644008.2016.1196664

Laméris, M., Jong-A-Pin, R., & Garretsen, H. (2017, maart 9). Kiezersvoorkeuren: links en rechts ingehaald. *Economie & Samenleving ESB, 102* (4747), 140-143.

Lanphen, J., & Van Berkestijn, T. (1995). [Brief van de Koninklijke Nederlandse Maatschappij tot Bevordering de Geneeskunst aan de leden van het Kabint en de leden vande Tweede Kamer der Staten Generaal]. *Dutch Tobacco Industry.*

Larsen, L. T. (2008). The political impact of science: Is tobacco control science- or policy-driven? *Science and Public Policy, 35*(10), 757–769. https://doi.org/10.3152/030234208x394697

Lelieveldt, H., & Princen, S. (2011). *The politics of the European Union.* Cambridge: Cambridge University Press.

Lenschow, A., Liefferink, D., & Veenman, S. (2005). When the birds sing. A framework for analysing domestic factors behind policy convergence. *Journal of European Public Policy, 12*(5), 797–816. https://doi.org/10.1080/13501760500161373

Leshner, A. L. (1997). Addiction is a brain disease, and it matters. *Science, 278*, 45–47. https://doi.org/10.1126/science.278.5335.45

Levine, C. H., Peters, B. G., & Thompson, F. J. (1990). *Public administration: Challenges, choices, consequences.* Glenview, IL: Scott, Foresman/Little Brown.

Lie, J., Willemsen, M. C., De Vries, N. K., & Fooks, G. (2016). The devil is in the detail: Tobacco industry political influence in the Dutch implementation of the 2001 EU Tobacco Products Directive. *Tobacco Control, 25*, 545–550. https://doi.org/10.1136/tobaccocontrol-2015-052302

Lijphart, A. (1999). *Patterns of democracy: Government forms and performance in thirty-six countries.* New Haven, CT: Yale University Press.

Liverani, M., Hawkins, B., & Parkhurst, J. O. (2013). Political and institutional influences on the use of evidence in Public Health Policy. A systematic review. *PLoS One, 8*(10), e77404. https://doi.org/10.1371/journal.pone.0077404

Lopez, A. D., Collishaw, N. E., & Piha, T. (1994). A descriptive model of the cigarette epidemic in developed countries. *Tobacco Control*, *3*(3), 242. https://doi.org/10.1136/tc.3.3.242

Loubeau, P. (2014). *An exploratory review of illicit tobacco trade in the Netherlands*. Den Haag: Alliantie Nederland Rookvrij.

Luyendijk, J., Verkade, T., & Heck, W. (2010). Het lobbywerk dat níét op de cv's van politici staat. Retrieved from https://www.nrc.nl/nieuws/2010/11/22/het-lobbywerk-dat-niet-op-de-cvs-van-politici-staat-11972720-a865044

Lynch, B. S., & Bonnie, R. J. (1994). *Growing up tobacco free: Preventing nicotine addiction in children and youths*. Washington, DC: National Academy Press.

Maarse, J. A. M. (2011). *Sturing op gezondheidsdoeleinden en gezondheidswinst op macroniveau. Achtergrondstudie bij RVZ-rapport: Sturen op gezondheid*. Den Haag: RVZ.

Mackay, C. (2017). Internationale samenwerking tegen tabak. *Columns NET*. Retrieved April 14, 2017, from http://columns-net.trimbos.nl/column-03-2017

Mackenbach, J. P. (2006). Antirookbeleid moet anders. *Medisch Contact*, *13*, 512–514.

Mackenbach, J. P. (2009). Echte minister van Gezondheid gezocht. *Volkskrant*.

Mackenbach, J. P. (2016). Nederland rookvrij: dokters spreken zich uit: Nu de politiek nog. *Nederlands Tijdschrift voor Geneeskunde*, *160*, D310.

Mackenbach, J. P., Klazinga, N. S., & Van der wal, G. (2004). Preventie vraagt ambitieuzere aanpak. Reactie op de kabinetsnota 'Langer gezond leven 2004–2007; ook een kwestie van gezond gedrag. *Nederlands Tijdschrift voor Geneeskunde*, *148*(15), 704–707.

Majone, G. (1992). *Evidence, argument, and persuasion in the policy process*. New Haven, CT: Yale University Press.

Malone, R. E. (2014). The symbolic and the material in tobacco control: Both matter. *Tobacco Control*, *23*(1), 1–2. https://doi.org/10.1136/tobaccocontrol-2013-051442

Mamudu, H., Dadkar, S., Veeranki, S. P., He, Y., Barnes, R., & Glantz, S. A. (2014). Multiple streams approach to tobacco control policymaking in a tobacco-growing state. *Journal of Community Health*, *39*(4), 633–645. https://doi.org/10.1007/s10900-013-9814-6

Mamudu, H., & Glantz, S. A. (2009). Civil society and the negotiation of the Framework Convention on Tobacco Control. *Global Public Health*, *4*(2), 150–168. https://doi.org/10.1080/17441690802095355

Mamudu, H., Gonzalez, M., & Glantz, S. (2011). The nature, scope, and development of the global tobacco control epistemic community. *American Journal of Public Health*, *101*(11), 2044–2054. https://doi.org/10.2105/AJPH.2011.300303

Mamudu, H. M., Cairney, P., & Studlar, D. T. (2015). Global public policy: Does the new venue for transnational tobacco control challenge the old way of doing things? *Public Administration, 93*(4), 856–873. https://doi.org/10.1111/padm.12143

Mandal, S., Gilmore, A. B., Collin, J., Weishaar, H., Smith, K., & McKee, M. (2009). Block, amend, delay: Tobacco industry efforts to influence the European Union's Tobacco Products Directive (2001/37/EC). Bath: University of Bath, School for Health.

Mantel, A., & de Wolf, P. (1983). Marktkoncentratie en internatialisatie in de Nederlandse tabaksindustrie. *Tijdschrift voor Politieke Ekonomie, 6,* 34–56.

Marks, G., & Hooghe, L. (2003). Contrasting visions of multi-level governance. In I. Bache & M. Flinders (Eds.), *Multi-level governance* (pp. 15–30). Oxford: Oxford University Press.

Marres, E. A. H., & Toet, R. L. J. (1987). Voorstellen van de SSI en de VNK ter aanpassing van de reclamecode. *Dutch Tobacco Industry Collection*, Bates No. JB2179. Retrieved from https://www.industrydocumentslibrary.ucsf.edu/tobacco/docs/tmdp0219

Martinez-Sanchez, J. M., Fernandez, E., Fu, M., Gallus, S., Martinez, C., Sureda, X., ... Clancy, L. (2010). Smoking behaviour, involuntary smoking, attitudes towards smoke-free legislations, and tobacco control activities in the European Union. *PLoS One, 5*(11), e13881. https://doi.org/10.1371/journal.pone.0013881

McCaul, K. D., Hockemeyer, J. R., Johnson, R. J., Zetocha, K., Quinlan, K., & Glasgow, R. E. (2006). Motivation to quit using cigarettes: A review. *Addictive Behaviours, 31*(1), 42–56. https://doi.org/10.1016/j.addbeh.2005.04.004

McCombs, M. (2005). A look at agenda-setting: Past, present and future. *Journalism Studies, 6,* 543–557.

McDaniel, P. A., Cadman, B., & Malone, R. E. (2016a). Shared vision, shared vulnerability: A content analysis of corporate social responsibility information on tobacco industry websites. *Preventive Medicine, 89,* 337–344. https://doi.org/10.1016/j.ypmed.2016.05.033

McDaniel, P. A., Smith, E. A., & Malone, R. E. (2016b). The tobacco endgame: A qualitative review and synthesis. *Tobacco Control, 25*(5), 594–604. https://doi.org/10.1136/tobaccocontrol-2015-052356

McNeill, A., Guignard, R., Beck, F., Marteau, R., & Marteau, T. M. (2015). Understanding increases in smoking prevalence: Case study from France in comparison with England 2000–10. *Addiction, 110*(3), 392–400. https://doi.org/10.1111/add.12789

Meeus, T.-J. (2015, November 7/8). Bericht uit Den Haag: Burger, u bent nog lang niet boos genoeg. *NRC Handelsblad,* 17.

Meijer, J. W., & Tjioe, B. K. (1990). *Maatschappelijke kosten alcoholmisbruik en tabaksgebruik.* Rotterdam: Nederlands Economisch Instituut (NEI).

Meijerink, R., & Vos, P. (2011). *Preventie van welvaartsziekten effectief en efficiënt georganiseerd.* The Hague: Raad voor de Volksgezondheid en Zorg.

Meinsma, L. (1969). *Roken en risico's.* Lochem: De Tijdstroom.

Meinsma, L. (1972). *Roken en gezondheid nu: Een nieuw rapport en samenvatting over het roken en de gevolgen daarvan voor de gezondheid van het Royal College of Physicians te London.* Naarden: Strengholt.

Meulblok, J. (1975). Advies inzake maatregelen tot beperking van de reclame voor sigaretten en shag en tot het aanbrengen van aanduidingen op de verpakkingen van sigaretten en shag. *Dutch Tobacco Industry Collection*, Bates No. JB2105. Retrieved from https://www.industrydocumentslibrary.ucsf.edu/tobacco/docs/ztbp0219

Mindell, J. S., & Whynes, D. K. (2000). Cigarette consumption in The Netherlands 1970–1995: Does tax policy encourage the use of hand-rolling tobacco? *European Journal of Public Health, 10*(3), 214–219. https://doi.org/10.1093/eurpub/10.3.214

Ministerie van Economische Zaken. (1982a). Ontmoedigingsbeleid tabaksgebruik. *Dutch Tobacco Industry Collection*, Bates No. JB2449. Retrieved from https://www.industrydocumentslibrary.ucsf.edu/tobacco/docs/#id=fyfp0219

Ministerie van Economische Zaken. (1982b). Ontmoedigingsbeleid tabaksgebruik en alcoholbeleid. *Dutch Tobacco Industry Collection*, Bates No. JB2447. Retrieved from https://www.industrydocumentslibrary.ucsf.edu/tobacco/docs/mfwp0219

Ministerie van Economische Zaken. (1984). Wetsontwerp ter verlaging van accijns op sigaretten i.v.m. eenmalige accijnsvrije prijsverhoging. *Dutch Tobacco Industry Collection*, Bates No. JB2221. Retrieved from https://www.industrydocumentslibrary.ucsf.edu/tobacco/docs/snfp0219

Ministerie van Economische Zaken. (1991). Nota Mondeling Overleg 17 oktober 1991 met vaste Commissie voor de Volksgezondheid van de Tweede Kamer inzake tabaksontmoedigingsbeleid. *Dutch Tobacco Industry Collection*, Bates No. JB2777. Retrieved from https://industrydocuments.library.ucsf.edu/tobacco/docs/lxfp0219

Ministerie van Economische Zaken. (1992). [Brief van het ministerie van EZ aan de NVS betreft sigarenaccijns]. *Dutch Tobacco Industry Collection*, Bates No. JB2464. Retrieved from https://www.industrydocumentslibrary.ucsf.edu/tobacco/docs/hgwp0219

Ministerie van Economische Zaken. (1995). Tussenrapportage Werkgroep Afspraken Tabaksbeleid. *Dutch Tobacco Industry Collection*, Bates No. JB1037.

Ministerie van Economische Zaken. (2009a). E-mails over plain packaging. *Dutch Tobacco Industry Collection*, Bates No. JB3821. Retrieved from https://www.industrydocumentslibrary.ucsf.edu/tobacco/docs/rrbn0217

Ministerie van Economische Zaken. (2009b). RE: Generieke verpakkingen voor tabaksproducten. *Dutch Tobacco Industry Collection*, Bates No. JB0505. Retrieved from https://www.industrydocumentslibrary.ucsf.edu/tobacco/docs/mtxb0191

Ministerie van Economische Zaken. (2009c). Stand van zaken invoering "plain packaging" in de Aanbeveling van de Raad inzake rookvrije ruimten. *Dutch Tobacco Industry Collection*, Bates No. JB0512. Retrieved from https://www.industrydocumentslibrary.ucsf.edu/tobacco/docs/nzxb0191

Ministerie van Economische Zaken. (2010). Dossier voor kennismakingsgesprek met tabaksindustrie. *Dutch Tobacco Industry Collection, Ministerie van Economische Zaken*, Bates No. JB0533. Retrieved from https://industrydocuments.library.ucsf.edu/tobacco/docs/lxxb0191

Ministerie van Financiën. (2011). Various e-mails. *Dutch Tobacco Industry Collection*, Bates No. JB0402. Retrieved from https://www.industrydocumentslibrary.ucsf.edu/tobacco/docs/mrhb0191

Moloughney, B. (2012). The use of policy frameworks to understand public health-related processes: A literature review. Retrieved from https://www.peelregion.ca/health/library/pdf/Policy_Frameworks.PDF

Monkhorst, T. (2002). Brief aan het ministerie van VWS over tabaksbeleid. *Dutch Tobacco Industry Collection*, Bates No. JB3528. Retrieved from https://www.industrydocumentslibrary.ucsf.edu/tobacco/docs/xncn0217

Morley, C. P., & Pratte, M. A. (2013). State-level tobacco control and adult smoking rate in the United States: An ecological analysis of structural factors. *Journal of Public Health Management Practice, 19*, E20–E27. https://doi.org/10.1097/PHH.0b013e31828000de

Moury, C. (2011). Coalition agreement and party mandate: How coalition agreements constrain the ministers. *Party Politics, 17*(3), 385–404. https://doi.org/10.1177/1354068810372099

Moury, C., & Timmermans, A. (2013). Case study three: The Netherlands. In *Coalition government and party mandate: How coalition agreements constrain ministerial action*. New York: Routledge.

Mudde, A. N., & De Vries, H. (1999). The reach and effectiveness of a national mass media-led smoking cessation campaign in the Netherlands. *American Journal of Public Health, 89*(3), 346–350. https://doi.org/10.2105/AJPH.89.3.346

Mulder, J., Bommelé, J., Branderhorst, D., & Hasselt, N. v. (2016). *De Rookvrije Generatie als kans voor gemeenten. Een needs-assessment onder gemeentelijke beleidsmakers en GGD-adviseurs*. Utrecht: Trimbos-instituut.

Nagelhout, G. E., de Vries, H., Fong, G. T., Candel, M. J., Thrasher, J. F., van den Putte, B., ... Willemsen, M. C. (2012). Pathways of change explaining the effect of smoke-free legislation on smoking cessation in The Netherlands. An application of the international tobacco control conceptual model. *Nicotine & Tobacco Research, 14*(12), 1474–1482. https://doi.org/10.1093/ntr/nts081

Nagelhout, G. E., & Fong, G. T. (2011). Netherlands: Plan to cut all health education. *Tobacco Control, 20*(4), 253–254.

Nagelhout, G. E., Levy, D. T., Blackman, K., Currie, L., Clancy, L., & Willemsen, M. C. (2012). The effect of tobacco control policies on smoking prevalence and smoking-attributable deaths. Findings from the Netherlands SimSmoke tobacco control policy simulation model. *Addiction, 107*(2), 407–416. https://doi.org/10.1111/j.1360-0443.2011.03642.x

Nagelhout, G. E., Mons, U., Allwright, S., Guignard, R., Beck, F., Fong, G. T., ... Willemsen, M. C. (2011). Prevalence and predictors of smoking in "smoke-free" bars. Findings from the International Tobacco Control (ITC) Europe Surveys. *Social Science & Medicine, 72*(10), 1643–1651. https://doi.org/10.1016/j.socscimed.2011.03.018

Nagelhout, G. E., Van den Putte, B., De Vries, H., Crone, M., Fong, G. T., & Willemsen, M. C. (2012). The influence of newspaper coverage and a media campaign on smokers' support for smoke-free bars and restaurants and on secondhand smoke harm awareness: Findings from the International Tobacco Control (ITC) Netherlands Survey. *Tobacco Control, 21*(1), 24–29. https://doi.org/10.1136/tc.2010.040477

Nagelhout, G. E., Willemsen, M. C., van den Putte, B., Crone, M., & de Vries, H. (2009). *Evaluatie 'in iedere roker zit een stopper' campagne: tweede nameting.* Den Haag: STIVORO.

Nathanson, C. A. (2005). Collective actors and corporate targets in tobacco control: A cross-national comparison. *Health Education & Behavior, 32*(3), 337–354. https://doi.org/10.1177/1090198105275047

National Cancer Institute. (2008). *The role of the media in promoting and reducing tobacco use.* NCI tobacco control monograph series (Vol. 19).

National Clearinghouse for Smoking and Health. (1969). Smoking and health programs in other countries. *Philip Morris Records,* Bates No. 2016003319–2016003331. Retrieved from http://legacy.library.ucsf.edu/tid/jdh68e00

National Research Council. (1986). *Environmental tobacco smoke: Measuring exposure and assessing health effects.* Washington, DC: National Academy Press.

Nederlands Economisch Instituut. (1991). *De evaluatie van het tabaksontmoedigingsbeleid nader beschouwd.* Rotterdam: NEI.

Nellen, M. E. A. H., & De Blij, B. A. I. M. (1999). The "success" of Philip Morris' campaign on environmental tobacco smoke in the Netherlands. *Tobacco Control, 8*(2), 221–222. https://doi.org/10.1136/tc.8.2.221a

Ngo, A., Cheng, K.-W., Chaloupka, F. J., & Shang, C. (2017). The effect of MPOWER scores on cigarette smoking prevalence and consumption. *Preventive Medicine.* Retrieved from May 11, 2017. https://doi.org/10.1016/j.ypmed.2017.05.006

Nguyen, L., Rosenqvist, G., & Pekurinen, M. (2012). *Demand for tobacco in Europe: An econometric analysis of 11 countries for the PPACTE project.* Tampere: National Institute for Health and Welfare.

Niemantsverdriet, T. (2011, November 9). Minister Edith Schippers: De vrouw van 75 miljard. *Vrij Nederland*. Retrieved from http://www.vn.nl/Archief/Politiek/Artikel-Politiek/Minister-Edith-Schippers-De-vrouw-van-75-miljard.htm

NKI-AVL. (2012). *Artsen zeggen NEE tegen tabak: Wij vragen de politiek om een effectief tabaksontmoedigingsbeleid*. Amsterdam: NKI-AVL.

NRC. (2010). Onderzoek: overheid faalt bij projecten gezondheid. *NRC Handelsblad*. Retrieved from https://www.nrc.nl/nieuws/2010/03/25/overheid-faalt-bij-projecten-gezondheid-11868351-a282303

Nuffield Council on Bioethics. (2007). *Public health: Ethical issues*. Cambridge: Cambridge Publishers Ltd.

NVK, NVS, SSI & Philip Morris Benelux. (2010). [Letter to Huijts]. *Dutch Tobacco Industry Collection*, Bates No. JB0562. Retrieved from https://www.industrydocumentslibrary.ucsf.edu/tobacco/docs/#id=hkxb0191

NVS, VNK & SSI. (1990). [Brieven van de NVS, VNK en SSI aan het ministerie van VWS en het ministerie van EZ]. *Dutch Tobacco Industry Collection*, Bates No. JB2347. Retrieved from https://www.industrydocumentslibrary.ucsf.edu/tobacco/docs/nqdp0219

O'NeillI, K., Brunnemann, K. D., Dodet, B., & Hoffmann, D. (1987). Passive smoking: Environmental carcinogens. *IARC scientific publications* (Vol. 9). Lyon: International Agency for Research on Cancer (IARC).

Obinger, H., & Wagschal, U. (2001). Families of nations and public policy. *West European Politics, 24*(1), 99–114. https://doi.org/10.1080/01402380108425419

OECD. (2014). *Health at a glance: Europe 2014*. Brussels: Organisation for Economic Co-operation and Development (OECD).

Okhuijsen, S. (2012). Fractiediscipline tweede kamer op 99,998%. Retrieved March 8, 2016, from http://sargasso.nl/fractiediscipline-tweede-kamer-op-99999/

Okkerse, W. D. (1997). *De sigarettenindustrie in Nederland: Uit (de) Balans?* Rijswijk: ITLC Associate.

Oliver, T. R. (2006). The politics of public health policy. *Annual Review of Public Health, 27*(1), 195–233. https://doi.org/10.1146/annurev.publhealth.25.101802.123126

Op de Weegh, J. M. J., & Willemsen, M. C. (2003). *Dat Kan Ik Ook!: De stoppen met roken millenniumcampagne*. Den Haag: STIVORO.

Oreskes, N., & Conway, E. M. (2010). *Merchants of doubt: How a handful of scientists obscured the truth on issues from tobacco smoke to global warning*. New York: Bloomsbury Press.

Oude Gracht Groep. (2015). Onderzoeks- en adviesrapportage m.b.t. de uitvoering van 'Artikel 5.3 van het WHO-Kaderverdrag inzake tabaksontmoediging (FCTC)' in Nederland.

Pacheco, J. (2012). The social contagion model: Exploring the role of public opinion on the diffusion of anti-smoking legislation across the American States. *Journal of Politics, 74*(1), 187–202.

Partnership Stop met Roken. (2004). *Beleidsaanbevelingen voor de behandeling van tabaksverslaving*. Den Haag: Partnership Stop met Roken.

Pasick, R. J., Onofrio, C. N., & Otero-Sabogal, R. (1996). Similarities and differences across cultures: Questions to inform a third generation of health promotion research. *Health Promotion Quarterly, 23*(Suppl 1), S142–S161.

Pauw, P. M. (1971). Televisiereclame en anti-reclame. *Dutch Tobacco Industry Collection*, Bates No. 2501265710–2501265713. Retrieved from http://legacy.library.ucsf.edu/tid/pwr22e00

Peeters, S., Costa, H., Stuckler, D., McKee, M., & Gilmore, A. B. (2016). The revision of the 2014 European tobacco products directive: An analysis of the tobacco industry's attempts to 'break the health silo'. *Tobacco Control, 25*(1), 108–117. https://doi.org/10.1136/tobaccocontrol-2014-051919

Philip Morris. (1979). Smoking & health—Five year plan. *Philip Morris Records*, Bates No. 2501020542-2501020686. Retrieved from https://www.industrydocumentslibrary.ucsf.edu/tobacco/docs/yfhl0000

Philip Morris. (1989). Several lobby letters about tax increase. *Dutch Tobacco Industry Collection*, Bates No. JB2223. Retrieved from https://www.industrydocumentslibrary.ucsf.edu/tobacco/docs/gydp0219

Philip Morris. (1993a). Marketing freedoms. *Philip Morris Records*, Bates No. 2501021740-2501021746. Retrieved from http://legacy.library.ucsf.edu/tid/wet19e00

Philip Morris. (1993b). Smoking restrictions 3 year plan. *Philip Morris Records*, Bates No. 2025497291–2025497303. Retrieved from http://legacy.library.ucsf.edu/tid/vlz88e00

Philip Morris. (1994). 1994 Action plans Benelux. *Philip Morris Records*, Bates No. 2501318291–2501318294. Retrieved from https://www.industrydocumentslibrary.ucsf.edu/tobacco/docs/pnbj0115

Philip Morris. (1996a). Corporate Affairs 1996/1997 The Netherlands. *Philip Morris Records*, Bates No. 2501076006–2501076023. Retrieved from https://www.industrydocumentslibrary.ucsf.edu/tobacco/docs/nzjl0112

Philip Morris. (1996b). Verhoging van de accijns op tabaksproducten. *Dutch Tobacco Industry Collection*, Bates No. JB2661. Retrieved from https://www.industrydocumentslibrary.ucsf.edu/tobacco/docs/hpwp0219

Prins, G. J. J. (2003). Verhoging tabaksaccijns. *Dutch Tobacco Industry Collection*, Bates No. JB0600. Retrieved from https://www.industrydocumentslibrary.ucsf.edu/tobacco/docs/mmxb0191

Rabe, B. (2013). Political impediments to a tobacco endgame. *Tobacco Control, 22*, i52–i54. https://doi.org/10.1136/tobaccocontrl-2012-050799

Radaelli, C. M. (1995). The role of knowledge in the policy process. *Journal of European Public Policy, 2*, 159–183.

Rathjen, H. (1999). *The coalition. How to build a coalition in connection with a public health campaign to obtain tobacco control measures.* Quebec: Coalition Québécoise pur le contrôle du tabac.

Raw, M., McNeill, A., & West, R. (1998). Smoking cessation guidelines for health professionals. *Thorax, 53*(Suppl 5, Part 1), S1–S18.

Reid, D. J., Killoran, A. J., McNeill, A. D., & Chambers, J. S. (1992). Choosing the most effective health promotion options for reducing a nation's smoking prevalence. *Tobacco Control, 1*(3), 185. https://doi.org/10.1136/tc.1.3.185

Reid, R. (2005). *Globalizing tobacco control: Anti-smoking campaigns in California, France, and Japan.* Bloomington, IN: Indiana University Press.

Remes, D. (1988). The PM EEC/EEMA ETS Project—Draft—20 Feb 1988. *Ness Motley Law Firm Documents*, Bates No. 2501474253–2501474259. Retrieved from https://www.industrydocumentslibrary.ucsf.edu/tobacco/docs/psly0042

Rennen, E., Nagelhout, G. E., Van den Putte, B., Janssen, E., Mons, U., Guignard, R., … Willemsen, M. C. (2014). Associations between tobacco control policy awareness, social acceptability of smoking and smoking cessation. Findings from the International Tobacco Control (ITC) Europe Surveys. *Health Education Research, 29*(1), 72–82. https://doi.org/10.1093/her/cyt073

Rennen, E., & Willemsen, M. C. (2012). *Dutch tobacco control: Out of control? FCTC shadow report 2011.* Amsterdam: KWF Kankerbestrijding.

Rijksen, W. (2005). Evaluatie van het tabaksontmoedigingsbeleid [letter KNMG]. *Dutch Tobacco Industry Collection*, Bates No. JB2971. Retrieved from https://www.industrydocumentslibrary.ucsf.edu/tobacco/docs/qsdn0217

Rijsterborgh, I. J. (2017). *The importance of the tobacco industry for the Dutch economy.* Maastricht: Maastricht University.

Rinnooy-Kan, A. H. G. (1994). Letter to VWS. *Dutch Tobacco Industry Collection*, Bates No. JB2591. Retrieved from https://www.industrydocumentslibrary.ucsf.edu/tobacco/docs/jmwp0219

Rinnooy-Kan, A. H. G. (1995a). Letter to Minister Wijers. *Dutch Tobacco Industry Collection*, Bates No. JB2589. Retrieved from https://www.industrydocumentslibrary.ucsf.edu/tobacco/docs/hkfp0219

Rinnooy-Kan, A. H. G. (1995b). Letter to VWS. *Dutch Tobacco Industry Collection*, Bates No. JB2590. Retrieved from https://www.industrydocumentslibrary.ucsf.edu/tobacco/docs/xmwp0219

RIVM. (1993). *Volksgezondheid Toekomst Verkenning: De gezondheidstoestand van de Nederlandse bevolking in de periode 1950–2010. Kernboodschappen.* Den Haag: SdU Uitgeverij.

RIVM. (1997). *Volksgezondheids Toekomst Verkenning 1991: De som der delen.* Bilthoven: Rijksinstituut voor Volksgezondheid en Milieu.

RIVM. (2002). *Gezondheid op koers? Volksgezondheid Toekomst Verkenning 2002.* Bilthoven: Rijksinstituut voor Volksgezondheid en Milieu.

RIVM. (2006). *Zorg voor gezondheid—Volksgezondheid Toekomst Verkenning 2006*. Bilthoven: Rijksinstituut voor Volksgezondheid en Milieu.

RIVM. (2010). *Van gezond naar beter. Volksgezondheid Toekomst Verkenning 2010*. Bilthoven: Rijksinstituut voor Volksgezondheid en Milieu.

RIVM. (2014). *A healthier Netherlands: Key findings from the Dutch 2014 Public Health Status and Foresight Report*. Bilthoven: Rijksinstituut voor Volksgezondheid en Milieu.

RIVM. (2017). Sterfgevallen door ziekten als gevolg van roken, 2013. Retrieved April 28, 2017, from https://www.volksgezondheidenzorg.info/onderwerp/roken/cijfers-context/oorzaken-en-gevolgen#node-sterfte-en-verloren-levensjaren-door-roken

RJ Reynolds. (1978). Chapter 1 smoking and health. *RJ Reynolds Records*, Bates No. 500534913–500534931. Retrieved from https://www.industrydocumentslibrary.ucsf.edu/tobacco/docs/llmf0099

RJ Reynolds. (1979). Summary of the PR Program of the Dutch Cigarette Manufactures Association. *RJ Reynolds Records*, Bates No. 500877429–500877431. Retrieved from https://www.industrydocumentslibrary.ucsf.edu/tobacco/docs/jrpj0096

Roelofs, W. J. (1996a). Letter to VWS. *Dutch Tobacco Industry Collection*, Bates No. JB2175. Retrieved from https://www.industrydocumentslibrary.ucsf.edu/tobacco/docs/pmdp0219

Roelofs, W. J. (1996b). Tabaksontmoedigingsbeleid. *Dutch Tobacco Industry Collection*, Bates No. JB2687. Retrieved from https://www.industrydocumentslibrary.ucsf.edu/tobacco/docs/pqwp0219

Roelofs, W. J. (1998). Tabaksontmoedigingsbeleid. *Dutch Tobacco Industry Collection*, Bates No. JB2391. Retrieved from https://www.industrydocumentslibrary.ucsf.edu/tobacco/docs/psdp0219

Roelofs, W. J. (2000a). [Letter to Minister Borst]. *Dutch Tobacco Industry Collection*, Bates No. JB2402. Retrieved from https://www.industrydocumentslibrary.ucsf.edu/tobacco/docs/xtdp0219

Roelofs, W. J. (2000b). [Letter to Prime Minister Kok]. *Dutch Tobacco Industry Collection*, Bates No. JB0349. Retrieved from https://www.industrydocumentslibrary.ucsf.edu/tobacco/docs/hyhb0191

Roelofs, W. J. (2001). Accijnskrediet. *Dutch Tobacco Industry Collection*, Bates No. JB1755. Retrieved from https://www.industrydocumentslibrary.ucsf.edu/tobacco/docs/xkcp0219

Roemer, R. (1982). *Legislative action to combat the world smoking epidemic*. Geneva: WHO.

Roessingh, H. K. (1976). *Inlandse tabak: Expansie en contractie van een handelsgewas in de 17e en 18e eeuw in Nederland* (Doctoral dissertation), Landbouw Hogeschool, Wageningen.

Rommetvedt, H., Thesen, G., Christiansen, P. M., & Nørgaard, A. S. (2012). Coping with corporatism in decline and the revival of parliament: Interest

group lobbyism in Denmark and Norway, 1980–2005. *Comparative Political Studies, 46*, 457–485.
Roos, M. J. (1985). Tabakswet. *Dutch Tobacco Industry Collection*, Bates No. JB2433. Retrieved from https://www.industrydocumentslibrary.ucsf.edu/tobacco/docs/pzdp0219
Roscam Abbing, E. W. (1992). Tabaksbeleid: rookgordijn voor massamoord. *Medisch Contact, 47*, 931.
Roscam Abbing, E. W. (1998). *Tabaksontmoedigingsbeleid: Gezondheidseffectrapportage*. Utrecht: Netherlands School of Public Health (NSPH).
Rose, G. (1992). *The strategy of preventive medicine*. Oxford: Oxford University Press.
Royal College of Physicians. (1962a). *Roken en gezondheid. Een rapport van de Koninklijk Genootschap van Londense artsen over roken in verband met longkanker en andere aandoeningen*. Amsterdam: Strengholt.
Royal College of Physicians. (1962b). *Smoking and health*. London: Royal College of Physicians of London.
Royal College of Physicians. (1971). Smoking and health now. A new report and summary on smoking and its effects on health. *Annals of Internal Medicine, 75*(1), 147–148. https://doi.org/10.7326/0003-4819-75-1-147
Royal College of Physicians. (2016). *Nicotine without smoke: Tobacco harm reduction*. London: Royal College of Physicians.
Ruiter, R., & Kok, G. (2006). Response to Hammond et al. showing leads to doing, but doing what? The need for experimental pilot-testing. *European Journal of Public Health, 16*, 225. https://doi.org/10.1093/eurpub/ckl014
Rutgers, M., Hanselaar, T., Stam, H., & Van Gennip, L. (2007). Letters to Klink. *Dutch Tobacco Industry Collection*, Bates No. JB0455. Retrieved from https://www.industrydocumentslibrary.ucsf.edu/tobacco/docs/rzhb0191
RVZ. (2010). *Perspectief op gezondheid 20/20*. Den Haag: Raad voor de Volksgezondheid en Zorg.
RVZ. (2011a). *Preventie van welvaartsziekten. Effectief en efficiënt georganiseerd*. Den Haag: Raad voor de Volksgezondheid en Zorg (RVZ).
RVZ. (2011b). *Sturen op gezondheidsdoelen*. Den Haag: Raad voor de Volksgezondheid en Zorg.
Sabatier, P. A. (1998). The advocacy coalition framework: Revisions and relevance for Europe. *Journal of European Public Policy, 5*(1), 98–130. https://doi.org/10.1080/13501768880000051
Sabatier, P. A. (2007). *Theories of the policy process* (2nd ed.). Cambridge, MA: Westview Press.
Sabatier, P. A., & Weible, C. M. (2007). The advocacy coalition framework: Innovations and clarifications. In P. A. Sabatier (Ed.), *Theories of the policy process* (2nd ed.). Cambridge, MA: Westview Press.

Sarewitz, D. (2004). How science makes environmental controversies worse. *Environmental Science and Policy, 7*, 385–403.
Sato, H. (1999). The advocacy coalition framework and the policy process analysis: The case of smoking control in Japan. *Policy Studies Journal, 27*(1), 28–44. https://doi.org/10.1111/j.1541-0072.1999.tb01951.x
Schama, S. (1987). *The embarrassment of riches: An interpretation of Dutch culture in the Golden Age*. New York: Vintage Books.
Scharpf, F. W. (1997). *Games real actors play: Actor-centred institutionalism in policy research*. Oxford: Westview Press.
Scheltema Beduin, A., & Ter Weele, W. (2015). *Lifting the lid on lobbying: Enhancing trust in public decisionmaking in the Netherlands*. Amsterdam: Transparency International Nederland.
Schipper, J. W. (1999a). [Brief van Philip Morris aan het ministerie van Economische Zaken betreft Overleg d.d. 14 juni 1999]. *Dutch Tobacco Industry Collection*, Bates No. JB2419. Retrieved from https://www.industrydocumentslibrary.ucsf.edu/tobacco/docs/ztdp0219
Schipper, J. W. (1999b). [Letter to Minister Jorritsma]. *Dutch Tobacco Industry Collection*, Bates No. JB2111. Retrieved from https://www.industrydocumentslibrary.ucsf.edu/tobacco/docs/gkdp0219
Schippers, E. J. (2010). Beleidsvoornemens tabaksontmoediging [letter to SSI and VNK]. *Dutch Tobacco Industry Collection*, Bates No. JB0562. Retrieved from https://www.industrydocumentslibrary.ucsf.edu/tobacco/docs/hkxb0191
Schraven, J. H. (2001a). [Letter VNO-NCW to Borst-Eilers]. *Dutch Tobacco Industry Collection*, Bates No. JB3560. Retrieved from https://www.industrydocumentslibrary.ucsf.edu/tobacco/docs/njwn0217
Schraven, J. H. (2001b). Regulier overleg tabaksontmoedigingsbeleid. *Dutch Tobacco Industry Collection*, Bates No. JB0271. Retrieved from https://www.industrydocumentslibrary.ucsf.edu/tobacco/docs/ljhb0191
Schraven, J. H. (2003a). [Letter VNO-NCW to Ross-van Dorp]. *Dutch Tobacco Industry Collection*, Bates No. JB3557. Retrieved from https://www.industrydocumentslibrary.ucsf.edu/tobacco/docs/sxdn0217
Schraven, J. H. (2003b). Regulier overleg tabaksontmoedigingsbeleid. *Dutch Tobacco Industry Collection*, Bates No. JB0269. Retrieved from https://www.industrydocumentslibrary.ucsf.edu/tobacco/docs/jjhb0191
Schwartz, R., & Johnson, T. (2010). Problems, policies and politics: A comparative case study of contraband tobacco from the 1990s to the present in the Canadian context. *Journal of Public Health Policy, 31*(3), 342–354.
Schwartz, R., & Rosen, B. (2004). The politics of evidence-based health policymaking. *Public Money & Management, 24*(2), 121–127. https://doi.org/10.1111/j.1467-9302.2004.00404.x

Schwartz, S. (2006). A theory of cultural value orientations: Explication and applications. *Comparative Sociology,* 5(2), 137–182. https://doi.org/10.1163/156913306778667357

Science & Strategy. (1996). Inventaristatie van de martketingactiviteiten van de tabaksindustrie. *Dutch Tobacco Industry Collection,* Bates No. JB1537. Retrieved from https://www.industrydocumentslibrary.ucsf.edu/tobacco/docs/jmbp0219

SCOTH. (1998). *Report of the Scientific Committee on tobacco and health.* London: Department of Health.

Shiffman, J., Quissell, K., Schmitz, H., Pelletier, D., Smith, S., Berlan, D., ... Walt, G. (2015). A framework on the emergence and effectiveness of global health networks. *Health Policy Plan, 31,* i3–i16. https://doi.org/10.1093/heapol/czu046

Siaroff, A. (1999). Corporatism in 24 industrial democracies: Meaning and measurement. *European Journal of Political Research, 36,* 175–205.

Sims, M., Salway, R., Langley, T., Lewis, S., McNeill, A., Szatkowski, L., & Gilmore, A. B. (2014). Effectiveness of tobacco control television advertising in changing tobacco use in England: A population-based cross-sectional study. *Addiction, 109*(6), 986–994. https://doi.org/10.1111/add.12501

Slama, K. (1995). Resolutions of the Ninth World Conference on Tobacco and Health. In K. Slama (Ed.), *Tobacco and Health* (pp. 1017–1018). New York: Springer.

Slob, M., & Staman, J. (2012). *Beleid en het bewijsbeest: Een verkenning van verwachtingen en praktijken rond evidence based policy.* Den Haag: Rathenau Instituut.

Smid, E. (2007). [Letter to Ministry of VWS]. *Dutch Tobacco Industry Collection,* Bates No. JB3477. Retrieved from https://www.industrydocumentslibrary.ucsf.edu/tobacco/docs/gffn0217

Smith, E. A. (2007). 'It's interesting how few people die from smoking': Tobacco industry efforts to minimize risk and discredit health promotion. *The European Journal of Public Health, 17*(2), 162–170. https://doi.org/10.1093/eurpub/ckl097

Smith, E. A., & Malone, R. E. (2007). We will speak as the smoker: The tobacco industry's smokers' rights groups. *European Journal of Public Health, 17*(3), 306–313. https://doi.org/10.1093/eurpub/ckl244

Smith, K. (2013). *Beyond evidence-based policy in public health: The interplay of ideas.* London: Palgrave Macmillan.

Smith, K. E. (2013). Understanding the influence of evidence in public health policy: What can we learn from the 'Tobacco Wars'? *Social Policy & Administration, 47*(4), 382–398. https://doi.org/10.1111/spol.12025

Smith, K. E., Fooks, G., Collin, J., Weishaar, H., Mandal, S., & Gilmore, A. B. (2010). "Working the System"—British American Tobacco's influence on the European Union treaty and its implications for policy: An analysis of internal tobacco industry documents. *PLoS Medicine,* 7(1), e1000202. https://doi.org/10.1371/journal.pmed.1000202

Smith, K. E., Fooks, G., Gilmore, A. B., Collin, J., & Weishaar, H. (2015). Corporate coalitions and policy making in the European Union: How and why British American Tobacco promoted "Better Regulation". *Journal of Health Politics, Policy and Law,* 40(2), 325–372. https://doi.org/10.1215/03616878-2882231

SNK & SSI. (1985). Jaaroverzicht 1984. *Dutch Tobacco Industry Collection,* Bates No. JB2269. Retrieved from https://www.industrydocumentslibrary.ucsf.edu/tobacco/docs/yfgp0219

Spijkerman, R., & van den Ameele, A. N. (2001). *Roken op het werk 2000 (een herhalingsonderzoek).* Den Haag: Arbeidsinspectie.

SRJ. (2017). Smokers bring case against the tobacco industry. Retrieved from http://www.stichtingrookpreventiejeugd.nl/over-rookpreventie-jeugd/english/item/86-smokers-bring-case-against-the-tobacco-industry

SSI. (1983). Ontmoedigingsbeleid tabak. *Dutch Tobacco Industry Collection,* Bates No. JB2225. Retrieved from https://www.industrydocumentslibrary.ucsf.edu/tobacco/docs/#id=hydp0219

SSI. (1984). [Letter to Ministry of Economic Affairs]. *Dutch Tobacco Industry Collection,* Bates No. JB3980. Retrieved from https://www.industrydocumentslibrary.ucsf.edu/tobacco/docs/zzwp0219

SSI. (1991). [Correspondence with Ministries of Economic Affairs and Finance]. *Dutch Tobacco Industry Collection,* Bates No. JB2354. Retrieved from https://www.industrydocumentslibrary.ucsf.edu/tobacco/docs/tqdp0219

SSI. (2001). [Letter to ministries of VWS and Economic Affairs]. *Dutch Tobacco Industry Collection,* Bates No. JB3498. Retrieved from https://www.industrydocumentslibrary.ucsf.edu/tobacco/docs/pmcn0217

SSI. (2002). Tabaksontmoedigingsbeleid [Letter to Bomhoff] *Dutch Tobacco Industry Collection,* Bates No. JB3526. Retrieved from https://www.industrydocumentslibrary.ucsf.edu/tobacco/docs/hncn0217

SSI & SNK. (1984). Jaaroverzicht 1983. *Dutch Tobacco Industry Collection,* Bates No. JB2268. Retrieved from https://www.industrydocumentslibrary.ucsf.edu/tobacco/docs/#id=nfgp0219

SSI, & Toet, R. L. (1972–1996). Collection of industry lobby letters about tobacco price and taxation. *Dutch Tobacco Industry Collection,* Bates No. JB2000. Retrieved from https://www.industrydocumentslibrary.ucsf.edu/tobacco/docs/fxfp0219

SSI & VNK. (2007). Overleg met VNO-NCW en de tabaksindustrie (SSI, VNK en NVS). *Dutch Tobacco Industry Collection,* Bates No. JB0454. Retrieved from https://www.industrydocumentslibrary.ucsf.edu/tobacco/docs/qzhb0191

SSI & VNK. (2009). [Letter to Klink concerning talks about WHO FCTC draft guidelines on December 11]. *Dutch Tobacco Industry Collection,* Bates No. JB0413. Retrieved from https://www.industrydocumentslibrary.ucsf.edu/tobacco/docs/hshb0191

Stewart, E., & Smith, K. (2015). 'Black magic' and 'gold dust': The epistemic and political uses of evidence tools in public health policy making. *Evidence & Policy, 11*, 415–437.
Stichting van de Arbeid. (1992). Aanbeveling over de bescherming van de niet-roker op het werk. *Dutch Tobacco Industry Collection*, Bates No. JB2035. Retrieved from https://www.industrydocumentslibrary.ucsf.edu/tobacco/docs/khdp0219
STIVORO. (1978). *Een gulden per jaar: Beleidslijnen van de Stichting Volksgezondheid en Roken*. Den Haag: STIVORO.
STIVORO. (1985). *Reclame als pacemaker van de tabaksindustrie*. Den Haag: STIVORO.
STIVORO. (1999). *25 jaar STIVORO: een goed begin [year report]*. Den Haag: STIVORO.
STIVORO. (2005). *Nationaal Programma Tabaksontmoediging 2006–2010*. Den Haag: STIVORO.
STIVORO. (2007). 7,4 miljoen te weinig om gewenste daling rokers te halen [press release 9 januari 2007]. In STIVORO (Ed.). Den Haag: STIVORO.
STIVORO. (2009). *Terugblik 2008 [Year report]*. Den Haag: STIVORO.
STIVORO. (2010a). Tabaksontmoediging moet anders [newsletter] *STIVORO. nl* (Vol. 14). Den Haag: STIVORO.
STIVORO. (2010b). *Van onderop en van bovenaf: De toekomst van tabaksontmoediging in Nederland 2011–2020*. Den Haag: STIVORO.
STIVORO. (2012). *Hoe ontmoediging verdween uit het tabaksontmoedigingsbeleid [Year Report 2011]*. Den Haag: STIVORO.
Stone, D. (2001). Learning lessons, policy transfer and the international diffusion of policy ideas. *CSGR Working Paper No. 69/01*.
Stronks, K., van de Mheen, H. D., Looman, C. W. N., & Mackenbach, J. P. (1997). Cultural, material, and psychosocial correlates of the socioeconomic gradient in smoking behavior among adults. *Preventive Medicine, 26*(5), 754–766. https://doi.org/10.1006/pmed.1997.0174
Studlar, D. T. (2002). *Tobacco control: Comparative politics in the United States and Canada*. Peterborough, ON, Canada: Broadview Press.
Studlar, D. T. (2006). Tobacco control policy instruments in a shrinking world: How much policy learning? *International Journal of Public Administration, 29*, 367–396. https://doi.org/10.1080/01900690500437006
Studlar, D. T. (2007a). Ideas, institutions and diffusion: What explains tobacco control policy in Australia, Canada and New Zealand? *Commonwealth & Comparative Politics, 45*(2), 164–184. https://doi.org/10.1080/14662040701317493
Studlar, D. T. (2007b). *What explains policy change in tobacco control policy in advanced industrial democracies?* Paper presented at the European Consortium of Political Research, Helsinki.

Studlar, D. T. (2015). Punching above their weight through policy learning: Tobacco control policies in Ireland. *Irish Political Studies, 30*, 41–78.

Studlar, D. T., & Cairney, P. (2014). Conceptualizing punctuated and non-punctuated policy change: Tobacco control in comparative perspective. *International Review of Administrative Sciences, 80*(3), 513–531. https://doi.org/10.1177/0020852313517997

Taylor, P. (1984). *The smoke ring: Tobacco, money & multinational politics.* London: Sphere Books.

Tesh, S. N. (1988). *Hidden arguments: Political ideology and disease prevention policy.* New Brunswick, NJ: Rutgers University Press.

Thieme, M., & Engelen, E. (2016). *De kanarie in de kolenmijn.* Amsterdam: Prometheus.

Thun, M., Peto, R., Boreham, J., & Lopez, A. D. (2012). Stages of the cigarette epidemic on entering its second century. *Tobacco Control, 21*(2), 96–101. https://doi.org/10.1136/tobaccocontrol-2011-050294

Thyrian, J. R., & John, U. (2006). Measuring activities in tobacco control across the EU. The MATOC. *Substance Abuse Treatment, Prevention, and Policy, 1*, 9. https://doi.org/10.1186/1747-597X-1-9

Timmers, R., & Van der Wijst, P. (2007). Images as anti-smoking fear appeals: The effects of emotion on the persuasion process. *Information Design Journal, 15*, 21–36.

TNS Opinion & Social. (2006). *Special Eurobarometer 239: Attitudes of Europeans towards tobacco.* Brussels: European Commission.

TNS Opinion & Social. (2010). *Special Eurobarometer 332: Tobacco.* Brussels: European Commission.

TNS Opinion & Social. (2012). *Special Eurobarometer 385: Attitudes of Europeans towards tobacco.* Brussels: European Commission.

Tobacco Free Initiative. (2003). *Tobacco industry and corporate responsibility…an inherent contradiction.* Geneva: WHO.

Tobacco Free Initiative. (2008). *Tobacco industry interference with tobacco control.* Geneva: WHO.

Tobacco Manufacturers' Assocation. (1971). Gentlemen's agreement. *Philip Morris Collection*, Bates No. 2501265714–2501265715. Retrieved from http://legacy.library.ucsf.edu/tid/qwr22e00

Toet, R. L. J. (1994). Reclamecode voor tabaksprodukten [letter]. *Dutch Tobacco Industry Collection*, Bates No. JB2533. Retrieved from https://www.industrydocumentslibrary.ucsf.edu/tobacco/docs/kjwp0219

Trappenburg, M. (2005). *Gezondheidszorg en democratie [inaugural lecture].* Rotterdam: Erasmus University.

Tubiana, M. (1994). [Letter from Tubiana to Borst-Eilers and Prime Minister Kok]. *Dutch Tobacco Industry Collection*, Bates No. JB2584. Retrieved from https://www.industrydocumentslibrary.ucsf.edu/tobacco/docs/hphp0219

U.S. Department of Health and Human Services. (1988). *The health consequences of smoking: Nicotine Addiction*. Washington: Public Health Service, Centers for Disease Control, Center for Chronic Disease Prevention and Health Promotion, Office on Smoking and Health.

U.S. Department of Health and Human Services. (2000). *Reducing tobacco use: A report of the Surgeon General*. Atlanta: U.S. Department of Health and Human Services, Centers for Disease Control and Prevention, National Center for Chronic Disease Prevention and Health Promotion, Office on Smoking and Health.

U.S. Department of Health, Education, and Welfare. (1964). *Smoking and health: Report of the Advisory Committee to the Surgeon General of the Public Health Service (Vol. DHEW publication no. (PHS) 64-1103)*. Washington, DC: Public Health Service.

UICC. (1996). Philip Morris campaign on passive smoking. *Dutch Tobacco Industry Collection*, Bates No. JB1186. Retrieved from https://www.industrydocumentslibrary.ucsf.edu/tobacco/docs/kkxp0219

Unger, J. B., Cruz, T., Baezconde-Garbanati, L., Shakib, S., Palmer, P., Johnson, C. A., … Gritz, E. (2003). Exploring the cultural context of tobacco use: A transdisciplinary framework. *Nicotine & Tobacco Research*, 5(Suppl 1), S101–S117. https://doi.org/10.1080/14622200310001625546

Unknown (Philip Morris). (1979). *Smoking & health—Five year plan*, Bates No 2501020542–2501020686. Truth Tobacco Industry Documents.

US Public Health Service. (1970). Smoking and health programs around the world. *American Tobacco Records*, Bates No. 968012023–968012038. Retrieved from http://legacy.library.ucsf.edu/tid/cob34f00

US Surgeon General. (1986). *The health consequences of involuntary smoking*. Rockville: USDHHS.

Van Aelst, P., & Vliegenthart, R. (2013). Studying the tango. *Journalism Studies*, 15(4), 392–410. https://doi.org/10.1080/1461670X.2013.831228

Van Baal, P. H. M., Brouwer, W. B. F., Hoogenveen, R. T., & Feenstra, T. L. (2007). Increasing tobacco taxes: A cheap tool to increase public health. *Health Policy*, 82(2), 142–152. https://doi.org/10.1016/j.healthpol.2006.09.004

Van Berkum, M. (2016). Pionieren met nieuwe filosofie. Retrieved April 29, 2017, from https://www.gezondin.nu/thema/roken/blog/43-pionieren-met-nieuwe-filosofie

Van Bladeren, F. (2011). Netherlands: Going backwards [news analysis]. *Tobacco Control*, 20, 4–7.

Van de Mortel, J. L. P. M. (1996). Reactie op de concept nota inzake tabaksontmoedigingsbeleid. *Dutch Tobacco Industry Collection*, Bates No. JB2518. Retrieved from https://www.industrydocumentslibrary.ucsf.edu/tobacco/docs/nxwp0219

Van de Mortel, P. M., & Roelofs, W. J. (1996). Concept-notitie interdepartementale werkgroep accijns. *Dutch Tobacco Industry Collection*, Bates No. JB2070.

Retrieved from https://www.industrydocumentslibrary.ucsf.edu/tobacco/docs/zxdp0219
Van de Wetering, C. (2010). Niek Jan van Kesteren, directeur VNO-NCW. De onzichtbare onderhandelaar. Retrieved from http://www.pm.nl/artikel/640/niek-jan-van-kesteren-de-onzichtbare-onderhandelaar
Van den Berg, P. J. C. M., & Kabel, D. L. (2010). Achtergrond en opzet van de brede heroverwegingen. *Tijdschrift voor Openbare Financieën, 42*(2), 69–75.
Van den Braak, B. H., & Van den Berg, J. T. J. (2017a). Historisch overzicht cijfers kabinetten. *Parlement & Politiek*. Retrieved July 20, 2017, from https://www.parlement.com/id/vht7jba3jsy6/historisch_overzicht_cijfers_kabinetten
Van den Braak, B. H., & Van den Berg, J. T. J. (2017b). Kabinetsformatie sinds 1945. *Parlement & Politiek*. Retrieved August 23, 2017, from http://www.parlement.com/id/vh8lnhrsr2z2/kabinetsformaties_sinds_1945
Van den Putte, S. J. H. M., Yzer, M. C., Ten Berg, B. M., & Steeveld, R. M. A. (2005). *Nederland start met stoppen/Nederland gaat door met stoppen. Evaluatie van de STIVORO campagnes rondom de jaarwisseling 2003–2004*. Amsterdam: Universiteit van Amsterdam, ASCOR.
Van der Bles, W. (1996). Boze Wijers treedt toe tot het gezelschap anti-rookmagiërs. Retrieved from http://www.trouw.nl/tr/nl/5009/Archief/article/detail/2632148/1996/09/06/Boze-Wijers-treedt-toe-tot-het-gezelschap-anti-rookmagiers.dhtml
Van der Kemp, S., & Bekker, B. (2007). Wat is effectief? De kruistocht van Kok. *TSG, 85*, 236–238.
Van der Laan, S. (2015). Politiek ziet rookverbod op terras (nog) niet zitten. Retrieved October 14, 2015, from http://www.elsevier.nl/Nederland/achtergrond/2015/9/Politiek-ziet-rookvrij-terras-nog-niet-zitten-2679393W/?masterpageid=158493
Van der Lugt, P. (Producer). (2016, May 20). Nieuwe tabaksregels dwingen industrie tot bezinning. [Written article]. Retrieved from https://www.ftm.nl/artikelen/nieuwe-sigarettenpakjes-doen-harde-tabakslobby-veranderen
Van der Meer, R., Spruijt, R., & De Beer, M. (2012). *Zoeken naar Nieuwe Kansen voor Lokaal Gezondheidsbeleid en Roken Project Structureel Aanbod Gemeenten Tabakspreventie Eindrapportage 2011*. The Hague: STIVORO.
Van der Poel, T., & Gutter, A. (2011). Transcripten interviews. *Dutch Tobacco Industry Collection*, Bates No. JB0561. Retrieved from https://www.industrydocumentslibrary.ucsf.edu/tobacco/results/#q=transcripten%20interviews&col=%5B%22Dutch%20Tobacco%20Industry%20Collection%22%5D&h=%7B%22hideDuplicates%22%3Atrue%2C%22hideFolders%22%3Atrue%7D&subsite=tobacco&cache=true&count=3
Van der Voet, G. W. (2005). *De kwaliteit van de WMCZ als medezeggenschapswet*. Den Haag: Boom Juridische Uitgevers.
Van der Wilk, E. A., Melse, J. M., Den Broeder, J. M., & Achterberg, P. W. (2007). *Leren van de buren: Beleid publieke gezondheid internationaal bezien: roken,*

alcohol, overgewicht, depressie, gezondheidsachterstanden, jeugd, screening. Houten: Bohn Stafleu Van Loghum.

Van Emst, A. J., & Willemsen, M. C. (2011). *Naar een nieuwe structuur voor tabaksontmoediging in Nederland: Verslag van een inspirational conference*. Den Haag: STIVORO.

Van Es, J. (1987). Roken. *Medisch Contact*, 42, 259.

Van Gelder, H. (1990). Rokers maken een vuist. Retrieved from http://www.nrc.nl/nieuws/1990/01/08/rokers-maken-een-vuist-6921081-a1190151

Van Gennip, E. M. S. J. (2007). Brief STIVORO aan Ministerie van Algemene Zaken over beleidsvoornemen om de horeca-rookvrij te maken. *Dutch Tobacco Industry Collection*, Bates No. JB0344. Retrieved from https://www.industrydocumentslibrary.ucsf.edu/tobacco/docs/snhb0191

Van Herten, L. M., & Gunning-Schepers, L. J. Targets as a tool in health policy. *Health Policy*, 53(1), 1–11. https://doi.org/10.1016/S0168-8510(00)00081-6

Van Hoogstraten, S. (1997a). Besluitenlijst overleg 'Aanscherping RvT'. *Dutch Tobacco Industry Collection*, Bates No. JB2196. Retrieved from https://www.industrydocumentslibrary.ucsf.edu/tobacco/docs/zxfp0219

Van Hoogstraten, S. (1997b). Gewijzigde definitieve verslag van de Hoordag op 2 September. *Dutch Tobacco Industry Collection*, Bates No. JB2079. Retrieved from https://www.industrydocumentslibrary.ucsf.edu/tobacco/docs/jpxp0219

Van Laar, M. W., & Van Ooyen-Houben, M. M. J. (2016). *Nationale Drug Monitor*. Utrecht: Trimbos-Institute.

Van Leeuwen, M. J., & Sleur, D. G. (1998). De economische effecten van maatregelen ter bestrijding van het roken. In E. Roscam Abbing (Ed.), *Tabaksontmoedigingsbeleid: Gezondheidseffectrapportage*. Utrecht: Netherlands School of Public Health (NSPH).

Van Londen, J. (1980). Voorstellen ICBT inzake beperking tabakreclame en verkooppunten tabaksproducten. *Dutch Tobacco Industry Collection*, Bates No. JB1801. Retrieved from https://www.industrydocumentslibrary.ucsf.edu/tobacco/docs/ffdp0219

Van Noije, L., Kleinnijenhuis, J., & Oegema, D. (2008). Loss of parliamentary control due to mediatization and Europeanization: A longitudinal and cross-sectional analysis of agenda building in the United Kingdom and the Netherlands. *British Journal of Political Science*, 38, 455–478.

Van Oosten, R. (1996). Introductie landelijke belangenvereniging van tabaksdustributeurs Nederland. *Dutch Tobacco Industry Collection*, Bates No. JB2671. Retrieved from https://www.industrydocumentslibrary.ucsf.edu/tobacco/docs/pggp0219

Van Outeren, E., & Pergrim, C. (2015, November 11). Weer zet de denaat er een streep door. *NRC Handelsblad*, 9.

Van Proosdij, C. (1957). *Smoking, its influence in the individual and its role in social medicine [Roken: Een individueel- en sociaalgeneeskundige studie]*. PhD thesis, University of Amsterdam, Amsterdam.

Van Rijn, M. (2014). Onderzoeken naar effecten verkooppunten en leeftijdverificatiesystemen tabaksproducten. *Kamerbrief 626288-122861-VGP*.
Van Ronkel, H. (1996). Overheid schendt gemaakte afspraken. *Dutch Tobacco Industry Collection*, Bates No. JB2174. Retrieved from https://www.industrydocumentslibrary.ucsf.edu/tobacco/docs/zqfp0219
Van Tulder, R. (1999). Small, smart and sustainable? Policy challenges to the Dutch model of governance (together) with multinationals. In R. Narula & R. van Hoesel (Eds.), *Multinational enterprises from the Netherlands*. London: Routledge.
Van Vliet, G. F. W. (1971). Gentlemen's agreement manufacturers on publicity vs. smoking and health. *Philip Morris Collection*, Bates No. 2501265716. Retrieved from http://legacy.library.ucsf.edu/tid/rwr22e00
Vandenbroucke, J. P., Kok, J. F. J., Matroos, A., & Dekker, E. (1981). Rookgewoonten van Nederlandse huisartsen vergeleken met die van de bevolking. *Nederlands Tijdschrift voor Geneeskunde, 125*(1), 406.
VARA. (2011). Minister of Tobacco [TV documentary]. *Zembla*. Retrieved July 26, 2017, from https://zembla.vara.nl/nieuws/minister-of-tobacco
Verdonk-Kleinjan, W. M. (2014). *Impact assessment of the tobacco legislation: Effects of the workplace smoking ban and the tobacco sales ba to minors*. PhD, Maastricht University, Maastricht.
Verdurmen, J., Monshouwer, K., & Van Laar, M. (2014). *Roken Jeugd Monitor 2013*. Utrecht: Trimbos-instituut.
Verdurmen, J., Monshouwer, K., & Van Laar, M. (2015). *Factsheet Continu Onderzoek Rookgewoonten 2014*. Utrecht: Trimbos-instituut.
Vermaat, H. (1995). *Een piece de résistance: De tabaksreclame en de lobby van de Nederlandse hartstichting voor een verbod* (Doctoral thesis), Vrije Universiteit Amsterdam.
Verschuuren, M. (2011). *International policy overview: Smoking*. Bilthoven: RIVM.
Vijgen, S. M. C., Gelder, B. M. v., Baal, P. H. M. v., Zutphen, M. v., Hoogenveen, R. T., & Feenstra, T. L. (2007). *Kosten en effecten van tabaksontmoediging*. Bilthoven: RIVM.
Visser, W. M. G. (2008). *Accijnzen : Een onderzoek naar de rechtsgronden van de Nederlandse accijnzen aan de hand van 200 jaar parlementaire geschiedenis (1805–2007) en naar de werking van het Europese accijnsregime binnen de interne markt in het licht van deze rechtsgronden*. PhD, University of Amsterdam, Amsterdam. Retrieved from http://dare.uva.nl/document/98972
VNK. (1991). [Brief van VNK aan het ministerie van EZ betreft Accijnsbrieven SSI/VNK]. *Dutch Tobacco Industry Collection*, Bates No. JB2780. Retrieved from https://www.industrydocumentslibrary.ucsf.edu/tobacco/docs/ltwp0219
VNK. (2011). [E-mails about visit to factory]. *Dutch Tobacco Industry Collection*, Bates No. JB3922. Retrieved from https://www.industrydocumentslibrary.ucsf.edu/tobacco/docs/mhcn0217

VNK & Ministry of Health. (2009). [various emails about VNK company day meeting]. *Dutch Tobacco Industry Collection*, Bates No. JB0066. Retrieved from https://www.industrydocumentslibrary.ucsf.edu/tobacco/docs/pmgb0191

VNK, NVS, SSI, & Philip Morris Benelux. (2010). Betreft: Gesprek 5 oktober jl. inzake ontwikkelingen tabaksbeleid. *Dutch Tobacco Industry Collection*, Bates No. JB0533. Retrieved from https://industrydocuments.library.ucsf.edu/tobacco/docs/lxxb0191

VNO-NCW. (2011a). alcohol en tabak [email from VNO-NCW to EZ]. *Dutch Tobacco Industry Collection*, Bates No. JB0539. Retrieved from https://www.industrydocumentslibrary.ucsf.edu/tobacco/docs/rxxb0191

VNO-NCW. (2011b). Economische impact tabaksector. *Dutch Tobacco Industry Collection*, Bates No. JB0537. Retrieved from https://www.industrydocumentslibrary.ucsf.edu/tobacco/docs/pxxb0191

Vogel, D., Kagan, R. A., & Kessler, T. (1993). Political culture and tobacco control: An international comparison. *Tobacco Control, 2*(4), 317–326.

Volkskrant. (1996, September 6). VVD en CDA tegen hogere tabaksaccijns. *Volkskrant*. Retrieved from http://www.volkskrant.nl/vk/nl/2844/Archief/archief/article/detail/425300/1996/09/06/VVD-en-CDA-tegen-hogere-tabaksaccijns.dhtml

Vonk, T. H. (1995). Verhoging Tabaksaccijns. *Dutch Tobacco Industry Collection*, Bates No. JB2657. Retrieved from https://www.industrydocumentslibrary.ucsf.edu/tobacco/docs/tywp0219

Voorlichtingsbureau Sigaretten en Shag. (1986). Jaaroverzicht. *Dutch Tobacco Industry Collection*, Bates No. JB2271. Retrieved from https://www.industrydocumentslibrary.ucsf.edu/tobacco/docs/qfgp0219

Vossenaar, T. (1997). Wetenschappelijke Adviesraad Roken en Gezondheid 1964–1997. *Dutch Tobacco Industry Collection*, Bates No. JB1390. Retrieved from https://www.industrydocumentslibrary.ucsf.edu/tobacco/docs/mhgp0219

VWA. (2005). *Evaluatie van de handhavingervaring van de Tabakswet 2002-2004: Een kwantitatieve en kwalitatieve analyse*. Utrecht: NVWA.

VWS. (1991). Zelfregulering tabaksreclame voldoet niet. *Press release 15 Oktober 1991, no 68*.

VWS. (1995). Volkgezondheidsbeleid 1995–1998 (Nota "Gezond en Wel"). *Handelingen II, 1994–1995, 24126, nr.2*.

VWS. (2001). Tabaksnota "Samen naar een rookvrije samenleving" *Truth Tobacco Industry Documents*, Bates No. JB2316. Retrieved from https://industrydocuments.library.ucsf.edu/tobacco/docs/rfgp0219

VWS. (2002). Jaarverslag van het ministerie van VWS over het jaar 2001. *Kamerstuk 28380, nr. 38*.

VWS. (2003a). *Langer Gezond Leven: Ook een kwestie van gezond gedrag*. Den Haag: Ministerie van VWS.

VWS. (2003b). Overleg 5/11/03 tabaksfabrikanten—VWS. *Dutch Tobacco Industry Collection*, Bates No. JB0266. Retrieved from https://www.industrydocumentslibrary.ucsf.edu/tobacco/docs/gjhb0191

VWS. (2005a). *Evaluatie Tabaksontmoediging.* Den Haag: Ministerie van VWS.

VWS. (2005b). *Tobacco Act: Tobacco control in the Netherlands* (International Publication Series Health, Welfare and Sport no. 22). The Hague.

VWS. (2006a). *Nationaal Programma Tabaksontmoediging.* Den Haag: Ministerie van VWS.

VWS. (2006b). *Preventienota Kiezen voor gezond leven. [Prevention Nota Choosing healthy life style].* Den Haag: Ministerie van VWS.

VWS. (2007a). *Gezond zijn, gezond blijven. Een visie op gezondheid en preventie.* Den Haag: Ministerie van VWS.

VWS. (2007b). Kaderbrief 2007-2011 visie op gezondheid en preventie. *Kamerstuk 22894, nr. 134.*

VWS. (2008). *Naar een weerbare samenleving: Beleidsplan aanpak gezondheidsverschillen op basis van sociaaleconomische achtergronden.* Den Haag: Ministerie van VWS.

VWS. (2011a). *Gezondheid dichtbij. Landelijke nota gezondheidsbeleid.* Den Haag: Ministerie van VWS.

VWS. (2011b). *Wet publieke gezondheid: De preventiecyclus.* Den Haag: Ministerie van VWS.

VWS. (2013). *Alles is gezondheid: Het Nationaal Programma Preventie 2014-2016.* Den Haag: Ministerie van VWS.

VWS. (2016). *Protocol over de wijze van omgang met de tabaksindustrie.* Den Haag: Ministerie van VWS.

Wakefield, M. A., & Chaloupka, F. J. (1998). Improving the measurement and use of tobacco control "inputs". *Tobacco Control, 7*(4), 333-335. https://doi.org/10.1136/tc.7.4.333

Wakefield, M. A., Durkin, S., Spittal, M. J., Siahpush, M., Scollo, M., Simpson, J. A., ... Hill, D. (2008). Impact of tobacco control policies and mass media campaigns on monthly adult smoking prevalence. *American Journal of Public Health, 98*(8), 1443-1450. https://doi.org/10.2105/ajph.2007.128991

Wakefield, M. A., Loken, B., & Hornik, R. C. (2010). Use of mass media campaigns to change health behaviour. *The Lancet, 376,* 1261-1271.

Walt, G. (1994). *Health policy: An introduction to process and power.* London: Zed Books.

Warner, K. E. (2005). The role of research in international tobacco control. *American Journal of Public Health, 95*(6), 976-984. https://doi.org/10.2105/AJPH.2004.046904

Warner, K. E., & Tam, J. (2012). The impact of tobacco control research and policy: 20 years of progress. *Tobacco Control, 21,* 103-109.

Wassink, W. F. (1948). Ontstaansvoorwaarden voor longkanker. *Nederlands Tijdschrift voor Geneeskunde, 92*, 3732–3747.
Weible, C. M., Sabatier, P. A., & McQueen, K. (2009). Themes and variations: Taking stock of the advocacy coalition framework. *Policy Studies Journal, 37*(1), 121–140. https://doi.org/10.1111/j.1541-0072.2008.00299.x
Weiss, C. H. (1980). Knowledge creep and decision accretion. *Science Communication, 1*(3), 381–404. https://doi.org/10.1177/107554708000100303
Weiss, J. A. (1989). The powers of problem definition: The case of government paperwork. *Policy Sciences, 22*(2), 97–121.
Werkgroep IBO Gezonde leefstijl. (2016). *IBO Gezonde leefstijl Eindrapportage van de werkgroep "IBO Gezonde leefstijl"*. Den Haag: Ministerie van Financiën.
Werkgroep IBO preventie. (2007). Gezond gedrag bevorderd. Eindrapportage van de werkgroep IBO preventie *Interdepartementaal beleidsonderzoek, 2006–2007*. Den Haag: Ministerie van VWS.
Wester, J. (1957). Roken en gezondheid. Rapport van de Gezondheidsraad. *Nederlands Tijdschrift voor Geneeskunde, 107*, 459–464.
Westerik, H., & Van der Rijt, G. A. J. (2001). *De millenniumcampagne 'Stoppen met roken 2000': Evaluatie van een campagne onder Nederlandse rokers*. Nijmegen: Katholieke Universiteit Nijmegen.
Wever, L. J. S. (1988). Proces SVR/Tabaksindustrie. *Dutch Tobacco Industry Collection*, Bates No. JB0981. Retrieved from https://www.industrydocumentslibrary.ucsf.edu/tobacco/docs/yscp0219
Wever, L. J. S. (1992). Beperking tabaksreclame. *Dutch Tobacco Industry Collection*, Bates No. JB2156. Retrieved from https://www.industrydocumentslibrary.ucsf.edu/tobacco/docs/zldp0219
WHO. (1975). *Smoking and its effects on health*. Report of a WHO expert committee No. 568, Technical Report Series. Geneva: World Health Organization.
WHO. (1979). *Controlling the smoking epidemic: Report of the WHO Expert Committee on Smoking Control*. WHO technical report series no. 636. Geneva: World Health Organization.
WHO. (1998). *Guidelines for controlling and monitoring the tobacco epidemic*. Geneva: World Health Organization.
WHO. (2001). *Evidence based recommendations on the treatment of tobacco dependence*. Geneva: World Health Organization.
WHO. (2003). *WHO framework convention on tobacco control*. Geneva: World Health Organization.
WHO. (2004a). *Building blocks for tobacco control: A handbook*. Geneva: World Health Organization.
WHO. (2004b). *Tobacco control legislation: An introductory guide* (2nd ed.). Geneva: World Health Organization.
WHO. (2006). *Legislating for smoke-free workplaces*. Copenhagen: WHO Regional Office for Europe.

WHO. (2008a). Elaboration of guidelines for implementation of Article 5.3 of the Convention *Conference of the Parties to the WHO Framework Convention on Tobacco Control Third session Durban, South Africa, 17–22 November 2008*. Geneva: World Health Organisation.
WHO. (2008b). *MPOWER*. Geneva: World Health Organisation.
WHO. (2012). *Technical Resource for Country Implementation of WHO FCTC Article 5.3*. Geneva: World Health Organization.
WHO. (2013). *Draft comprehensive global monitoring framework and targets for the prevention and control of noncommunicable diseases*. Geneva: World Health Organisation.
Wigand, J. S. (2005). Expert report on tobacco additives and validity of the Dutch decree on lists of tobacco ingredients. *Dutch Tobacco Industry Collection*, Bates No. JB0836. Retrieved from https://www.industrydocumentslibrary.ucsf.edu/tobacco/docs/glbp0219
Wijers, G. J. (1996). Tabaksontmoedigingsbeleid. *Dutch Tobacco Industry Collection*, Bates No. JB2701. Retrieved from https://www.industrydocumentslibrary.ucsf.edu/tobacco/docs/mrwp0219
Willemsen, M. C. (2005). Tabaksgebruik: trends bij de Nederlandse bevolking. In L. Knol, C. Hilvering, D. J. T. Wagener, & M. C. Willemsen (Eds.), *Tabaksgebruik: Gevolgen en bestrijding*. Utrecht: Lemma.
Willemsen, M. C. (2006). *Rokers onder vuur? Invloed van de gewijzigde Tabakswet op rokers, met speciale aandacht voor verschillen tussen sociaal-economische klassen*. Den Haag: STIVORO.
Willemsen, M. C. (2010). Tabaksverslaving: de impact van gezondheidsvoorlichting en hulpverlening op de totale populatie rokers. *Psychologie en Gezondheid, 38*, 119–130.
Willemsen, M. C. (2011). *Roken in Nederland: De keerzijde van tolerantie [inaugural lecture]*. Maastricht: Maastricht University.
Willemsen, M. C. (2012). Pak de tabakslobby keihard aan. *de Volkskrant*, 31.
Willemsen, M. C. (2017). Het Nederlandse tabaksontmoedigingsbeleid: Mijlpalen in het verleden en een blik op de toekomst. *Nederlands Tijdschrift voor Geneeskunde, 161*, D949.
Willemsen, M. C., & De Vries, H. (1996). Saying "no" to environmental tobacco smoke: Determinants of assertiveness among nonsmoking employees. *Preventive Medicine, 25*(5), 575–582. https://doi.org/10.1006/pmed.1996.0092
Willemsen, M. C., De Vries, H., & Genders, R. (1996). Annoyance from environmental tobacco smoke and support for no-smoking policies at eight large Dutch workplaces. *Tobacco Control, 5*(2), 132–138.
Willemsen, M. C., De Vries, H., & Van Schayck, O. (2009). Wat ging er mis met rookverbod in de horeca? [Why only the Dutch resist the smoking ban?]. *NRC Handelsblad*.

Willemsen, M. C., De Zwart, W. M., & Mooy, J. M. (1998). Effectiviteit van overheidsmaatregelen om het tabaksgebruik terug te dringen. In E. Roscam Abbing (Ed.), *Tabaksontmoedigingsbeleid: Gezondheidseffectrapportage*. Utrecht: Netherlands School of Public Health.

Willemsen, M. C., Kiselinova, M., Nagelhout, G. E., Joossens, L., & Knibbe, R. A. (2012a). Concern about passive smoking and tobacco control policies in European countries: An ecological study. *BMC Public Health, 12*, 876. https://doi.org/10.1186/1471-2458-12-876

Willemsen, M. C., & Nagelhout, G. E. (2016). Country differences and changes in focus of scientific tobacco control publications between 2000 and 2012 in Europe. *European Addiction Research, 22*, 52–58.

Willemsen, M. C., van Kann, D., & Jansen, E. (2012b). Stoppen met roken: ontwikkeling, implementatie en evaluatie van een massamediale campagne. In J. Brug, P. v. Assema, & L. Lechner (Eds.), *Gezondheidsvoorlichting en gedragsverandering*. Assen: Van Gorcum.

Wipfli, H., Stillman, F., Tamplin, S., e Silva, L. d. C. V., Yach, D., & Samet, J. (2004). Achieving the Framework Convention on Tobacco Control's potential by investing in national capacity. *Tobacco Control, 13*, 433–437.

Wirthlin Group. (1996). *ETS perceptions and attitudes: A review of available studies*, Bates No. 2065210430–2065210477. Retrieved from http://legacy.library.ucsf.edu/tid/txf83c00

Wolfson, M. (2001). *The fight against big tobacco: The movement, the state, and the public's health*. New York: Aldine de Gruyter.

World Bank. (1999). *Curbing the epidemic: Governments and the economics of tobacco control*. Washington: The World Bank.

World Bank. (2003). *Tobacco control at a glance*. Washington, DC: World Bank.

WRR. (2017). *Weten is nog geen doen. Een realistisch perspectief op redzaamheid*. Den Haag: Wetenschappelijke Raad voor het Regeringsbeleid.

WVC. (1984). Volksgezondheid bij beperkte middelen. *Kamerstuk 18108, nrs 1–2*.

WVC. (1986). Over de ontwikkeling van gezondheidsbeleid: feiten, beschouwingen en beleidsvoornemens (Nota 2000). *Handelingen II, 1985–1986, 19500, nr 1–2*.

WVC. (1991a). Gezondheid met beleid. *Handelingen II, 1991–1992, 22459, nr 2*.

WVC. (1991b). Scherpere aanpak van tabaksontmoedigingsbeleid. *Press release 16 Oktober 1991, no 69*.

Wynder, W. L., & Graham, E. A. (1950). Tobacco smoking as a possible etiological factor in bronchiogenic carcinoma: A study of six hundred and eighty-four proved cases. *Journal of the American Medical Association, 143*, 329–336.

Young, D., Borland, R., & Coghill, K. (2010). An actor-network theory analysis of policy innovation for smoke-free places: Understanding change in complex systems. *American Journal of Public Health, 100*(7), 1208–1217. https://doi.org/10.2105/AJPH.2009.184705

Youth Smoking Prevention Foundation. (2014). *Five years of action for a smoke-free country*. Amsterdam: Youth Smoking Prevention Foundation.
Youth Smoking Prevention Foundation. (2015). Huge progress made thanks to court case against Dutch State Retrieved May 26, 2017, from http://www.stichtingrookpreventiejeugd.nl/over-rookpreventie-jeugd/english/item/67-huge-progress-made-thanks-to-court-case-against-dutch-state
Zahariadis, N. (2007). The multiple streams framework: Structure, limitations, prospects. In P. Sabatier (Ed.), *Theories of the policy process* (2nd ed.). Boulder, CO: Westview Press.
Zatoński, W., Przewoźniak, K., Sulkowska, U., West, R., & Wojtyła, A. (2012). Tobacco smoking in countries of the European Union. *Annals of Agricultutal Environmental Medicine, 19*, 181–192.
Zeeman, G., & De Beer, M. A. M. (2012). 50 jaar GVO en Gezondheidsbevordering: Geschiedenis van de tabaksontmoediging in Nederland; succesverhaal met een droevig einde. *Tijdschrift voor Gezondheidswetenschappen, 90*, 253–261.
Zeeman, G., Willemsen, M. C., & Van Gennip, L. (2007). Foto's op pakjes passen in overheidsbeleid om tabaksgebruik te denormaliseren. *Tijdschrift voor Gezondheidswetenschappen, 85*, 234. https://doi.org/10.1007/BF03078670

Index[1]

NUMBERS & SYMBOLS
2002 Tobacco Act, 308

A
Acquis communautaire, 146
ACTAL, *see* Adviescollege Toesting Administratieve Lasten
Adema, Nienke Hora, 43
Administrative burden, 132, 137
Adolescent smoking, 101
Adoption of smoking bans, 177
Advertising and promotion ban, 79
Advertising bans, 35, 171
Advertising code, 37, 210
Advertising Code Committee, 254, 255
Advertising Code Foundation (*Stichting Reclame Code*, SRC), 21
Advertising code of conduct, 32, 34, 35, 209
Advertising directive, 148, 150
Advertising restrictions, 37
Adviescollege Toesting Administratieve Lasten (ACTAL), 132
Advocacy coalition, 6
Advocacy Coalition Framework (ACF), 5, 307
 theory, 312
Age limit, 62
Age limit for the sale of tobacco, 127
Agema, Fleur, 56
Agenda setting, 9, 166, 271
Ambiguity, 165
Amended Tobacco Act, 127
American Stop Smoking Intervention Study for Cancer Prevention (ASSIST), 243
Andriessen, Koos, 35, 196
Anti-smoke magician (*Anti-rook magiër*), 232
Article 5.3, 157, 158, 216, 218, 306, 309

---

[1] Note: Page numbers followed by 'n' refer to notes.

© The Author(s) 2018
M. C. Willemsen, *Tobacco Control Policy in the Netherlands*,
Palgrave Studies in Public Health Policy Research,
https://doi.org/10.1007/978-3-319-72368-6

Article 5.3 Framework Convention on Tobacco Control (FCTC), 129, 202, 220n42, 251
Associates for Research into the Science of Enjoyment (ARISE), 187
Association for Dutch Cigarette and Fine Cut Tobacco Manufacturers (*Vereniging Nederlandse Sigaretten- en Kerftabakfabrikanten*, VSK), 184
Astroturfing, 195
Australia, 97, 129, 145

B
Baan, Ben, 253
Balkenende II cabinet, 46
Balkenende, Jan Peter, 53, 116, 192
Banning smoking in bars and restaurants, 298
Banning tobacco advertising, 199
Ban on advertising and promotion, 81
Ban on advertising on radio and television, 29
Ban on sales through vending machines, 81
Ban on sales to those under 16, 81
Ban on sale to those under 18, 81
Ban on the display of tobacco products at point of sale, 62
Ban on tobacco advertising, 198
  in cinemas, 81
  on radio and television, 32
  on television, 81
  on the radio, 81
Ban on tobacco display, 81
Ban on tobacco sales to those under 16, 79
Ban on tobacco sale to those under 18, 79
Ban on tobacco vending machines, 127
Ban smoking in public places, 29, 30
Ban tobacco advertising, 26, 257
Ban vending machines, 39, 256
Bar smoking ban, 55
Better regulation, 132
  agenda, 132
Blocking minority, 201, 256
Blocking position, 149
Bomhoff, Eduard, 45, 46, 151, 214, 292
Borgman, 32
Borst, Els, 36, 37, 39, 126, 198, 199, 210–213, 248, 257, 258, 278, 280, 285, 291, 298, 307
Bouwmeester, Lea, 129
Brinkman, Elco, 129, 192, 193
British American Tobacco (BAT), 203
Brundtland, Gro Harlem, 40
Buijs, Siem, 52, 116

C
Cafes, 157
California-inspired activist model, 261
CAN, *see* Clean Air Netherlands
Canada, 99
Cancer Society, 233, 248
Christian Democratic Party (Christen-Democratisch Appèl, CDA), 191, 192
Christian democratic principles, 152
Christian Democratic values, 115
Christian Democrats, 114
Citizen participation, 135
Clean Air Netherlands (CAN), 62, 130, 157, 236–237, 259, 309
Clinical guidelines for the treatment of tobacco addiction, 241, 291
Clinical guidelines for the treatment of tobacco dependence, 241
Coalition agreements, 58, 119, 121, 137, 259, 260, 298, 307, 308, 313
Coalition-building, 312
Coalitions, 312–314

INDEX 365

Coffee shops, 48
Commission Van der Grinten, 131, 198
Common courtesy, 286
Compromise, 306
Confederation of Netherlands Industry and Employers (*Verbond van Nederlandse Ondernemingen en Nederlands Christelijk Werkgeversverbond*, VNO–NCW), 32, 191, 192, 200, 203, 210, 213–215, 218, 261
Conference of the Parties (COP), 156
Confrontational media campaigns, 171
Consensual knowledge, 173
Consensus democracy, 117
Consensus seeking, 117–120, 313
Consultation, 115, 211
   meetings, 209
Consulting, 216
Context and Institutions, 305–309
Convergence, 114
   of tobacco control policies, 315
Cookies campaign, 189–190
Coordination of tobacco control policy across the EU, 153
Corporate social responsibility programmes, 292
Corporatism, 114–117, 306
Corporatist, 137
   system, 115
Corporatist political environments, 312
Corporatist tradition of policymaking, 305
Council for Public Health and Health Care (*Raad voor de Volksgezondheid en Zorg*, RVZ), 135, 279
"Courtesy of choice" programmes, 188
Cruquiushoeve, 43
Cultural values, 92–93, 173, 174, 306, 310, 315

D
Danger of passive smoking, 286
De Blij, Boudewijn, 211, 256, 258, 313
De Goeij, Hans, 216
De Jager, Jan-Kees, 208
De Jong, Roch, 252–256
de Kanter, Wanda, 251
Death in the West (documentary), 252
Decentralisation, 133, 135, 138, 308, 310
Dees, Dick, 32, 168
Dekker, Pauline, 251
Delegated legislation, 126
Den Uyl, Joop, 24, 27, 284
Den Uyl cabinet, 283
Denormalisation, 95
   of smoking, 94
Deregulation, 131–132, 284, 310
Deregulation commission, 131
Deregulation committee, 31
Deregulation operations, 137
Devil shift, 6
Diffusion of ideas, 9
Diffusion of knowledge and ideas, 309–311
Directive on Tobacco Advertising, 256
Disease burden, 275, 278
Documentary, 252
Dutch Alliance for a Smokefree Society (*Alliantie Nederland Rookvrij*, ANR), 157, 250, 293, 312
Dutch Cancer Institute, 185
Dutch Cancer Society, 21, 167, 177, 231, 234
Dutch Cigarette Manufacturers Association (*Stichting Sigaretten Industrie*, SSI), 184, 185, 207
Dutch Cigar Industry Association (*Nederlandse Vereniging voor de Sigarenindustrie*, NVS), 184

Dutch Cigar Sale Organisation (*Nederlandse Sigarenverkopers Organisatie*, NSO), 185
Dutch Fine Cut Tobacco Industry Association (*Vereniging Nederlandse Kerftabakindustrie*, VNK), 184, 261
Dutch General Practitioners Association (*Landelijke Huisartsen Vereniging*, LHV), 239
Dutch golden age, 183
Dutch Heart Association, 255
Dutch Heart Foundation, 231, 255
Dutch Smoking or Health Foundation (*Stichting Volksgezondheid en Roken*, STIVORO), 26, 33, 58, 60, 169, 190, 231, 234–236, 243, 246, 247, 250, 259, 262, 285, 310, 313, 315
Dutch tobacco control advocacy movement, 231
Dutch tobacco control coalition, 231

E
ECToH, *see* European Conference on Tobacco or Health
Educational programmes, 79
Effect of smoking bans, 170
Electronic cigarettes, 293
Employability in the tobacco sector, 203–204
Employment, 207
Environmental tobacco smoke (ETS), 168
Epistemic communities, 172, 174
EU, *see* European Union
Europe against cancer programme, 146, 147
European advertising directive, 82, 149
European Conference on Tobacco or Health (ECToH), 174
European health council, 153
European Network of Smoking Prevention (ENSP), 147
European tobacco control, 174
policy, 146–147
European tobacco directive, 39
European Union (EU), 146, 174
advertising ban, 39, 152, 257
advertising legislation, 149
competence in tobacco control, 147–151
governance, 308
public health competence, 147
recommendation, 151–152
tobacco advertising ban, 149–150
EU Tobacco Product Directive, 44–46, 214
EU-wide advertising ban, 36
Evidence base, 171
for tobacco control policy, 170–172
Evidence-based movement, 165
Evidence-based smoking cessation, 245
Evidence-based tobacco control, 310
Exempt small cafés from the smoking ban, 60

F
Fact-free politics, 176
Families of nations, 113, 173
FCTC, *see* Framework Convention on Tobacco Control
FCTC's Article 5.3, 157–158
Fear appeals, 172
Feeling of urgency, 281, 311
Finance STIVORO, 235
Financial reimbursement to smokers for smoking cessation, 285
First Balkenende (CDA) cabinet (2002–2003), 45, 285
First Lubbers Cabinet (1982–1986), 131
First Purple cabinet Kok (Labour) (1994–1998), 285

First Rutte (VVD) cabinet (2010–2012), 58, 285
First, second, and third order policy changes, 64
Flywheel model, 90, 97
 of tobacco control, 280
Formula 1 races in Zandvoort, 209
Frames, 298
Framework Convention Alliance (FCA), 156
Framework Convention on Tobacco Control (FCTC) treaty, 154–156, 170, 171, 308, 309, 315
 measures, 171
Framing, 194, 272, 313
 the smoking problem, 286
 of tobacco control, 286

G
Goals for tobacco control, 277–278
Golden years for Dutch tobacco control, 315
Golden years of STIVORO, 246
Government (1973–1977), 284
Governmental agencies, 242–243
Governmental decrees (orders-in-council), 126
Grootveld, Robert Jasper, 232, 233

H
Health awareness media campaigns, 105
Health Council, 20, 23, 25, 33, 47, 166–168, 170, 172, 177, 234, 309
 passive smoking, 33, 47
Health Council report *Measures to Reduce Smoking*, 217
Health differences between the high and low educated, 275
Health inequalities, 282, 294
A Health Inequality Frame, 294–295
Health warnings, 28, 36, 52, 61, 79, 81, 127, 167, 168, 170, 201
Heart Foundation, 234
Heat-not-burn products, 293
Hendriks, Jo, 27, 235
Hermann, Corrie, 42
Higher-order legislative act, 126
High politics, 280
Hillen, Hans, 191
Hofstede, Geert, 92
Hoogervorst, Hans, 46, 47, 50, 59, 60, 215, 279, 292, 308
Hospitality sector, 48
Huijts, Paul, 216

I
IBO reports, 299n4
Ideological grounds, 310
Ideological nature, 307
Ideological pillar, 117
Ideological preferences, 176, 308
Ideology, 307
Implementation of the smoking ban in cafés, 260
Importance of the legal system, 130
Increase tobacco taxation, 258
Increasing taxation levels, 257
Industry influence, 198
Industry interference, 202
Industry lobby, 200, 202, 218
Industry lobbyists, 215, 311
Information asymmetry, 218
Insider groups, 312
Institutional factors, 113
Institutional memory, 122
Intellectual property, 204
Interactive governance, 114
Interdepartmental Committee for Reducing Tobacco Use (*Interdepartementale Commissie Beperking Tabaksgebruik*, ICBT), 27, 29, 80, 167, 197
 committee, 29
 report, 30
Internal market, 149

International levels, 146
International Tobacco Control (ITC), 173
International tobacco control epistemic community, 310
Intersectoral approach, 133
Introductory dossiers, 123, 260
Involuntary smoking, 169
Iron triangles, 217
Issue expansion, 314
Issue framing, 166, 294

J
Jorritsma, Annemarie, 124, 199
Judicial system, 130

K
Kant, Agnes, 42, 57, 193
Kingdon's multiple streams analysis, 298
Klink, Ab, 53, 54, 56, 57, 93, 116, 173, 201, 216, 249, 260, 292, 298, 307
Knowledge creep, 175
Kok, Wim, 36, 208
Kranenburg, 20
Kruisinga, Roelof, 167

L
The Labour Foundation (*Stichting van de Arbeid*, STAR), 35, 41, 43, 44, 47
Last Balkenende cabinet (2007–2010), 285
Leadership, 310
Left–right orientation of the government, 283
Legitimacy, 281–282
Legitimise governmental interference, 282

"Light" and "mild,", 81, 82, 151
Limit tobacco sales to specialty shops, 256
Lobbying, 124–130, 149, 191, 217, 306
  capacity of STIVORO, 247
  transparency, 129
Lobbyism, 115
Lobbyists, 129, 137
Local government, 134
Local level, 134–136
Local tobacco control policy, 136
Low politics, 280
Lubbers cabinet, 30
Lubbers (CDA) cabinet (1982–1986), 284
Lubbers cabinets (1982–1994), 133
Lubbers, Ruud, 192
Lung cancer, 20
Lung cancer rates, 166
Lung cancer risk of non-smokers, 168
Lung Foundation, 234
Lung Foundation Netherlands, 231

M
Maessen, Wiel, 195
Marijnissen, Jan, 39, 42, 124, 127
Mass media campaigns, 43, 49, 60, 91, 170, 172
Mass media cessation campaigns, 245
Media advocacy, 272, 295–296
Media awareness campaigns, 167
Media campaigns, 96, 128
Medical Alliance Against Smoking (*Medische Alliantie tegen het Roken*), 239, 255, 257
Medical community, 309
Medical sector, 238–240
Meinsma, Lenze, 116, 232–234, 236
Meulblok, J., 22, 26
Meulblok Committee, 30
Ministerial decrees, 126

Minister of tobacco, 293
Ministry of Economic Affairs, 195, 197, 198, 200, 202–204
Ministry of Finance, 204–208
Ministry of Health, 198, 200, 208–210, 212, 310
Monitoring data, 279
Morris, Philip, 41
MPOWER, 78, 171
Multicomponent programmes, 170
Multi-level governance, 146
Multi-party nature, 118
Multiple Streams Approach (MSA), 5, 6
Municipalities, 134–136, 138, 295
Municipal level, 138

N
Nannyism, 292, 293
National Association for Tobacco Distributors (*Landelijke Belangenvereniging van Tabaksdistributeurs Nederland*, LBT), 185
National culture, 92
National expert centre, 259
National Institute for Public Health and the Environment (*Rijksinstituut voor Volksgezondheid en Milieu*, RIVM), 135, 136, 153, 174, 242, 272, 310
National Institute of Health and the Environment, 274–276
National prevention policy documents, 277–278, 311
National Prevention Program (NPP), 135
National Program of Tobacco Control (*Nationaal Programma Tabaksontmoediging,* NPT), 50–53, 58, 80, 245, 248, 249, 278

National targets for tobacco control, 273–280
National tobacco control goals, 136
Nelissen, Jean, 252, 253
Neo-liberal, 284
Neo-liberalist, 131
  agenda, 137
Netherlands Food and Consumer Product Safety Authority (*Nederlandse Voedsel en Waren Autoriteit*, NVWA), 55, 153, 243
Netherlands ratified FCTC, 155
Netherlands School of Public Health (NSPH), 39, 40, 42, 176
Nicotine addiction was an addictive disorder, 290
Nixon, President, 22
Non-governmental organisations (NGOs), 156
Nooijen, Nanny, 43, 130, 259
Nooijen case, the, 41
Normative factors, 94
Nota 2000, 133, 273
Nota Tabaksontmoedigingsbeleid, 38
NPT programme, 58, 249, 259, 279
Nypels, Erwin, 32

O
Occupational health and safety legislation, 35
Oppose the EU advertising ban, 258
Organise health education, 235
Oudkerk, Rob, 39, 57, 116, 193, 211
Outsider groups, 312

P
Parallel interests, 53
Parliament, 126–128, 191
Parliamentarians, 128
Parliamentary questions, 296

Partnership Stop Smoking (*Partnership Stop met Roken*), 240, 241, 249, 291
Party discipline, 119, 126
Passive smoking, 33, 47, 168, 187, 254, 255
Paternalism, 57, 176
People's Party for Freedom and Democracy (*Volkspartij voor Vrijheid en Democratie*, VVD), 192
Percolation, 175
Philip Morris, 149, 185, 189, 192, 194, 196, 201–203, 208
Picture warnings on cigarettes packs, 81
Plain packaging, 152, 201, 202
Platform Prevention of Youth Smoking, 199, 292
Pluralist systems, 115
Polderen, 118, 212, 306
Polder model, the, 118, 285
Policy brokers, 6, 306
Policy core beliefs, 307
Policy cycle, 78–80
Policy diffusion, 173
Policy Evaluation Project, 173
Policy goal, 277
Policy instrument, 170
Policy learning, 174
Political commitment, 279
Political will, 279
Pontfoort, Albert, 235
Population impact, 170
Prevention cycle, 134, 135
Prevention policy, 53, 136
Prins, Trudy, 258
Problem identification, 271–273, 311
Professional lobbying, 262
Provo youth counter movement, 232
Public health act (*Wet Publieke Gezondheidszorg*, WPG), 134

Public Health Collective Prevention Act (*Wet Collectieve Preventie Volksgezondheid*, WCPV), 133
Public Health Status and Foresight, report (*Volksgezondheid Toekomst Verkenning*, VTV), 135, 272, 311
Public Health Status Forecasts reports, 274–276
Public opinion, 102
  about passive smoking, 188
  on the risks of passive smoking, 189
Public support, 97, 102–104
  for smoking bans, 190
Purple cabinet, 36

Q

Qualified majority voting, 149
Quantifiable targets for smoking, 279
Quit & Win contests, 248

R

Raising tobacco prices, 170
Reader's Digest, 20
Reclame Code, 30
Recommendation on smoke-free environments, 200, 201
Recommendations on tobacco control, 151
Reduce sales to specialised tobacco retailers, 198
Reducing the number of tobacco selling points, 257
Reduction of tobacco selling points, 197
Regulate tobacco advertising, 257
Regulatory impact assessment, 131
Regulatory reforms in the EU, 132
Reimbursement, 50, 128
  for smoking cessation, 50, 57, 60, 79, 241
  for smoking cessation support, 259

Restricting sales to minors, 82
Restrict the sale of tobacco to specialty shops, 127
Restrict tobacco sales to specialty shops, 30, 42, 52
Restrict tobacco to specialty shops, 198
Retreating government, 308
Revised Tobacco Act, 41, 44, 126, 176, 246, 263, 273, 298
Revise the Tobacco Act, 218
Revision of the Tobacco Act, 41, 79, 213
Rights of non-smokers, 236
Rinnooy-Kan, Alexander, 191, 210
Risk awareness campaigns, 307
Role of ideology, 176
Rookspectrum, 238
Ross-van Dorp, Clémence, 46, 214, 215, 292
Routes of influence, 218
Royal College of Physicians, 20, 23
Royal Dutch Medical Association (*Koninklijke Nederlandsche Maatschappij tot bevordering der Geneeskunst*, KNMG), 238, 239, 257
Rules of the game, 113

S

Sale of cigarettes restricted to specialty shops, 41
Save the small hospitality entrepreneur (*Stichting Red de kleine horecaondernemer*), 194
Schipper, Jan, 193
Schippers, Edith, 48, 52, 55, 59–61, 176, 216, 217, 251, 261, 293, 296, 307
Scientific Advisory Council on Smoking and Health (*Wetenschappelijke Adviesraad Roken en Gezondheid*, WARG), 185
Scientific community, the, 241–242
Scientific evidence, 166, 309
Second Balkenende cabinet, 131
Second-hand smoke, 168–170
Second Kok cabinet (1998–2002), 285
Second Lubbers cabinet (1986–1989), 32, 284
Second Purple Cabinet, 39
Second Rutte cabinet (2013–2017), 285
Second (amended) Tobacco Act, 125
Self-regulation, 35, 43, 47, 48, 54, 79, 82, 119, 131, 137, 191, 198, 209, 210, 218, 285, 305
Self-regulatory agreements, 118
Shadow reports, 156
Simons, Hans, 33, 35, 196, 209, 210, 247, 289
Single European Act, 147
Smoke-free bars, 309
Smoke-free generation, 293
Smoke-free hospitality sector, 237, 259, 260
Smoke-free public places, 79
Smoke-free public transport, 44
Smoke-free work environment, 254
Smoke-free workplaces, 44, 79
Smoke ring, 217
Smokers' rights group (*Stichting Rokers Belangen*, SRB), 194, 260
Smoking
an addiction, 290
cessation quitline, 246
cessation support, 128
and health, 274
in health-care facilities, 49
prevalence, 274
prevalence in the Netherlands, 99
in pubs, 58
rates, 97–102, 274, 311

Smoking ban, 157
  in bars, 296
  in bars and restaurants, 55, 57, 308
  in the hospitality sector, 81
  in private workplaces, 42, 81
  in public places, 38, 81
  in pubs, 307
  in pubs and restaurants, 79, 295
  in small bars, 81
  for workplaces and public transport, 48
Social acceptability, 94
Social acceptance of smoking, 49
Social gradient in smoking, 294
Social norms, 93–97
Societal support for most tobacco control, 105
Sprenger, Mark, 136
Stages heuristics approach, 78
Stages of the policy process, 78
Stakeholder consultation, 137
State income that comes from tobacco, 205
Statistical indicators, 272
STIVORO, 33, 169, 285
  budget, 246
  campaigns, 243
  lobbying accomplishments, 252
  lobbying activities, 247
Subsidiarity, 115, 118, 137, 152–153, 158
  principle, 36
Support for tobacco control, 103
Support smoking restrictions, 187
System thinking in tobacco control, 89

T
Tabaksnota II, 42, 44, 46
TAD-2, *see* Tobacco Advertising Directive
Targets in tobacco control, 279
Tax increases, 206, 207, 259

Terpstra, Erica, 127
Third Lubbers cabinet (1986–1989), 285
Third Lubbers cabinet (1989–1994), 33
TNO, 185
Tobacco Act, 41, 79, 82, 308
Tobacco addiction, 241
Tobacco advertising, 39, 209
  and promotion ban, 252
Tobacco Advertising Directive (TAD-2), 150, 255
Tobacco a "low politics" Issue, 280–281
Tobacco commercials on cinema screens, 37
Tobacco control advocacy coalition, 252–262
Tobacco control building blocks, 171, 315
Tobacco control coalition, 313
  several important lobbying successes, 263
Tobacco control expert centre, 262
Tobacco control in times of economic recession, 284–286
Tobacco control measures, 91
Tobacco control policies, 77
  convergence, 174
  cycles, 79
  goals, 278
  in the Netherlands and in the United Kingdom, 81
Tobacco Control scale (TCS), 83, 250
Tobacco Education Bureau (*Bureau Voorlichting Tabak*, BVT), 238
Tobacco epidemic, 97
Tobacco industry
  demonising, 293
  influence, 183–218
  lobbyists, 208
  tolerance campaigns, 104, 188
Tobacco lobbyists, 184

Tobacco manufacturing sector, 204
Tobacco Memorandum, 19, 27, 235
Tobacco Product Directive (TPD-1), 44–46, 147, 150
Tobacco Product Directive (TPD-2), 61, 150
Tobacco selling points, 31
Tobacco tax, 38
  increase, 261
  revenues, 205
Tobacco taxation, 85, 206
Tobacco vending machines, 30
Tolerance to smoking, 188
Trade balance, 204
Trimbos Institute, 60, 174, 250
Truth Tobacco Industry Documents database, 13
TT motorcycle events in Assen, 209

U
Uncertainty reduction, 166
United Kingdom, 81–83, 99, 145
United States, 145
US Environmental Protection Agency (EPA) report, 169, 186

V
Van Agt, Dries, 28
Van Agt (CDA) cabinets (1977–1982), 284
Van den Bergh, Sidney, 23
van den Doel, Hans, 22
van der Reijden, Joop, 30, 102, 175, 198, 253
Van Gennip, Lies, 259, 260
van Kesteren, Niek-Jan, 192
Van Oort & Van Oort Public Affairs, 259
van Rey, Jos, 207
Van Rijn, Martin, 61, 251, 293
van Veen, Anne Marie, 251

van Zeil, Piet, 30
Veder-Smit, Els, 29
Vending machines, 39, 131, 198
Ventilation, 56, 128
  technology, 188
Venue shopping, 130
Verhagen, Maxim, 203
Voluntary advertising agreements, 35
Voluntary agreements, 118

W
Wassink, W. F., 20
Werner, 128, 246
Werner, Jos, 43, 46
WHO, *see* World Health Organisation
Wiegman, Esmé, 157
Wijers, Hans, 36, 198, 199, 285
Wilders, Geert, 59, 151
Window of opportunity, 298, 307
Working Group on Agreements about Tobacco Policy (*Werkgroep Afspraken Tabaksbeleid*, WAT), 197
Workplace smoking, 258
  ban, 82, 126, 263
Worksite smoking ban, 127
World Bank published its influential report *Curbing the Epidemic*, 289
World Conferences on Tobacco or Health (WCToH), 174
World Health Organisation (WHO), 154–157, 171
Wurtz, Ton, 194

Y
Youth smoking, 101
Youth Smoking Prevention Foundation (*Stichting Rookpreventie Jeugd*, SRJ), 158, 217, 251–252, 293, 309, 312

Printed by Printforce, the Netherlands